To Robert

John Robbins

ALSO BY JOHN ROBBINS

*Diet for a New America: How Your Food Choices Affect
Your Health, Happiness, and the Future of Life on Earth*

*Reclaiming Our Health: Exploding the Medical Myth
and Embracing the Source of True Healing*

*The Food Revolution: How Your Diet Can Help
Save Your Life and the World*

*May All Be Fed: Diet for a New World*

*The Awakened Heart* (with Ann Mortifee)

# HEALTHY AT 100

# HEALTHY AT
# 100

The Scientifically Proven Secrets

of the World's Healthiest

and Longest-Lived Peoples

## JOHN ROBBINS

RANDOM HOUSE / NEW YORK

Published in the United States by Random House, an imprint of The Random House Publishing Group, a division of Random House, Inc., New York.

RANDOM HOUSE and colophon are registered trademarks of Random House, Inc.

Grateful acknowledgment is made to the following for permission
to reprint previously published material:

ALFRED A. KNOPF, A DIVISION OF RANDOM HOUSE, INC.: Excerpt from *The Prophet* by Kahlil Gibran, copyright © 1923 by Kahlil Gibran and renewed 1951 by Administrators C.T.A. of Kahlil Gibran Estate and Mary G. Gibran. Reprinted by permission of Alfred A. Knopf, a division of Random House, Inc.

HEALTH COMMUNICATIONS, INC.: "The Travelers" by Bobbi Wilkinson from *Chicken Soup for the Caregiver's Soul* edited by Jack Canfield, Mark Victor Hansen and LeAnn Thieman, copyright © 2002 by Bobbi Wilkinson. Reprinted by permission of Health Communications, Inc., www.hcibooks.com.

RUTH HEIDRICH: "Racing for Life" by Ruth Heidrich. Reprinted by permission of Ruth Heidrich.

THE MCGRAW-HILL COMPANIES: Excerpts from *Young in Old Age* by Alexander Leaf and John Launois, copyright © 1975. Reprinted by permission of The McGraw-Hill Companies.

ROCHELLE PENNINGTON: "For Richer or Poorer" by Rochelle Pennington from *Stories for the Heart* (Multnomah Publishing), copyright © 1999 by Rochelle Pennington. Rochelle Pennington is the author of *Highlighted in Yellow, The Golden Formula, Reach for the Stars, The Christmas Tree Ship*, and *The Historic Christmas Tree Ship*. Contact her at 1-800-503-5507. Reprinted by permission of Rochelle Pennington.

PENGUIN GROUP (USA) INC.: Excerpts from *Kitchen Table Wisdom* by Rachel Naomi Remen, M.D., copyright © 1996 by Rachel Naomi Remen, M.D. Reprinted by permission of Riverhead Books, an imprint of Penguin Group (USA), Inc.

READER'S DIGEST: "A Family for Freddie" by Abbie Blair from the December 1964 issue of *Reader's Digest,* copyright © 1964 by The Reader's Digest Assn., Inc. Reprinted by permission of *Reader's Digest.*

RIVERHEAD BOOKS, AN IMPRINT OF PENGUIN GROUP (USA), INC., AND ANNE LAMOTT: Adapted excerpt from *Plan B: Further Thoughts on Faith* by Anne Lamott, copyright © 2005 by Anne Lamott. Reprinted by permission of Riverhead Books, an imprint of Penguin Group (USA), Inc., and Anne Lamott.

ELIZABETH SONGSTER: "Engraved in His Heart" by Elizabeth Songster. Reprinted by permission of Elizabeth Songster.

LIBRARY OF CONGRESS CATALOGING-IN-PUBLICATION DATA
Robbins, John.
Healthy at 100: the scientifically proven secrets of the world's healthiest and longest lived peoples /
John Robbins.
p.   cm.
ISBN 1-4000-6521-6
1. Longevity.   2. Health.   3. Aging.   4. Diet.   5. Exercise.   6. Mind and body.
7. Centenarians.   I. Title: Scientifically proven secrets of the world's healthiest
and longest lived peoples.   II. Title.
RA776.75.R63 2006       613.2—dc22       2005057710

The author is committed to preserving ancient forests and natural resources and wishes to acknowledge Random House for printing this book on paper that is 100 percent postconsumer-recycled fibers and processed chlorine free. For more information about Green Press Initiative and the use of recycled paper in book publishing, visit www.greenpressinitiative.org.

www.atrandom.com

2   4   6   8   9   7   5   3   1

FIRST EDITION

*Book design by Casey Hampton*

*I wish you health.*
*I wish you wealth*
*That passes not with time,*
*I wish you long years.*
*May your heart be as patient as the earth*
*Your love as warm as the harvest gold.*
*May your days be full, as the city is full*
*Your nights as joyful as dancers.*
*May your arms be as welcoming as home.*
*May your faith be as enduring as God's love*
*Your spirit as valiant as your heritage.*
*May your hand be as sure as a friend*
*Your dreams as hopeful as a child.*
*May your soul be as brave as your people*
*And may you be blessed.*

—Wigglier Blessing

# Contents

# Introduction

"Every young man," wrote Ernest Hemingway, "believes he will live forever." And the same could be said for every young woman. But whatever our beliefs and thoughts about life, there remains an undeniable and ever-present fact: We are, each and every one of us, growing older.

This is true in every country and among every people throughout the world, but the way different cultures have responded to this reality has varied widely.

For many of us in the industrialized world today, our aging is a source of grief and anxiety. We fear aging. The elderly people we see are for the most part increasingly senile, frail, and unhappy. As a result, rather than looking forward to growing old, we dread each passing birthday. Rather than seeing our later years as a time of harvesting, growth, and maturity, we fear that the deterioration of our health will so greatly impair our lives that to live a long life might be more of a curse than a blessing.

When we think of being old, our images are often ones of decrepitude and despair. It seems more realistic to imagine ourselves languishing in nursing homes than to picture ourselves swimming, gardening, laughing with loved ones, and delighting in children and nature.

In 2005, the famed American author Hunter S. Thompson took his life. He was only sixty-seven, and had no incurable disease. He was wealthy and famous, and his thirty-two-year-old wife loved him. But according to the literary executor of Thompson's will, "he made a conscious decision that he . . . wasn't going to suffer the indignities of old age."[1]

It doesn't help to live in a society where there is so little respect for the elderly. Television shows and movies frequently portray older people as feeble, unproductive, grumpy, and stubborn. Advertisements selling everything from alcohol to cars feature beautiful young people, giving the impression that older people are irrelevant. Colloquialisms such as "geezer," "old fogey," "old maid," "dirty old man," and "old goat" demean the elderly and perpetuate a stereotype of older people as unworthy of consideration or positive regard.

Greeting card companies routinely sell birthday cards that mock the mobility, intellect, and sex drive of the no longer young. Novelty companies sell "Over-the-Hill" products such as fiftieth-birthday coffin gift boxes containing prune juice and a "decision maker to assist in planning daily activities" (a large six-sided die, with sides labeled "nap," "TV," "shopping," etc.). Gifts for a man's sixtieth birthday include a "lifetime supply" of condoms (one), Over-the-Hill bubble bath (canned beans), and "Old Fart" party hats.

We may chuckle at such humor, but negative stereotypes about aging are insidious. They attach a social stigma to aging that can affect your will to live and even shorten your life. In a study published by the American Psychological Association, Yale School of Public Health professor Becca Levy, Ph.D., concluded that even if you are not aware of them, negative thoughts about aging that you pick up from society can undermine your health and have destructive consequences.

In the study, a large number of middle-aged people were interviewed six times over the course of twenty years and asked whether they agreed with such statements as "As you get older, you are less useful." Remarkably, the perceptions held by people about aging proved to have more impact on how long they would live than did their blood pressure, their cholesterol level, whether they smoked, or whether they exercised. *Those people who had positive perceptions of aging lived an average of 7.5 years longer than those with negative images of growing older.*[2]

Negative images not only lead to compromised health and shortened lives—they also are distressing in the present. Dr. Levy's study found that people with negative perceptions of aging were more likely to consider their lives worthless, empty, and hopeless, while those with more positive perceptions of aging were more likely to view their lives as fulfilling and hopeful.

When we are disrespectful to older people and make them invisible, we attempt to ignore the aging process we are experiencing. We hide its signs and look away from the longer-term consequences of our lifestyles. As a result, we make lifestyle choices that may make sense in the short term but take a heavy toll in the end.

I asked a friend recently how he thought he might age. "I'll probably end up in a nursing home somewhere," he replied with some bitterness, "with a feeding tube in my nose, staring at the acoustic squares in the ceiling, incontinent, impotent, and impoverished." Sadly, such views are not unusual. I've seen bumper stickers that say "Avenge Yourself: Live Long Enough to Become a Burden to Your Children." When you distrust the aging process, it's hard to imagine yourself enjoying your older years, doing things like dancing, jogging, or hiking. It can be difficult even to consider the possibility that you might, during every phase of your lifetime, have the capacity for growth, change, and creativity.

In the last hundred years we've added nearly thirty years to the average life expectancy in the industrialized world, but for many older adults the later years are not a time of happiness and well-being. *A century ago, the average adult in Western nations spent only 1 percent of his or her life in a morbid or ill state, but today's average modern adult spends more than 10 percent of his or her life sick.* People are living longer today, but all too often they are dying longer, too—of chronic diseases that cause debility and cognitive impairment.

By 2025, the annual cost of managing chronic conditions in the United States will exceed a trillion dollars. Already, half of those age sixty-five and over have two or more chronic diseases, and a quarter have problems so severe as to limit their ability to perform one or more activities of daily living. Meanwhile, the average age of the chronically ill is continually getting younger. *Throughout the industrialized world, people are living longer, but they are getting sick sooner, so the number of years they spend chronically ill is actually increasing in both directions.*

Sometimes I think we have not so much prolonged our lives as prolonged our dying. While we have extended the human *life* span, we have not extended the human *health* span.

## THE AGE WAVE

As our older people are getting less and less well, their numbers are growing, and this process is about to shift into hyperdrive. As author Ken Dychtwald has described in his seminal book *Age Power,* there are at this very moment approximately eighty million baby boomers in the United States barreling toward old age.[3] (The term "baby boomer" generally refers to people born between 1945 and 1960.)

In 1900, there were only 3 million people in the United States who were sixty-five or older. By 2000, the number had leaped to 33 million.

A century ago in the United States, the odds of living to the age of 100 were less than one in five hundred. Now the Census Bureau expects that one in twenty-six baby boomers will reach that age. Today, the likelihood that a twenty-year-old American will have a living grandmother (91 percent) is higher than the likelihood that a twenty-year-old in 1900 had a living mother (83 percent).[4]

This advancing age wave is the most significant demographic event of our lifetime, and it is taking place in every industrialized nation in the world. *About half of all people who have ever lived past the age of sixty-five are alive today.*

In Chile, Costa Rica, Mexico, and Venezuela, the percentage of elderly persons in the population is projected to double between 2000 and 2025.[5] China is expected to be home to 332 million oldsters by midcentury. That's more elderly people in a single country than inhabited the entire planet as recently as 1990.[6]

According to the United Nation's Population Division, roughly 10 percent of the world's 6.4 billion people are today over sixty. By 2050, 20 percent of the planet's 10 billion human beings will be over sixty. By then there will be nearly 2 billion people in the world sixty years of age and older. This is a number roughly equal to one-third of the entire current global human population.

This increased longevity would be a blessing if it were accompanied by increased health and wisdom, but sadly it often is not. Close to half of all Americans over the age of eighty-five have Alzheimer's disease. The toll taken by Alzheimer's and other chronic diseases on the old is increasing so much today that *the average twenty-first-century American will likely spend more years caring for parents than for children.*

By 2040, it is estimated that 5.5 million Americans—more than the entire current population of Denmark—will live in nursing homes. Another 12 million—equal to the combined populations of Israel, Singapore, and New Zealand—will require ongoing homecare services. Many will spend their final decades struggling with loneliness and depression.

Although modern medicine is eminently equipped to prolong life, it seems to be far less able to promote healthy aging. What good will it do us, asked a comedian in 2004, if at some point in the future, the human life span is extended to two hundred years, but the last hundred and fifty years are spent in unremitting pain and sadness?

An ancient Greek fable tells of Aurora, the beautiful goddess of the dawn, falling deeply in love with a human being—the warrior Tithonus. Distraught over his mortality, Aurora requests a special favor from Zeus, the supreme ruler of Mount Olympus and of the pantheon of gods who reside there. She begs Zeus to grant her lover eternal life.

Zeus, foreseeing trouble, asks her if she is certain that this is what she wants. "Yes," she responds.

At first, Aurora is delighted that Zeus has granted her request. But then she realizes that she neglected to ask that Tithonus also remain eternally young and healthy. With each passing year, she looks on with horror as her lover grows older and sicker. His skin withers, his organs rot, his brain grows feeble. As the decades pass, Tithonus's aging body becomes increasingly decrepit, yet he cannot die. Ultimately the once proud warrior is reduced to a wretched collection of painful, foul, and broken bones—but he continues to live forever.

Like Tithonus, ever more of us are living longer, but our added years are too often years of suffering and disability.

## MORE LIFE, MORE HEALTH

It has been said that we can destroy ourselves with negativity just as effectively as with bombs. If we see only the worst in ourselves, it erodes our capacity to act. If, on the other hand, we are drawn forward by a positive vision of how we might live, we can shrug off the cynicism that has become fashionable today and build truly healthy lives.

It is extraordinarily important for us today to replace the prevailing image and reality of aging with a new vision—one in which we grasp the possibility of living all our days with exuberance and passion. There are few things of greater consequence today than for us to bring our lives into alignment with our true potential for health and our dreams for a better tomorrow.

It is a sad loss that our medical model has been so focused on illness rather than wellness. Until recently, there has been so much preoccupation with disease that little attention has been paid to the characteristics that enable people to lead long and healthy lives and to be energetic and independent in their elder years. As a result, few of us in the modern world are aware that there have been, and still are, entire cultures in which the majority of people live passionately and vibrantly to the end. Few of us realize that there are in fact societies of people who look forward to growing old, knowing they will be healthy, vital, and respected.

There are many people today who want to live in harmony with their bodies and the natural forces of life. You may be one of them. If so, it's helpful to understand that you are not alone, and that you have elders from whom you can learn how to accomplish your goals. There are cultures whose ways have stood the test of time that can stand as teachers on the path of wellness and joy. There are whole populations of highly spirited, vigorous people who are healthy in their seventies, eighties, nineties, even healthy at a hundred. What's more, they have a great deal in common, and their secrets have been corroborated and to a large extent explained by many of the latest findings in medical science. New research is showing that we have all the tools to live longer lives and to remain active, productive, and resourceful until the very end.

This is good and hopeful news. It offers us a much-needed paradigm of aging as a period of wisdom and vitality. Through these healthy cultures, we can find a compelling vision of how to mature with pleasure, dignity, purpose, and love. We are being shown that something precious is possible—a far brighter future in which aging is enjoyable and desirable. And we are being shown the practical steps we can take to achieve it.

Aging, of course, is not something that begins on your sixty-fifth birthday. Who you will become in your later years is shaped by all the choices you make, all the ways you care for yourself, how you manage your life, even how you think, from your earliest years, about your future. I have written *Healthy at 100* because I have seen too many people grow old in agony and bitterness while others grow old with vitality and beauty, and I know it is possible to age with far more vigor, happiness, and inner peace than is the norm in the Western world today.

No one familiar with my earlier work will be surprised that I am interested in how our diets and exercise can help us to live long and healthy lives. But they may be surprised by some of my findings, including the great emphasis I am now placing on strong social connections. I have learned that the quality of the relationships we have with other people makes a tremendous difference to our physical as well as emotional health. Loneliness, I discovered in my research, can kill you faster than cigarettes. And by the same token, intimate relationships that are authentic and life-affirming can have enormous and even miraculous healing powers. In this book you will find why this is so, and gain clarity about the various essential steps you can take to extend both your life span and your health span dramatically. Reading this book will not only help you add many years to your life, but also help make those added years—and indeed all your remaining years—ones in which you experience the blossoming of your finest and wisest self.

Even if you've eaten poorly and have not taken very good care of yourself, even if you've had more than your share of hardships and pain, this book will show you how the choices you make today and tomorrow can greatly improve your prospects for the future. It will give you a chance to right any wrongs you've committed against your body. You'll see how to regain the strength and passion for life that you may have thought were gone forever.

Whether you are in your twenties or your eighties or somewhere in between, whether you consider yourself superbly fit or hopelessly out of shape, I believe you'll find in these pages what you need in order to regenerate rather than degenerate as the years unfold. This book will show you how to regain, and to retain, more mental clarity, physical strength, stamina, and joy.

I have written *Healthy at 100* to offer you ways to enhance and improve both the quality and quantity of your remaining years. In this book are steps you can take to shatter stereotypes and misconceptions about aging and to rejuvenate your mind and body. Here are practices you can start today in order to live with greater health and joy no matter what your age.

In our youth-oriented culture, aging is often a source of great suffering. Older people frequently start to see themselves as collections of symptoms rather than whole human beings. But it doesn't have to be that way. It is within your grasp to realize the opportunities for beauty, love, and fulfillment that occur at every stage of your life. It is possible to live your whole life with a commitment to your highest good. I have written *Healthy at 100* so that you can learn how to make each and every one of the years of your life more full of vitality and joy, and more worth living, than you may ever have imagined.

# PART

# 1

# THE WORLD'S HEALTHIEST AND LONGEST LIVED PEOPLES

# 1

# Abkhasia: Ancients of the Caucasus

*People don't grow old. When they stop growing, they become old.*
—Anonymous

In the early 1970s, *National Geographic* magazine approached the world-renowned physician Alexander Leaf, asking him to visit, study, and write an article about the world's healthiest and most long-living people. Dr. Leaf, a professor of clinical medicine at Harvard University and Chief of Medical Services at Massachusetts General Hospital, had long been a student of the subject and had already visited and studied some of the cultures known for the healthy lives of their elderly people. Now, *National Geographic* commissioned him to continue these travels and investigations and to share with the world his observations and comparisons of those areas of the planet which were famous for the longevity and health of their inhabitants. It was a time, unlike today, when these regions and their cultures were still somewhat pristine.

As a scientist, Dr. Leaf did not believe in a mythical fountain of youth in which anyone can bathe and be miraculously restored to eternal youth; nor did he believe in magic potions that can instantly heal all afflictions. But he did believe it was possible that there existed certain places on earth where people actually lived longer and healthier lives than is considered normal in the modern West. His goal was not to identify the oldest living individual, but rather to locate and study those societies—if they did in fact exist—where a large percentage of elder citizens retained their faculties, were vigorous, and enjoyed their lives. Rather than being interested in mythology or panaceas, his goal was to understand the key factors that influence human prospects for long and healthy life.

Dr. Leaf undertook a series of journeys that he subsequently described in an influential series of articles that appeared in *National Geographic* magazine beginning in 1973.[1] His writings were among the first authoritative efforts to bring practical medical knowledge and research to our desire to know what we can do to impact the future of our lives.

When Dr. Leaf began his study and his travels, three regions of the world were famous for the longevity of their inhabitants: the valley of Vilcabamba in Ecuador, the Hunza region of Pakistan, and certain portions of the Caucasus mountains in what was then the Soviet Union. These three locales had long been the subject of claims that they were home to the longest living and healthiest people on earth. According to the stories swirling around these high mountainous regions, people in these communities often lived spectacularly long lives in vibrant health.

Dr. Leaf and prizewinning *National Geographic* photographer John Launois traveled to these remote areas to meet, photograph, examine, and appraise for themselves the longevity and health of those who were reputed to be the world's oldest and healthiest people. Dr. Leaf listened to their hearts, took their blood pressure, and studied their diets and lifestyles. He watched them dance and saw them bathe in ice-cold mountain streams. He spoke with them about their daily lives, their hopes, their fears, their life histories. His goal was to separate fact from fallacy and determine the truth about longevity.

## LONGEVITY IN ABKHASIA

"Certainly no area in the world," Leaf wrote, "has the reputation for long-lived people to match that of the Caucasus in southern Russia."[2] And in all the Caucasus, the area most renowned for its extraordinary number of healthy centenarians (people above the age of 100) was Abkhasia (pronounced "ab-KAY-zha"). A 1970 census had established Abkhasia, then an autonomous region within Soviet Georgia, as the longevity capital of the world. "We were eager to see the centenarians," Leaf said, "and Abkhasia seemed to be the place to do so."[3]

Abkhasia covers three thousand square miles between the eastern shores of the Black Sea and the crestline of the main Caucasus range. It is bordered on the north by Russia, and on the south by Georgia.

Prior to Dr. Leaf's visit, claims had been widely circulated for life spans reaching 150 years among the Abkhasians. Just a few years earlier, *Life* magazine had run an article with photos of Shirali Muslimov, said to be 161 years old.[4] In one of the photos, Muslimov was shown with his third wife. He told the reporter that he had married her when he was 110, that his parents had both lived to be over 100, and that his brother had died at the age of 134.

Muslimov had passed away by the time of Leaf's studies. But a woman named Khfaf Lasuria had also been featured in the *Life* article. Leaf wanted to meet her, and he found her in the Abkhasian village of Kutol, where she sang in a choir made up entirely, he was told, of Abkhasian centenarians.

> I had a long talk with this diminutive—she stands not five feet tall—sprightly woman who claimed to be 141 years old. . . . Although she carried a handsomely carved wooden walking stick, her nimbleness belied need of it. Her memory seemed excellent. . . . She spoke lucidly and easily about events recent and past. At the age of 75 to 80 as a midwife she assisted more than 100 babies into the world. . . . She described the life of women: "Women had a very difficult time before the Revolution; we were practically slaves." And she ended our talk with a toast, "I want to drink to women all over the world . . . for them not to work too hard and to be happy with their families."[5]

Though he was greatly impressed by this elderly lady's charm and spirit, Leaf did not simply take her word for her age. To the contrary, he went to significant efforts to assess it objectively. Such a task is harder than it might sound, for there are no signs in the human body, like the annual rings of a tree, that tell us a person's age.

After laborious investigations, Leaf concluded that Mrs. Lasuria was close to 130 years old. He wasn't certain about that, saying only that he had arrived at a degree of confidence and this was his best estimate. But he was sure of one thing. She was one of the oldest persons he had ever met.[6]

Everywhere he went in Abkhasia, Leaf met elders in remarkable health. The area seemed to warrant its reputation as the mecca of superlongevity. Like others who have studied the elders of Abkhasia, Leaf had colorful stories to tell. He wrote of one elder, nearly 100, whose hearing was still good and whose vision was still superb.

"Have you ever been sick?" Leaf asked.

The elder thought for some time, then replied, "Yes, I recall once having a fever, a long time ago."

"Do you ever see a doctor?"

The old man was surprised by the question, and replied, "Why should I?"

Leaf examined him and found his blood pressure to be normal at 118/60 and his pulse to be regular at 70 beats per minute.

"What was the happiest period of your life?" Leaf asked.

"I feel joy all my life. But I was happiest when my daughter was born. And saddest when my son died at the age of one year from dysentery."[7]

Among the others Leaf met were a delightful trio of gentlemen who, like many elderly Abkhasians, were still working despite their advanced age. They were Markhti Tarkhil, whom Leaf believed to be 104; Temur Tarba, who was apparently 100; and Tikhed Gunba, a mere youngster at 98. All were born locally. Temur said his father died at 110, his mother at 104, and an older brother just that year at 109. After a short exam, Leaf said that Temur's blood pressure was a youthful 120/84, and his pulse was regular at a rate of 69.[8]

The old fellows clowned around constantly, joking and teasing each other and Leaf. While he was checking pulses and blood pressures the other two would shake their heads in mock sadness at the one being examined, saying "Bad, very bad!" They never seemed to tire of friendly joking, always finding new ways to have fun. Leaf was impressed by their sharp minds, high spirits, and relentless sense of humor.

Like many of the elders in Abkhasia, regardless of the weather, these men swam daily in cold mountain streams. One day, Leaf accompanied Markhti Tarkhil on his morning plunge and was astonished by the vitality and physical agility of the 104-year-old.[9] It was a steep and rugged half-mile climb down from the road to the river, but Markhti moved with confident speed and agility. Seeing Markhti take off down the slope, Leaf, a physician coming from a society where elders have thin and fragile bones, was concerned that the older man might fall, and thought he should accompany Markhti down the hill and see to it that he didn't slip. But he was unable to do so, because he couldn't keep up with the pace of the far older man, who as it turned out never lost his footing. Later, Leaf learned from the regional doctor that there is no osteoporosis among the active elders, and that fractures are rare.

When Markhti arrived at the riverbank, he stripped and waded out into the stream, immersing his entire body in the cold water. A young guide Leaf had brought with him from Moscow also stripped and began wading into the water, but immediately jumped out, exclaiming that the water was far too cold.

After bathing in the cold water for some time, Markhti got out, dried himself off, put on his clothes, and proceeded to climb swiftly back up the rugged slope, with Leaf, who was a half-century younger and who considered himself physically fit, once again struggling to keep up.

## ARE THEY REALLY *THAT* OLD?

After Leaf's articles in *National Geographic* appeared, however, a heated controversy developed over the validity of the ages claimed by some Abkhasians. When people say they are 140 or 150 years old, this naturally raises eyebrows. When the Soviet press announced that Shirali Muslimov was 168 years old, and the government commemorated the assertion by putting his face on a postage stamp, knowledgeable scientists around the world were skeptical. There is a reason that, until recently, *The Guinness Book of World Records* introduced its section on longevity with the warning: "No single subject is more obscured by vanity, deceit, falsehood and deliberate fraud than the extremes of human longevity." Currently, the longest fully documented and irrefutably authenticated age ever reached by a human being is 122, by a Frenchwoman named Jeanne Louise Calment.

How old, in fact, are the oldest Abkhasians? No one knows with absolute certainty. In the days when these elders were born, probably less than one-tenth of 1 percent of the world's population was keeping written birth records. When birth records are lacking or questionable, as they are in almost all cases of people born prior to 1920 in regions like the Caucasus, contemporary researchers have had to be creative in developing methods to appraise the ages of elders. Many volumes have been written about the enterprising techniques that have been employed in the effort, and probably an equal number of scholarly volumes have been written critiquing these techniques. It has been a difficult task.

Probably the foremost skeptic about the extremely old ages sometimes claimed for elders in the Caucasus was a geneticist from Soviet Georgia named Zhores A. Medvedev, an expert in the methodologies used in the effort to arrive at accurate age verifications in Abkhasia and elsewhere in the Caucasus. Medvedev's articles expressing his doubts received a great deal of attention when they were published in the scientific journal *The Gerontologist* shortly after Leaf's articles appeared in *National Geographic*. (Gerontology is the study of the changes and associated problems in the mind and body that accompany aging.) In these articles, Medvedev presented convincing evidence that the claims that people were regularly living past the age of 120 were not to be trusted.[10] At the same time, though, he recognized that unusual longevity in the region was a genuine reality, and that the area was indeed home to an inordinate number of extremely healthy elders.

As the controversy was unfolding, the legend of extraordinarily healthy and long-lived people in the Caucasus was being heavily promoted by U.S. corporations that manufactured and sold yogurt, attempting to connect the phenomenal longevity of people in the region to their consumption of yogurt. The Dannon yogurt company marketed a widely seen commercial showing a 110-year-old mother pinching the cheek of her 89-year-old son and telling him to eat his yogurt. This clever ad and others featuring Soviet centenarians were fabulously successful in the American market. They produced a generation of Americans who associated yogurt with extreme longevity, and who naïvely believed that people regularly lived to 140 and beyond in the Caucasus.

Unfortunately, it was the inflated claims for supercentenarians living to extreme ages that got most of the attention in the 1970s and 1980s. What made Abkhasians so interesting to the Western world at the time was not their lifestyle and the wondrously healthy way they aged, but the exotic phenomenon of people supposedly living to unbelievable ages. When these extreme claims for superlongevity were found to be false, there was a regrettable tendency to dismiss everything about Abkhasian longevity as a hoax.

My interest in longevity in Abkhasia, however, doesn't depend on whether any specific individuals have reached ages beyond 120. Perhaps none have, but I don't find the question to be particularly important. What makes these people fascinating to me is the fact that an extraordinary percentage of Abkhasians have lived to ripe old ages while retaining their full health and vigor. What I find remarkable is the high degree of physical and mental fitness commonly found among the elders in Abkhasia, and their obvious joy in life.

## WHAT IS THEIR SECRET?

What I want to know is how they've done it. How have they managed to maintain their vitality and strength to the very ends of their long lives? What can we learn from how they've lived that will make our lives longer in health and greater in joy? What are the key factors that have produced such exceptionally healthy aging? What can we learn from their lifestyles, and from the ways of life in other areas of the world that have also produced extraordinary numbers of extremely healthy old people?

It's not that I think the elders of Abkhasia are perfect, or that we should in all ways model our lives after theirs. Nothing is served by unduly romanticizing these people. They are human, and they have their idiosyncrasies and flaws. But the fact remains that they can provide a positive and valuable counterbalance to the images most of us have of aging today.

Very few people in modern Western society look forward to growing old. We lack models that speak to us of the possibilities and opportunities of our elder years. The Abkhasians and the other peoples of the world who have consistently enjoyed vibrant and lengthy lives have something important to show us.

Shoto Gogoghian, M.D., is one of the world's leading authorities on Abkhasian longevity. He was director of public health in Abkhasia for twenty-three years, and subsequently became director of the Institute of Gerontology, a part of the prestigious Soviet Academy of Medical Science. Like almost all gerontologists today, he recognizes that most (if not all) of the extreme claims for hyperlongevity have been inflated.[11] But after personally visiting, interviewing, and appraising the ages of almost all the most elderly people in Abkhasia, Dr. Gogoghian wrote that the people of Abkhasia most certainly do have unusual rates of longevity and remarkable health in old age. About 80 percent of all Abkhasians over the age of ninety, he said, are mentally healthy and outgoing. Only 10 percent have poor hearing, and fewer than 4 percent have poor eyesight.[12] These are staggering statistics when compared to the health of elders in the United States and other fully industrialized nations.

One part of the Abkhasian formula for exceptionally healthy aging is the great amount of regular exercise built into the routines of their daily lives. One gerontologist who had studied longevity in the Caucasus for many years speculated in the 1970s that the constant physical activity required of the Abkhasians develops the function of their hearts and lungs to such a degree that an enhanced amount of oxygen is supplied to their hearts. Such suppositions were confirmed in 2005, when the *Journal of Epidemiology and Community Health* published a new study that found mountain dwellers live longer than their lowland counterparts.[13] The reason? Their hearts get a better workout on a daily basis. The researchers pointed to the increased physical activity from walking on rugged terrain with less oxygen in the surrounding air to explain the extended life spans and lower rate of heart disease among those living in the mountains.

For the Abkhasians, a high level of physical fitness is both required and produced by the steep terrain on which they live and work. Simply going through their normal day requires a great deal of physical exertion. No one sits at a desk or rides to and from work. Even the elders think nothing of hiking several miles up and down steep hillsides to get from one dwelling to the next, or from a village to the surrounding fields and back.

Retirement is an unknown concept in Abkhasian thinking. The Abkhasians never, at any stage of life, become sedentary. Most of the elderly still work regularly, many in the orchards and gardens, pruning the fruit and nut trees, removing dead wood, and planting young trees. Some still chop wood and haul water.

They work hard, but they are fortunate in that their work does not entail the emotional stress we often associate with work. Their work tempos are natural expressions of biological rhythms, and they have no sense of the drivenness and hurry that predominate in most industrialized nations. In fact, Abkhasians distinctly dislike being rushed and have no concept of a deadline. The only time they feel a sense of urgency is during rare actual emergencies, such as when a house is on fire. Other than that, they are remarkably relaxed, and often joke and sing while working.[14]

How many of us in the modern world can say the same thing about our work environment? Some of us fear that unless we are driven by a sense of urgency and competition we will become lazy. But the Abkhasians are anything but lazy. In fact, they are astoundingly fit. When Dr. Alexander Leaf learned of an old man, Kosta Kashig, said to be 106 years old, who spent the summers with his goats in the high alpine pastures, he wanted to meet the elder in that setting to learn firsthand the level of physical exertion involved in his daily activities. Leaf set out early one morning with two companions and a young local guide to climb to where the elder could be found. The trail, however, proved so steep and muddy that his two companions gave up about one-third of the way up and headed back downhill. Only Leaf and the young guide continued on.

After six hours of arduous climbing, they came out of the woods and onto a grassy slope where Kosta Kashig was spending the summer tending his goats. Leaf proceeded to have a lengthy discussion with the old man, after which he concluded Kashig was not 106, but probably "only" 90. Whichever age was correct, Leaf wrote that for Kashig "to be able to spend four months of the year bounding over the hillside from dawn until dusk in pursuit of his agile goats was remarkable."[15]

Eventually, Leaf made the long and difficult climb down from the high pastureland. When he arrived back in town, he was exhausted, but also elated to have accomplished the trek and proud of how fast he had been able to make it down. Then he learned to his amazement that Kosta Kashig, be he 106 or only 90, regularly made the same trek in just half the time it had taken Leaf. Such is the level of physical fitness commonplace among the elderly in Abkhasia.

## A TOAST TO SWEET OLD AGE

Our capacity to understand the lifestyles of the Abkhasians owes much to the work of Dr. Sula Benet. A professor of anthropology at Hunter College, City University of New York, she was fluent in Russian, which all Abkhasians understand, and she spent several years living in Abkhasia, doing fieldwork under the auspices of Columbia University, the Social Science Research Council, the Research Institute for the Study of Man, and the Wenner-Gren Foundation for Anthropological Research. Her book, *Abkhasians: The Long-Living People of the Caucasus,* is considered one of the finest case studies in cultural anthropology ever written.[16]

As to the controversy over the ages of the oldest of the old, Benet felt it didn't matter that much. "If a person lives to 120 rather than 130 in health and vigor," she said, "the fact of old age is barely diminished."[17] Though not knowing the exact age of any particular elder, she pointed out the remarkable fact that people in Abkhasia have specific terms or expressions for great-grandparents going back six generations. These expressions are used to refer to the living, not to those who have died.[18] Very few languages contain expressions for so many generations of living relatives.

Benet was also impressed by the physical condition of even the very elderly in Abkhasia. Only the oldest people have wrinkles, she noted. Only the very elderly have gray hair. Baldness is extremely rare.[19] More than a third of those over ninety do not need glasses for any kind of work, including reading or threading a needle.[20] Most have their own teeth. And Benet was particularly affected by the beautifully erect posture elderly Abkhasians maintain, even to very advanced ages.[21]

Most tellingly, she found that "sickness is not considered a normal or natural event even in very old age."[22]

To Benet, the reasons for the remarkable health and longevity in Abkhasia are many. One factor that she highlighted in particular was the tremendous respect for the aged that is a defining feature of Abkhasian culture. In Abkhasia, a person's status increases with age, and he or she receives ever more privileges with the passing years. This deference does not depend on wealth or occupation. Elders are respected, even revered, simply by virtue of being old. Elders who are poor and known only to their families have greater social standing in Abkhasian society than someone who may have become rich and famous but is not yet an elder. There is nothing elders have to do to earn this respect. They are never required to compete with younger people.[23]

When one U.S. researcher explained to a group of Abkhasians that in the wealthy United States, old people are sometimes left homeless and hungry, he was met with total disbelief. Nothing he said could overcome their inability to grasp such a reality.

The Abkhasian respect for the aged is clear from their vocabulary. They do not even have a phrase meaning "old people." Instead, those over 100 are called "long-living people."[24] And all Abkhasian villages celebrate a holiday in their honor called "the Day of the Long-Living People." On this day each year, the elders dress in elaborate costumes and parade before the rest of the villagers, who gather to pay them homage.[25]

## IN CONTRAST

The more I have learned about Abkhasian culture, the more I've been struck by the contrast with the modern industrialized world, and the more I've become aware of how youth-obsessed we are. In Abkhasia, people are esteemed and seen as beautiful in their old age. Silver hair and wrinkles are viewed as signs of wisdom, maturity, and long years of service.

In the West, on the other hand, we tend to associate old age with ugliness and youth with beauty, so much so that an increasing number of people today are willing to spend a great deal of money and undergo a considerable degree of pain in order to have facelifts, that they might look younger.

Are these people putting themselves through the agony of a procedure that includes skull drains, titanium screws, bloody eyes with lashless lids, tightened skin, painfully slow recoveries, and eating tiny bites of baby food because they are vain and unable to accept nature and life's realities?[26] Or is it because they are fighting to ward off the invisibility that all too often comes with aging in a culture where looking older is equated with a loss of beauty and value? Some say that only people who hate themselves would be willing to undergo such an ordeal, but I wonder. Living in a youth-obsessed culture, maybe they hate the way they are treated because of how they look.

Popular television programs like *The Swan* and *Extreme Makeover* have contributed greatly in recent years to the rise in cosmetic surgery. At the climax of one show, a participant (having received a million dollars' worth of plastic surgery) was finally revealed. Her elated husband beamed at the camera. "I had a forty-year-old wife," he said, "and now I have a twenty-five-year-old wife." Deliriously happy with the change in his wife's appearance, he described the improvement entirely as a matter of her looking younger. I'm sure he meant it as a compliment, but his comment reflected something about our culture that I find troubling. Is it really better to have a twenty-five-year-old wife than a forty-year-old wife? Is younger always better?

*The Simpsons* television show often satirically portrays cultural trends that are all too real. In one episode, a children's hospital was torn down so the new Springfield Plastic Surgery Clinic could be built. Mayor Quimby gave a speech at the ribbon-cutting ceremony. "Thanks to this clinic," he said, "we will no longer be terrorized by the spectacle of women aging naturally."

*American Idol* is another television program that reflects the perspectives of mainstream Western culture. The show has phenomenal ratings. In 2004, more than forty-nine million viewers tuned in to watch the finale. When the *American Idol* judges were asked whether they would consider getting plastic surgery, one of the judges, Simon Cowell, said he would make it mandatory for every woman over forty.

He probably thought he was being funny. I don't think he had any idea what the impact of his remark was on every woman over forty, and indeed on younger women, too, each of whom will likely be over forty someday herself.

This kind of thing takes a terrible toll on women's self-image, which is none too high in the modern world in the first place. A worldwide 2004 survey by Dove soap found that only 2 percent of women consider themselves "beautiful." And it gets worse as women get older. Among women over sixty, almost none consider themselves even "average-looking."[27]

In my eyes, this is cruel. But it's the norm wherever women are beset by unobtainable media images of beauty and by a cosmetics industry that encourages women to be terrified of aging. One cosmetics ad shows a woman in her forties fiercely proclaiming, "I don't intend to grow old gracefully. I'm going to fight it every step of the way."

I do take heart, though, from the fact that modern Western culture is not the only way people can live and its prevailing assumptions are not the only way people can think. Moreover, there are signs, even in the modern world, that things could be changing. A new ad campaign from Dove skin care products, for example, features Irene Sinclair, a ninety-six-year-old woman with a luminous smile who was discovered at a nursing home in London. The ad asks, "Will society ever accept that old can be beautiful?"

## WHERE AGE IS BEAUTY

In Abkhasia, it would be considered an insult to be told that you are "looking young" or that the years have barely changed you. People there compliment others by saying "You're looking old today," meaning that the person is wise and beautiful in their maturity. In Abkhasia, when older people lie about their age, they do not give a younger age, as is common in the West. Instead, they exaggerate how old they are, for this gives them greater standing in their culture.

Researcher Dan Georgakas sought to explain the exalted social status of the aged in Abkhasia:

> Old age is the crown of a successful life. . . . The psychological climate for the old is so positive that rest homes available through government auspices are rarely utilized, as even in the smallest of families there are many relatives who covet the honor of housing an elder.[28]

Abkhasians expect a long and useful life, and they look forward to old age with good reason. In a culture which so highly values continuity in its traditions, the elders are indispensable. They are never thought of as—or experienced as—burdens. Quite the contrary, they are the society's most treasured resources. An oft-repeated Abkhasian proverb is "Besides God, we also need the elders."[29]

In the modern Western world, older men who show an interest in sex are sometimes disparaged as "dirty old men." In Abkhasia, on the other hand, continuation of an active sex life into old age is considered to be as natural as maintaining a healthy appetite or sound sleep. Abkhasians do not think there is any reason why increased years should strip them of so human a function.

Almost everyone who visits Abkhasia ends up remarking on the importance of song, music, and dance in Abkhasian life. People of all ages in Abkhasia love to sing, and there are songs for every occasion. There are lullabies, there are work songs, and there are healing songs. There are special songs for weddings and other rituals. Each chore has a special song. While working in the fields, people often divide into groups for choral singing.

In Abkhasian culture, songs are used like medicine. There is a song called "the Song of the Wounded One" which is sung by friends and relatives to support the recovery of someone who has been hurt. Sometimes the injured one may also sing along.[30] When someone falls ill, his or her friends and relatives, in addition to assuming the sick person's responsibilities, surround the bedside. They tell jokes and stories, and they sing and dance. When someone is about to die, friends and relatives sing quietly at the bedside, and also at the memorial services.

Singing may not seem to have anything to do with health, but I think it might. When people celebrate and enjoy life, is it possible they are sending life-affirming messages to their cells? Could this help explain why long-living people everywhere tend to be those who live with gusto? They dance, they sing, and they celebrate life as it unfolds.

## CHILDREN

I also think the way children are raised in Abkhasia has much to do with the kind of elders they eventually grow up to become. Having lived many years in the United States and several years in Abkhasia, Sula Benet was struck by the way Abkhasian children behave and the way they are treated:

> I never heard a child cry in protest or a parent raise his voice or threaten spanking. A command is never repeated twice. As a teacher of fidgety American youth, I marveled at Abkhasian schoolchildren who . . . sit at attention for hours. Such miraculous results are not motivated by fear."[31]

Abkhasian parents never scold or nag, and they never criticize or punish their children. How, you may wonder, do they get their children to behave properly? Benet explains:

> Abkhasian parents express disapproval by withholding praise, which is otherwise very generously dispensed. The Abkhasian concept of discipline, considered necessary and good for children, is not intertwined with the concept of punishment. Abkhasians feel that physical punishment induces disrespect. . . . The Abkhasian method of discipline does not allow for the development and expression of even the mildest forms of sadistic impulse. . . . With no threat of punishment . . . the young never express resentment. It gradually became apparent to the author that they do not *feel* resentment.[32]

It's different, unfortunately, in the United States today, a nation in which 565,000 children are killed or seriously injured by their parents or guardians each year.

How much better would life be in the modern world if all children were raised with the kind of respect they are offered in Abkhasia? In Abkhasian schools, children are never made to feel inferior. Ridicule is never used to "teach" children. Scorn and rejection are not part of the curriculum. And neither is any kind of physical coercion.[33]

Abkhasians are consistently respectful of their bodies and the bodies of others. They never physically punish children, adults, or animals.[34] This may help explain why domestic violence is almost entirely unknown in Abkhasia, as is rape.

Friendships are extremely important to Abkhasians. When guests arrive at an Abkhasian home, they are embraced and kissed, and the host makes a circular motion above the guest's head and says, "Let all the evil spirits who may be hovering around you come to me instead."[35]

## THE FOOD THEY EAT

What, then, of the Abkhasian diet?

Thanks to the Dannon yogurt ads, people in the United States and elsewhere often believe that it is the consumption of yogurt which is responsible for the unusually long lives of the Abkhasians and others in the Caucasus. Actually, though, the Abkhasians do not eat yogurt. They drink one or two glasses a day of a fermented beverage called *matzoni*, made from the milk of goats, cows, or sheep. This variety of fermented milk has been used in the Caucasus for centuries, and most likely originated in this part of the world. The traditional Abkhasian diet is essentially lacto-vegetarian, with a rare serving of meat, and with the dairy component consisting primarily of the fermented matzoni.

According to Benet, the Abkhasians usually begin breakfast with a salad of green vegetables freshly picked from the garden. During the spring, it is made up of pungent vegetables such as watercress, green onions, and radishes. In summer and autumn, tomatoes and cucumbers are more popular, while the winter salad consists of pickled cucumber and tomatoes, radishes, cabbage, and onion. Dill and coriander may be added, but no dressings are used. Many plants that grow wild in Abkhasia also end up in their salads. Breakfasts also often include a glass of matzoni. At all three meals, the people eat their "beloved abista," a cornmeal porridge, always freshly cooked and served warm.

If they get hungry between meals, Abkhasians typically eat fruit in season from their own orchard or garden. Thanks to the mild climate, fresh fruit is available seven or eight months of the year. During these months, the Abkhasians enjoy large quantities of fruit eaten fresh from the tree or vine. There are cherries and apricots in the spring. Throughout the summer, there are pears, plums, peaches, figs, and many kinds of berries. In the fall, there are grapes and persimmons, as well as apples and pears, both of which grow wild in great abundance. Wild pears are cooked into a thick syrup, with no added sweeteners—something like apple butter. The fruit that is not eaten fresh is stored or dried for winter use. Thus many fruits are used all year round.

With rare exceptions, vegetables are eaten raw, or cooked in only a very small amount of water. Abkhasians do not traditionally eat any fried food. And the freshness of food is considered paramount. Vegetables are picked just prior to serving or cooking, and leftovers are discarded, because food that is not totally fresh is considered harmful. While modern urbanites may scoff at such fastidiousness, there is a good reason for it. Such a heightened concern for freshness ensures that food is never eaten that has become spoiled and might be carrying pathogenic microorganisms. It also guarantees that foods are eaten at the height of their nutritional value, with a minimal loss of nutrients.

Nuts play a major role in Abkhasian cuisine and are the primary source of fat in the Abkhasian diet. Almonds, pecans, beechnuts, and hazelnuts are cultivated, and chestnut trees grow wild and profusely, as do many other wild nut trees. Virtually every meal contains nuts in one form or another.

Abkhasians eat relatively little meat, and when they do, the meat is always from animals who have been healthy and who have been freshly slaughtered. Even then, the fat from the meat or poultry is never used. When meat is served, even the smallest pieces of fat are removed. The Abkhasians do not care at all for fatty dishes. They also consume no sugar, little salt, and almost no butter.

This may help explain why the average cholesterol level among Abkhasian centenarians is 98.[36] This compares extremely favorably to the cholesterol levels common in people in the United States, where nearly everyone's is over 200, and where until recently levels as high as 250 were sometimes considered "normal."

One of the most definitive features of the Abkhasian diet is that in comparison with Americans, Abkhasians eat very little. Most Abkhasians consume less than two thousand calories a day, while many people in the United States eat literally twice that much.[37] And unlike most of the world, the Abkhasian diet does not change significantly with an increase in wealth. Regardless of how poor or how affluent Abkhasians are, they still consume protein in moderation, fat mainly from nuts, and carbohydrates primarily from vegetables, fruits, and whole-grain cereals such as their cornmeal abista.

In fact, people almost never overeat in Abkhasia, because overeating is considered both socially inappropriate and dangerous.[38] This no doubt contributes to the fact that Abkhasians are universally very strong and slender people, with no excess fat on their bodies. They eat slowly and chew thoroughly, savoring each moment and deeply enjoying one another's company.

When an Abkhasian host invites a guest for dinner, the wording of the invitation says a great deal about the priorities of these remarkable people. The invitation always says, "Come and be our guest." It never says, "Come for dinner."[39] Of course dinner is served, and it is prepared and shared with joy. But the emphasis is never on the food, but rather on the pleasures of being together. These are a people who relish the joys of friendship above all others.

## LEARNING FROM THEIR WISDOM

Of course, people in Abkhasia have always struggled with the trials and crises that exist in all human life. In addition, the modern world has been encroaching in recent years, and there have been particularly challenging events since the breakup of the former Soviet Union in the early 1990s. I will speak more about these later, but I want to focus now on what those of us in the more modern world can learn from these friendly, long-living, happy, and extraordinarily healthy people.

Not long ago, I unconsciously equated aging with the loss of mental agility, sensory acuity, physical limberness, sexual desire, and a host of other human abilities. I thought it almost certain that we will all become more frail and disease-prone as we get older. I thought that the best we could do was to be satisfied to accept these "inevitable" losses with dignity. But the more I have learned from the people of Abkhasia, the more hopeful I have become. They seem to suggest that there might be another possibility for us entirely. If we choose wisely, maybe we, too, can live long lives in good health and spirits. Maybe our wisdom years can, after all, be rich with vitality, joy, and fulfillment. Particularly when, as we shall now see, the Abkhasians are far from the only culture representing this fascinating possibility.

## 2

# Vilcabamba: The Valley of Eternal Youth

*A society's quality and durability can best be measured by the re-
spect and care given to its elder citizens.*

—Arnold Toynbee

The second people famous for their longevity and health who
were visited and studied by Dr. Alexander Leaf for *National Geographic* were the Vilcabambans.

Vilcabamba is a small, extremely inaccessible town tucked away
in Ecuador's Andes mountains. Perched serenely at an altitude of
some 4,500 feet, the Vilcabamban valley is not far from the Peruvian
border, and about a hundred miles inland from the Pacific Ocean. In
the language of the Inca Indians, Vilcabamba means "Sacred Valley,"
and there is indeed something magical about the place. For one thing,
the climate could hardly be more benign. With an average year-round
temperature of 68 degrees and almost no seasonal variation, Vilcabamba is an idyllic land of lush, subtropical agriculture where a
wide variety of grains, fruits, and vegetables can be easily cultivated,
and many grow wild for the picking.

In 1981, the physician and medical journalist Morton Walker
conducted a series of studies of Vilcabambans' health and wrote effusively of what he found:

In the Western Hemisphere, a place exists where degenerative diseases seldom if ever affect the population. The people have no heart disease, no cancer, no diabetes, no stroke, no cirrhosis, no senility, no arteriosclerosis, nor any other morbid conditions connected with an interruption in blood flow that are commonly responsible for illness, disability, and death among industrialized people. Since they don't die of degenerative diseases, the inhabitants of this place are able to live the full complement of mankind's years—more than a century. . . .

Vilcabamba is a veritable paradise on earth. . . . Over the years the Sacred Valley has been variously called "The Land of Eternal Youth," "The Valley of Peace and Tranquility," and "The Lost Paradise." It has been given these labels because of the valley's solitude, serenity, clean air, dazzling sun, nearly constant blue sky, pure mineral drinking water, helpful neighbors, lack of illness, and a kind of ubiquitous beauty that penetrates to one's soul and provides a sense of well-being.[1]

Dr. Leaf, ever the careful scientist, was not inclined to use such lyrical prose. But he was impressed by the considerable number of active oldsters whose lifestyles he and his medical associates were able to examine. These included a 103-year-old woman whom Leaf watched thread a sewing needle without the aid of eyeglasses, and a 95-year-old woman he found happily at work in the local bakery. After examining the elderly woman in the bakery, Leaf commented, "Her health through her long life has been excellent. She has a good heart and is in excellent condition."[2]

## A REPUTATION FOR LONG LIFE

Vilcabamba first began to come to international attention in 1954, when a U.S. physician, Eugene H. Payne (clinical investigator for Parke Davis Pharmaceuticals), wrote a *Reader's Digest* article saying he had found little or no evidence of cardiac or circulatory diseases in the area.[3]

A year later, another American doctor, Albert Krammer, went to

Vilcabamba to recuperate from a heart attack, then returned home feeling "better than I could ever remember."[4] He described his experience in a series of widely read articles. Soon stories were becoming common of heart patients from Mexico and Japan who after a few weeks in the valley found themselves bounding up steep mountains.

In 1956, a very elderly Vilcabamban named Javier Pereira, said to be 167, was brought to New York City and presented to the public by the owners of the syndicated newspaper feature "Believe It or Not."[5]

Before long, serious scientists began to investigate. In 1969, a team of Ecuadorian physicians headed by Dr. Miguel Salvador, a Quito cardiologist, undertook one of the first major studies of the health of people living in Vilcabamba. Salvador and his team studied 338 Vilcabambans and found that they were free not only of arteriosclerosis and heart disease, but also of cancer, diabetes, and degenerative diseases such as rheumatism, osteoporosis, and Alzheimer's. The researchers called the general standard of fitness among the old "amazing." The Vilcabamban valley, the Ecuadorian doctors concluded, somehow provided immunity to the physical problems that shorten lives elsewhere.[6]

In the 1970s, a British gerontologist named Dr. David Davies made four separate visits to the valley, studying the health of the old people and their way of life. In a series of articles published in scientific journals and in a book he wrote for the public titled *The Centenarians of the Andes,* he asserted that the elders of Vilcabamba

> may die as the result of an accident, or from a sickness introduced by visitors from the outside, but never from the major killing diseases that afflict the rest of the world.[7]

After Dr. Leaf's article extolling the health and longevity in Vilcabamba was published in *National Geographic* in 1973, the elders of Vilcabamba were beset by a swarm of gerontologists and other researchers who were examining their teeth, eyes, and ears, measuring their blood pressure, and connecting them to cardiac and chest monitors. The scientists took samples of their hair, saliva, and urine, took notes on their diet, and interviewed them about their sex lives.

In 1978, the National Institute of Aging and the Fogerty International Center for Advanced Study in Health Science cosponsored an international conference focused on the health of the elderly in Vilcabamba. Dr. Leaf was co-chairman of the event, which included scientists, physicians, and researchers from Japan, Canada, France, Ecuador, and the United States, all of whom had worked in Vilcabamba. The participants agreed that the over-seventy population in Vilcabamba had spectacular cardiovascular health, including almost no incidence of high blood pressure and only one third of the cardiac abnormalities usually found in the same age categories in developed nations. Researchers linked the Vilcabamban elders' extraordinary cardiovascular health with their leanness, their diet, their low cholesterol levels, and their high levels of physical activity.[8]

As the years went along, Japanese researchers began studying sleep patterns in the Vilcabamban elderly. In the modern world, sleep apnea, or difficulty in breathing while at rest, is very common among people over 65. The Japanese used portable respiratory monitoring devices to record breathing patterns of Vilcabambans aged 84 to 94 and found that nearly all participants enjoyed healthy and peaceful sleep.[9]

In 1993, an article in the Los Angeles Times enthusiastically summed up the picture:

> Folks in Vilcabamba have a reputation for long life. Very long life. More than a few say they have passed the century mark; people in their 80s and 90s appear almost common. And the Ancient Ones, as they are called, maintain their health and vitality right to the end.[10]

## HOW OLD ARE THEY REALLY?

As in Abkhasia, though, there has been a great deal of controversy over the actual ages of the elders in Vilcabamba and serious doubt about the most extreme of the superlongevity claims. Claiming an age of 167 when the oldest fully authenticated human age known to modern science is 122 is not the quickest route to credibility.

Verifying the ages of old people in places like Abkhasia and Vilcabamba is never as simple as it sounds. Unlike the case in Abkhasia, where there are hardly any records to speak of, there are baptismal records in Vilcabamba that have been kept by the local church and birth records kept by the Civil Registry that go back as far as 1860. But the records are old and incomplete. There are pages missing, and pages so worn they cannot be read. What is more, Vilcabamban parents have not always registered the births of their children. And to make things even more confusing, cousins and other close relatives in Vilcabamba have often been given the same names.

Several years after the excitement about longevity in Vilcabamba had grown to a worldwide phenomenon, two American scientists— Dr. Richard B. Mazess, a radiologist, and Dr. Sylvia H. Forman, an anthropologist—sought to arrive at as much certainty as possible about the ages of the elders in Vilcabamba. They performed a meticulous house-by-house census, then checked all the birth, death, and marriage records that they could find, and finally cross-checked the various documents against one another. It was a bewildering maze of documentation, but Mazess and Forman eventually concluded that there had been a consistent pattern of age inflation.

For example, in the case of a man who had claimed to be 132 shortly before his death, they found that the man had actually been only ninety-three at the time of his death. Apparently, the man had attempted to appear older than he actually was by adopting as his own the baptismal certificate of an older deceased relative who shared the same name. It turned out that his mother had in fact been born five years after his own stated birth date, something that even the heroic modern advances in reproductive technology have not been able to replicate.[11]

Mazess and Forman ultimately came to believe that this kind of thing was common, and that none of the twenty-three self-proclaimed centenarians then living in the village of Vilcabamba had actually reached the age of 100. When they published their findings in *The*

*Journals of Gerontology* in 1979, they titled their article "Longevity and age exaggeration in Vilcabamba, Ecuador," and declared that "extreme ages were either incorrect or unsubstantiated."[12] As a result, many in the scientific community came to believe that longevity in Vilcabamba had been totally discredited.

At that time, Vilcabamba had only about a thousand residents. Mazess said that in a population that small, it would be out of the ordinary if even a single person over the age of 100 were to be found, and truly remarkable if there were two people of such an age. He listed ten people who claimed to be centenarians, but who he considered to be between 85 and 95.

Presumably, Mazess and Forman were correct in their evaluations. However, fifteen years later, two of the ten people Mazess had listed were still alive, which would mean that based on the ages he attributed to them, there were in 1994 at least two centenarians in a population of one thousand—a number that Mazess himself had said would be extraordinary.

Dr. Leaf had been aware, of course, of the tendency for old people to exaggerate their ages. He and his team had also spent long, painstaking hours studying the available records, and they had eventually concluded that the elder Vilcabambans probably did not actually know their ages, and so the ages they gave were almost completely useless. He was struck, nevertheless, by the fact that the very oldest people were remarkably fit for their age, even if they might actually be a decade or two younger than they claimed.

In 1990, the Ecuadorian physician Guillermo Vela Chiriboga, who headed one of the scientific expeditions organized by Dr. Leaf to explore longevity and health in Vilcabamba, published *The Secrets of Vilcabamba (Secretos de Vilcabamba para vivir siempre joven)*. Having done further study after Leaf had left, he also could find no evidence to substantiate the claims for particular individuals living to extreme ages. And, like Leaf, he recognized that in a culture where people don't actually have a very good idea of how old they are and where there is much respect for the elderly, there can be an incentive to exaggerate. But he continued to find numerous oldsters whose later years were filled with health and vitality and who did not suffer from the cardiovascular ailments so common among elders in the modern world. He wrote:

> Even if Gabriel Erazo, who claimed to be 130 years old, and others who claim to be over 100, are 20 or 30 years younger (than they claim), that does not invalidate the reality. . . . In Vilcabamba I found very elderly people with healthy bodies and souls.[13]

Dr. Chiriboga also found that even the most elderly of the residents of Vilcabamba rarely suffer from fractures, osteoporosis, or arthritic ailments, which are common among older people elsewhere. His trained medical eyes could find no evidence of cancer, diabetes, obesity, heart disease, arthritis, or dementia, even among the very eldest of the population. He wrote that local inhabitants, even in extreme old age, "are agile and mentally lucid, with a sense of humor and admirable physical health. . . . [They] enjoy tranquility without a competitive spirit, and spurn the accumulation of wealth."[14]

## GRACE HALSELL

Of the many perspectives on the people of Vilcabamba, one that I find particularly fascinating is that of an American woman named Grace Halsell, who lived in Vilcabamba for two years in the 1970s and subsequently wrote a book about the people there, titled *Los Viejos (The Old Ones)*.[15]

To say that Grace Halsell was an amazing human being is an understatement. She died in 2002 after living what the writer Gore Vidal called "the most interesting and courageous life of any American in our time." A distinguished journalist, she worked for three years in the White House as a speechwriter for President Lyndon Johnson. Her newspaper articles for the *New York Post,* the *New York Herald Tribune, The Christian Science Monitor,* and other major newspapers were filed from war zones in Korea, Vietnam, and Bosnia, as well as Russia, China, Macedonia, and Albania.

She was also the author of twelve books, including *Soul Sister,* in which she related her experiences, after taking a medication to turn her skin black, living as an impoverished African American in

Harlem and Mississippi.[16] Her book *Bessie Yellowhair* tells the story of the years she spent living with the Navajo on an isolated reservation in Arizona, and then, with their approval, dyeing her skin ochre and passing as an Indian among white people, including working as a live-in Navajo maid in Los Angeles.[17]

In researching her book about illegal immigrants in the United States, Halsell, who spoke fluent Spanish, became an illegal and undocumented "wetback," swimming across the Rio Grande to enter the United States, dodging border patrol guards, crawling through sewers, and hiding from Customs in the dreaded Smugglers Canyon. Then, presenting herself as the journalist she also was, she interviewed the whites of the Sun Belt who fear the rising tide of Hispanic immigration, and also interviewed armed border patrolmen, riding with them as they vainly attempted to seal the porous U.S.–Mexico border.[18]

Grace Halsell had an almost unworldly ability to connect with people and see the world through their eyes. The title of her autobiography is, aptly, *In Their Shoes.*[19]

During the two years she lived in Vilcabamba, Grace Halsell was one of Alexander Leaf's interpreters and assistants. Apparently, Leaf never realized that the resident of Vilcabamba who was such an outstanding translator, whose English and Spanish were both impeccable, who seemed to know so much not only about Vilcabambans but also about Americans, was not in fact a penniless Vilcabamban peasant but a world-renowned American journalist who had regularly flown on Air Force One (the U.S. president's personal plane), and who had interviewed presidents, prime ministers, movie stars, and kings.[20]

Unlike Leaf and the other scientists, though, Grace Halsell had not come to the valley to peer, probe, and analyze the people. She had not come to take their blood pressure or measure their cholesterol. She had come to be one with them:

> I have always gone to other lands with one idea: to meet people and come to know them. I learn to sing their songs, dance their jigs, eat their food. I try to be one among the people in whose land I am living.[21]

Doctors, scientists, and researchers have come up with many explanations for the marvels of Vilcabamba. Some have credited the pure mountain air that is uniquely rich with negative ions. Others have pointed to the natural, healthful diet and the great amount of exercise inherent in the Vilcabamban lifestyle. A few have pointed to the soil and its high levels of selenium and other minerals. Others have suggested that Vilcabamban drinking water holds the secret. (Vilcabamba is apparently one of the few places in South America where you not only can but should drink the water. Not surprisingly, several companies have sought to capitalize on this fact by marketing the water in Europe.)

Grace Halsell understood and appreciated these viewpoints, particularly the ones about diet and exercise. She loved the fresh fruits of every variety and the fresh garden vegetables. She loved the tremendous amount of walking she and all the others did up and down the verdant hills in the course of a day. And she loved the magnificent scenery, the pristine air, and the crystal-clear water. But what caught her eye and heart most of all was the quality of human relationships in Vilcabamba. To her, the sense of connectedness that people had with one another was paramount, and was, if anything, more important than the other explanations for their notable health in old age. Like the researchers and doctors who visited Vilcabamba, she, too, sought to understand the underlying reasons for the health and longevity of the people. But what made her unique was that rather than trying to remain dispassionate, Grace Halsell met the Vilcabamban people with love.

> I went to visit them because I had heard they were old. But I stayed with them because they were themselves, a most lovable people, from whom I wanted to learn. Each one seemed to believe that he would become all that he had given away. I never before experienced a people who had so little and gave so much. Without any material possessions, they somehow assert their personalities, their individuality, their right to be giving. Of all the Biblical injunctions they had heard from the Spanish priests, the *viejos* [old ones] seemed to have taken "It is more blessed to give, than to receive" as their maxim in life.[22]

## SHE WHO LAUGHS, LASTS

Halsell was accustomed to the luxuries we take for granted in the modern industrialized world, yet she found the far more simple life in Vilcabamba not to be a burden, but in many ways to be a freedom.

> I had no mirror, no running water with which to brush my teeth. I was liberated from the time-consuming feminine activities such as shaving my legs and under my armpits, spraying deodorant under my arms, and plucking my eyebrows, painting my nails, curling my hair. Living in the Sacred Valley was like being a child again. I awoke each morning at sunrise, brushed my hair into a ponytail, slipped on my every-day-of-the-week clothes, and I was ready to greet the day, the Vilcabamban way.[23]

The people of Vilcabamba are poor in material things by modern standards, but Grace Halsell found them to be rich in other ways, for they radiated a sense of self-confidence and security in themselves that people in the modern world, with all its material abundance, often find themselves endlessly seeking. As she reflected on the underlying reasons for their remarkable health and longevity, she came back again and again to the way she saw them treat each other:

> Living among the *viejos,* I never heard them quarrel or fight or dispute with each other. They had what I would consider a "high" culture in this regard. They spoke beautifully, elegantly, with ample flourishes of tenderness. Their words themselves were often caresses.[24]

She asked one of the two local policemen what kinds of crimes were committed in the valley. "Not much," he replied. "We don't have any real crimes."[25]

Halsell believed that a key to the health and harmony in Vilcabamba was that people of all ages were intimately interwoven with one another. Living in close-knit families, they enjoyed all the benefits and comforts that come from sharing one's life with loved ones. She saw no separation of people by ages.

I often reflected on the needs that the old and the young have for each other as I sat on a bench outside the stucco house with Angel Modesto. His great-grandson, Luis Fernando, not yet two, usually was at his side. They seemed sewn from the same bolt of cloth. They walked at the same pace, with the gait of kinship. They had time and love and attention for each other. For long stretches, I would watch the tireless Luis Fernando romping and running and laughing, testing his legs and his arms and his place in the world, and daily growing more secure in the knowledge that the loving eyes of his great-grandfather countenanced with enormous approbation his every move. Each was aware of the other and shared their love with an unaffected ease. I felt having his great-grandfather in his life was as important for Luis Fernando's sense of well-being, now and in his future, as his having nursed from his mother's breast.[26]

Like the Abkhasians, the Vilcabambans dwell in a society that is suffused with respect for the elderly. No elder ever fears being abandoned or isolated. In a dramatic contrast with modern American culture, old people are loved simply for who they are, regardless of whether they have any wealth. Their wisdom is admired, their seniority respected. The younger people flock to be around them, enjoying their company and appreciating the opportunity to learn from them. Older people are not treated with any condescension or false deference. The respect of the younger people for the elders is genuine and potent. The elders are fully present, involved, and responsive. Halsell said she never saw a single case of senility.[27]

Halsell knew American culture inside and out. She knew that in a youth-obsessed culture, the elderly are often seen as obsolete, as standing in the way of "progress." With profound empathy for those who are left out, she was poignantly aware of the differences in how those who are most vulnerable, including the very young and the very old, were treated in Vilcabamba as compared to the United States:

Living among these people, I learned that it isn't a bank account that can give an old person a sense of security so much as the assurance that he or she never will live alone, nor die alone. Regardless of his age in the Sacred Valley the *viejo* never fears being abandoned or being put away in an institution, unwanted, neglected, left to wither and die. . . . In the U.S. a person can work hard all of his or her life, only to reach the heap of obsolescence. The reality is that the old in the U.S. have every right to feel depressed. A *viejo* will never know that kind of desolation, that kind of abandonment and depression.[28]

One visiting doctor who had come to study the health of the elderly in Vilcabamba was aware that depression is extremely common among the aged in the United States. He asked a very old man named Ramon, "Are you often depressed?"

Ramon replied, quite simply, "Only if I have reason to be."

The doctor asked for a recent example of a time the elder had been depressed, but Ramon could not think of one. The last time, he said, was many years ago, when his house had burned down. "Then, I was depressed," he said. "But with the help of others I built it back again and felt happy to be alive."[29]

In the modern world, in contrast, when people are depressed, for whatever reason, they're often given Prozac or other antidepressant drugs. I know, of course, that these drugs have helped some people to get through very difficult times. But when someone has experienced a disheartening loss or defeat, how much better it would be to have a community of support and love in which to find our healing rather than having to rely only on a drug.

One of the great strengths of both the Abkhasian and Vilcabamban cultures lies in how deeply people are in touch with one another. Not only do they plant and harvest and eat together, but people share with their neighbors the experiences of birth and bereavement, of children marrying and parents dying. In this way, the community is able to take part together in the most joyous and most frightening moments of life. No one has to face them alone.

It is inspiring to know that this way of living is possible, but I do not want to be overly sentimental about life in these regions. It's true that there is no record of there having ever been a suicide in Vilcabamba. It's true that none of the old people wear glasses or hearing aids, and that few of them, even at the most advanced ages, need a cane or crutch to help them walk. But the people in what is called the Sacred Valley certainly have their share of suffering. The poverty is serious, and infant mortality is high by our standards. There are accidents and deaths in Vilcabamba, there are broken marriages and disappointments.

And yet somehow the people have not armored themselves against the pain, and have not withdrawn from one another into shells. If they are hurt, they cry; when a loved one dies, they grieve. The very act of grieving is considered part of life, part of learning and loving. Then they usually go on, their spirits connected to each other, their smiles all the deeper for all they have known and shared.

"What pleases me most about the Vilcabambans," Grace Halsell wrote, "is that they spend a lot of their time laughing."[30]

## THEIR SECRETS

There is much we can learn from the Vilcabambans, and I admire their ability to be so joyful with so few possessions, but I don't believe there is anything ennobling about poverty. In the modern world, a lack of money prevents many from meeting their most basic human needs and reduces them to a squalid existence. An empty purse can be heavy baggage to carry through life. It's crucial that we work to abolish poverty so that every human being has food, clothing, housing, healthcare, education, employment, and a lifetime of peace.

At the same time, I think it's a shame that we in the modern world have made the acquisition of money so important that we often define ourselves and our value by how much we can spend. We've made money into the measure of our success. A satirical poet once said that the two most beautiful words in the English language are "check enclosed."

The Reverend Dale Turner tells of a mystic from India who was introduced to New York City. His guide took him to the Times Square subway station at the peak of morning rush hour. The visitor was appalled at what he saw—people with briefcases pushing hard and driving madly. Not understanding what was causing people to behave so frantically, he asked, "Is there a wolf behind them?"

"No," said the guide, "there's a dollar in front of them."[31]

A life devoted to the acquisition of wealth is useless unless we know how to turn it into joy. This is an art that requires wisdom and unselfishness, qualities the Vilcabambans, who have little in material possessions, seem to have in abundance. Perhaps they can remind us that our fulfillment does not lie in clamoring for ever more of life's goods. Perhaps they can help us recall the wisdom of simplicity, the importance of our relationships with one another, and help us appreciate the teachings of Gandhi, who urged us to "live simply so others may simply live."

As difficult as it may be for many of us in the modern world to accept, there may actually be some advantages to not having a surfeit of material things in your life. Grace Halsell noted,

> The *viejos* of Vilcabamba have never been handicapped by the wheel as a mode of transport. They own no cars or bicycles. Nor do they have horses or burros to move them over the rugged landscape of the Sacred Valley. They simply walk. They walk to work and they walk home from work. That necessity enriches and strengthens them.[32]

She contrasted this with sedentary Americans who say "Let's take a walk" as if it were a challenge, a novelty, a course for which they deserve some credit. In the modern world, we drive our cars everywhere. We drive to a drive-in cleaner, a drive-in bank, the drive-in window at a fast-food restaurant. To some of us, getting exercise means driving to a golf course and then riding around in an electric cart.

In Vilcabamba, as in Abkhasia, even the oldest people are very active. There is always physical work to do in the household or garden, and both males and females are involved in it all from earliest childhood until their final days on earth. They have no need of exercise equipment, for simply traversing the hilly terrain during each day's activities sustains a high degree of cardiovascular fitness as well as general muscular tone.[33]

Perhaps as a result of the great amount of walking and other exercise, even the oldest Vilcabambans have extremely healthy bones. Unlike elders in the industrialized world, they almost never fall and break an arm, leg, or hip. Even at the most advanced ages, they rarely limp or become disabled.

In the modern world, when people are feeling down they are often told to "take it easy," to simply lie in bed and relax. In both Vilcabamba and Abkhasia, however, people experiencing "the blues" typically respond by becoming active and involved with others. Rather than withdrawing and becoming sedentary, they will walk great distances for the joy of visiting one another. So great is the recognition of the healing power of walking to visit a friend that there is a saying in Vilcabamba that each of us has two "doctors"— the left leg and the right leg.

## WHAT THEY EAT

What kinds of foods, you may wonder, make up the Vilcabamban diet?

They have nothing remotely comparable to food stores or markets as we know them, with selections of packaged goods. There are no canned foods in their homes, and they never open a box of breakfast cereal, pancake mix, or crackers. For the vast majority of their lives, the old people in Vilcabamba have had no experience of processed food. They have known nothing of the artificial preservatives and other chemical additives that are found in so many modern foods.

Vegetables are picked fresh from the gardens, with their full nutritional value intact. Fruits are eaten the same day they are plucked, often on the spot. The Vilcabamban diet is almost entirely vegetarian, made up primarily of whole grains, vegetables, fruits, seeds, beans, and nuts. Once in a while they will consume milk or eggs, but these are usually quite scarce. The *viejos* eat almost no meat, and never any butter. Their overall diet is very low (by contemporary

American standards) in calories. There are no overweight people in Vilcabamba.

Their protein comes from vegetables, whole grains, and a variety of beans. Their carbohydrates are always unrefined and come primarily from whole-grain cereals such as corn, quinoa, wheat, and barley, and from tubers including potatoes, yucca, and sweet potatoes. Their fat comes mostly from avocados, seeds, and nuts.

The diets of the Vilcabambans are remarkably similar to the diets of the Abkhasians. In the Vilcabamban diet as in the traditional Abkhasian diet, protein and fat are almost entirely of vegetable origin. The diets of both regions are low in calories. And both cultures depend almost entirely on natural foods rather than processed and manufactured ones.

Desserts as we know them in the modern world do not exist in Vilcabamba. When the *viejos* in Vilcabamba want a sweet taste, they eat fresh fruit such as figs, pineapples, watermelons, oranges, bananas, *naranjillas* (a type of small orange), papayas, or mangos. Fruits of all kinds are plentiful year-round. When Vilcabambans go visiting their neighbors, they often bring fresh fruit as a present.

Coming from the United States, Grace Halsell was used to a far more complex and varied diet. But she noticed something interesting.

In Vilcabamba . . . my mind never dwelled on food. I wasn't frustrated, and didn't yearn for chocolate. It may be that [the unavailability of sugary and processed foods] had disciplined my appetite. But I suspected other reasons for this absence of the usual cravings. The stress was missing. Traffic never jangled my nerves, and decisions about food were simply unnecessary. No compulsions were generated by the bombardment of television commercials exhorting me to bite into a particular brand of potato chips. . . .[34]

Walking up and down mountains, the *viejos* and I never stopped to talk about food. Our minds were occupied with love stories or other thoughts more interesting than food. And when we sat down to eat, everyone was courteous, and still more interested in talking than eating. I never saw anyone greedy for food, or afraid he would not get his share. I never saw any *viejo* overeat. I saw families with one plate of maize to share who were less greedy than a group of gringos eating a five-course meal. I ate less because they were a good influence.[35]

## THE CONTRAST IS STRIKING

It's hard not to see the contrast with the modern industrialized world. If you live in the modern West today, you live in a very different food environment than do the Vilcabambans. Most likely, you are surrounded by fast-food chain restaurants and are continually exposed to ads for junk foods. In many neighborhoods, it's easier to find a Snickers bar, a Big Mac, or a Coke than it is to find an apple.

If you go to a doctor in the United States for health tips, you may find in the waiting room a glossy 243-page magazine titled *Family Doctor: Your Essential Guide to Health and Wellbeing*. Published by the American Academy of Family Physicians and sent free to the offices of all fifty thousand family doctors in the United States in 2004, it's full of glossy full-page color ads for McDonald's, Dr Pepper, chocolate pudding, and Oreo cookies.

Meanwhile, kids in U.S. schools are learning arithmetic by counting M&M's, using lesson plans supplied by candy companies. When they walk though the hallways of their high schools, they may see a series of brightly colored mini-billboards, cheerfully telling them that "M&M's are better than straight A's" and instructing them to "satisfy your hunger for higher education with a Snickers."

Government figures show that American children now obtain an incredible 50 percent of their calories from added fat and sugar. Many health-conscious people criticize official U.S. dietary guidelines for not taking a stronger stand for more nutritious foods, but even as it is, less than 1 percent of U.S. kids regularly eat diets resembling the guidelines.

A few weeks ago I had dinner with relatives of mine who are in their seventies. They typically eat lots of meat and sugar, and their dinner that evening was no exception. Meanwhile, their conversation consisted primarily of complaining about a long list of aches and pains and about how bleak their lives were becoming. Finally, trying to look on the bright side, one of them said, "Well, old age isn't so bad, I guess, when you consider the alternative." He meant, of course, that it is better to grow old, even if you are miserable, than to die.

I appreciated that he was trying to be positive, but I found myself wondering how much more satisfying life could be if we could understand that there really *is* another alternative, if we could recognize that there are ways of living and eating that lead toward a more healthful and fulfilling life than many of us have ever thought to be possible.

## WHAT WE CAN LEARN ABOUT OURSELVES

There are, of course, real challenges in Vilcabamba, as there are in Abkhasia, and as indeed there are wherever human beings exist. It would be a mistake to be blinded by our nostalgia for a pure and unspoiled way of life and to romanticize life in these regions. Neither Abkhasia nor Vilcabamba is a Garden of Eden. It would be both emotionally self-indulgent and intellectually indefensible to project our own fantasies of an ideal society onto these people.

But at the same time we would be remiss if we failed to notice that there is indeed something inspiring and beautiful about life in these special places. If we want to understand ourselves better, if we want to understand why some people grow old in sickness and despair while others grow old with vitality and inner peace, then we have much to learn from the simplicity and good-heartedness with which the residents of these places live. If we want to understand the factors that are at play in our lives that can produce on the one hand a person who at the age of sixty is already debilitated, defeated, and depressed, or on the other hand someone who at ninety is energetic, alert, and happy, then I am sure their examples have something to teach us.

As in Abkhasia, there is in Vilcabamba an abiding and profound appreciation for the natural transitions of life. Aging is celebrated, and elderly people are held in great respect. How different this is from the modern world's youth-obsessed culture, where we tend to look with horror upon aging, as if the goal of life were to remain perpetually twenty-five.

All too often, we seem as a culture to be at war with life's transitions, viewing death as the failure to stay alive, and aging as the failure to remain young. We do something grievous to ourselves when we buy into this cultural ideology.

The myths and stereotypes we have about old age are so deeply entrenched in American society that they can insinuate themselves into our psyches without our even knowing what they are. It is difficult to escape the messages that our culture sends about the aging process. From birthday cards that decry the advance of age to the widespread use of demeaning language about the elderly ("geezer," "old fogey," "old maid," "dirty old man," "old goat," etc.) to the lack of positive images of the elderly in ads and on television programs, each of us is continually imbued with feelings of aversion toward those who are old.

I am fifty-nine, and I consider myself fairly aware of the pernicious nature of how our society views aging, and how we damage ourselves by buying into that view. One morning not too long ago, however, I wandered into the bathroom after an all-too-short night of sleep. Gazing into the mirror, I was shocked by how old the guy was who was staring back at me. My instinct was to recoil, and immediately I saw the man in the mirror grow even more difficult to like as his eyebrows drew together toward the middle of his forehead in a scowl of displeasure. I felt awful, and it took me some time to understand what had happened and what I had done.

I had greeted the signs of aging not with cheerful acceptance, but with trepidation and disdain. I had taken on the widespread cultural repugnance for what can be a natural and beautiful stage of life, and I had looked upon my tired self with contempt rather than with compassion and respect.

When I understood what I had done, I went back to the mirror and actually apologized out loud to the man looking back at me. I resolved, as well, to remember this learning experience, and from now on to greet the signs of aging and vulnerability, wherever I might meet them, with a smile rather than a frown, and with tenderness instead of contempt.

In countless ways, the dominant Western culture teaches us to value younger people and devalue older ones. How often do we notice when movie roles that should be played by mature actresses are played instead by hot young babes? In the 2005 film *Alexander,* for example, the mother of Alexander the Great (played by Colin Farrell) is portrayed by Angelina Jolie, who in fact is all of eleven months older than Colin Farrell.

Occasionally, however, a film is made that dares to convey the message that aging is a normal and healthy aspect of life. In 2003, *Calendar Girls,* based on a true story, told of a group of older women in Yorkshire, England, who belong to the local Women's Institute, which is staid and traditional and is boring them silly. When the beloved husband of one of the women dies of cancer, she decides to raise money for a new sofa in the hospital waiting room. In previous years, they had raised money for various causes through calendars with pictures of cakes, jams, flowers, and the like, but none of these calendars had ever raised more than a few dollars. Realizing that they need to do something different this year, something that would make more money, they recall a speech the dying husband had written. He had proclaimed that "the flowers of Yorkshire are like the women of Yorkshire. Every phase of their growth is more beautiful than the last, and the last phase is always the most glorious."

Inspired by the now dead man's words, the elderly women decide to sell a calendar featuring themselves (tastefully) in the nude.

*Calendar Girls* has now been seen by many millions of people, and has done much to publicize the actual events on which it was based. Meanwhile, the actual calendar has in fact raised more than $1.6 million for a new cancer hospital wing (including the new sofa).

Inspired by the film, older women throughout the world produced more than a thousand such calendars in the years 2003 and 2004 to raise money for worthy causes. In almost every case, they found the experience a joyful one, enabling them to celebrate the unique beauty of older women and to defy any cultural assumption that as women age they necessarily become unattractive.

## AGEISM

The term "ageism" was coined in 1969 by Robert Butler, the founding director of the National Institute on Aging. He likened it to other forms of bigotry such as racism and sexism, defining it as a process of systematic stereotyping and discrimination against people because they are old.[36]

The consequences of ageism are similar to those associated with discrimination against other groups. People who are subjected to prejudice and intolerance often internalize the dominant group's negative image and then behave in ways that conform to that negative image. Thus older people often hold ageist views about their contemporaries, about those who are slightly older than they are, and even about their own worth.

From our culture, we learn what is expected of us, and to a considerable extent we then conform to those expectations. When the prevailing image of aging expects older people to be asexual, intellectually rigid, forgetful, and invisible, many elderly people will take on these characteristics even though doing so may run counter to the way they have previously lived their lives. If society's view is that an appropriate solution to the health problems of very old people is to warehouse them in nursing homes and exile them from the mainstream of society, then sure enough, many old people will end up languishing in short-staffed and soulless institutions.

*Ageism represents a prejudice against a group that all people will inevitably join if they live long enough. As a result, an ideology that equates aging with deterioration steals hope from everyone, and from every stage of our lives.*

We can acquiesce in our society's script for our later years, succumbing to a perspective that defines those years as ones of loss and defeat. But I would rather challenge the assumptions of a culture that has lost touch with what aging really is: a transformational process as full of wonder and beauty as any other stage of the human journey.

If we want to create a healthy relationship to aging, then cultures like Abkhasia and Vilcabamba have much to offer us in how we understand our place in the life cycle. In these cultures, elders are looked up to and appreciated for their wisdom. They feel socially useful and needed, and even the oldest people typically retain their mental faculties and physical abilities. In the modern industrialized world, on the other hand, older people often feel useless and disconnected. As we grow older we are put out to pasture where we are left with only our ailments to think about and with ever fewer opportunities to contribute to the well-being and happiness of others. After a long life we may have learned a few things, but the prevailing social context provides us ever fewer ways to express what we have learned for the benefit of our community. From the Vilcabambans, as from the Abkhasians, we can learn a more fulfilling and joyful way to experience our aging and a better way to inhabit our lives.

While I have several friends who have moved to Vilcabamba, and I understand why they have done so, I don't plan to move there for my own final years. And I certainly don't want to go back to a way of life as devoid of modern technologies as the Vilcabambans have traditionally known. I've lived without having a soft place to sleep and I've lived without food refrigeration, so I know it is possible to be happy without them, but I enjoy such comforts and am grateful for them. I do not want to live in a barely heated house with a mud floor, and I'd rather not live without running water and indoor plumbing. I also treasure the low rates of infant mortality that have ensued from advances in public health and sanitation, and I appreciate many of the complexities and challenges of the modern world. I love my life in the modern Western world, and even with all its faults and limitations, I still cherish it as my home. I recognize as well that some of the toxicities of the modern world are beginning to encroach upon and alter the traditional Vilcabamban way of life, a development I'll discuss more fully later on.

No, I don't want to move to Vilcabamba, but I do want to bring something of the Vilcabamban spirit and wisdom into life here in the modern world. I want to understand and incorporate the principles that have enabled these people, even in the midst of primitive conditions, to live with so much vitality and beauty.

I do not want to imitate the *viejos,* the old ones of Vilcabamba, but I want to honor them, and to hold them as guides, as reminders, as friends. Their lives, like those of the Abkhasians, can show us that aging is not a disease, that growing old need not be a calamity, and that people can, when we love each other, look forward to lives that are rich at every stage with vitality, presence, and joy.

# 3

## Hunza: A People Who Dance
## in Their Nineties

*Exuberance is beauty.*
—William Blake

The Abkhasians and the Vilcabambans are not the only people who have long been the topic of stories attributing to them extraordinary longevity and health. There is yet another region that has if anything been the subject of even more fabulous claims, and that also was visited and studied by Dr. Alexander Leaf for *National Geographic*. This is the fabled land of Hunza.

Hunza lies at the northernmost tip of Pakistan, where Pakistan meets Russia and China. The setting is awe-inspiring in its majesty, for here no fewer than six mountain ranges converge. The average height of the peaks in these mountain ranges is twenty thousand feet, with some, such as Mount Rakaposhi, soaring as high as twenty-five thousand.

The people of Hunza live in an extraordinarily fertile valley that is nestled between rocky ramparts that reach toward the stars. This valley has sustained a population of from ten thousand to thirty thousand people for two thousand years in almost complete isolation from the rest of the world. Until recently, it was almost totally inaccessible, the only entry or exit for most of the year being an extremely

hazardous trail winding through the towering mountains which en-
circle the Hunza valley. In some places, the trail was only two feet
wide. In other places, there were perilously frayed rope bridges to
cross. In yet other places, the trail was actually cantilevered out from
sheer rock walls on platforms of creaking timbers.[1] The historical degree of isolation is reflected in the fact that the Hunzans, as the people of the region are sometimes called, speak Burushaski, a language
with no known relatives.

One of the first things Leaf noticed after he arrived in Hunza was
the remarkable good cheer and vitality of the elders he had come to
study. Everywhere he went he kept meeting elderly people who were
extraordinarily vigorous and who hiked up and down the steep hillsides with what seemed to him amazing ease and agility.[2]

Leaf wrote of one elderly gentleman he believed to be 100 years
old. The elder

> appeared lean and agile and still works breaking rocks for the
> road. He showed us the iron sledgehammer which he . . . flour-
> ished with ease with one hand. . . . Coming up the hill from our
> guest house we were overtaken by three elders who walked up the
> twenty- or thirty-degree incline without pause or difficulty while
> we stopped every few steps to catch our breath and quiet our
> pounding hearts. . . . [Another elder] served as our porter, shoul-
> dering a heavy box of photographic equipment and bounding
> with it over the forbidding terrain like an agile mountain goat.[3]

## UNSURPASSED IN FREEDOM FROM DISEASE

One of the first scientists to comment on the health of the people of
Hunza was the British physician Dr. Robert McCarrison. A major
general in the Indian Health Service who was later to become India's
director of nutritional research, Dr. McCarrison lectured frequently
to the British College of Surgeons and wrote for the *British Medical
Journal.* He became world renowned for his discovery that a disease
then inflicting an enormous amount of suffering in India, called
"three-day fever," was caused by the bite of the sand fly.

Shortly after making this historic discovery in the early twentieth century, Dr. McCarrison was assigned by the British Army to establish a hospital and healthcare system for the Hunzans. He lived among them for seven years, tracing family records, conducting daily interviews, performing physical examinations, and keeping meticulous records. The more he learned, the more impressed he was by the health and robustness of the Hunzans.

In particular, he was astounded by the physical and mental status of the very elderly. Dr. McCarrison's years of careful scrutiny inspired him to describe the health of the Hunzan people in rhapsodic terms:

> My own experience provides an example of a (people) unsurpassed in perfection of physique and in freedom from disease in general. . . . The people of Hunza . . . are long-lived, vigorous in youth and age, capable of great endurance, and enjoy a remarkable freedom from disease in general. . . . Far removed from the refinements of civilization, [they] are of magnificent physique, preserving until late in life the character of their youth; they are unusually fertile and long-lived, and endowed with nervous systems of notable stability. . . . Cancer is unknown.[4]

In 1964, another prominent Western physician studied the Hunzans and gave his impressions. The heart specialist Dr. Paul Dudley White had become internationally famous during the 1950s when he was the cardiologist chosen to treat U.S. president Dwight Eisenhower after the nation's chief executive suffered a heart attack. This forward-thinking physician was also a founder of the American Heart Association.

Dr. White went to visit the Hunzans, to see for himself whether the claims were true that these people lived to exceedingly old ages without any heart disease, bringing along a portable battery-operated electrocardiograph. Owing to a lack of documentation, he was not able to verify the actual ages of the elderly Hunzans he studied, but he did blood pressure, blood cholesterol, and electrocardiogram studies and found not a trace of heart disease, even in the oldest people he examined. Writing in the *American Heart Journal* and elsewhere, Dr. White described examining a group of twenty-five Hunzan men he believed

on fairly good evidence, to be between 90 and 110 years old. . . .
Not one of them showed a single sign of coronary heart disease,
high blood pressure, or high cholesterol levels. They have 20-20
vision and no tooth decay. In a country of 30,000 people, there is
no vascular, muscular, organic, respiratory, or bone disease.[5]

Hearing such reports, the U.S. National Geriatrics Society asked
Dr. Jay Hoffman to go to Hunza to investigate the health and
longevity of this unique and isolated people. When Hoffman returned home, he was utterly enthralled with what he had seen. He
wrote,

> Down through the ages, adventurers and utopia-seeking men
> have fervently searched the world for the Fountain of Youth but
> didn't find it. However unbelievable as it may seem, a Fountain of
> Youth does exist high in the Himalayan Mountains. . . . Here is a
> land where people do not have our common diseases, such as
> heart ailments, cancer, arthritis, high blood pressure, diabetes, tu-
> berculosis, hay fever, asthma, liver trouble, gall bladder trouble,
> constipation, or many other ailments that plague the rest of the
> world. Moreover, there are no hospitals, no insane asylums, no
> drug stores, no saloons, no tobacco stores, no police, no jails, no
> crimes, no murders and no beggars.[6]

## EXTRAORDINARY MOUNTAINEERS

If these and other physicians who have made similar reports are to be
believed, the health of the Hunzans has long been nothing short of
spectacular. And certainly, mountaineers have been greatly impressed
by the strength, agility, and hardiness of the Hunzan people. The
mountaineering legend Eric Shipton, who was the only man to be
part of all of the first four Mount Everest expeditions, often employed Hunzans as porters on his adventures in the region. He said
the Hunzans were even better mountain men than the legendary
Sherpas of Nepal.[7]

Shipton was not alone in this judgment. Many mountaineers consider the Hunzans to be the world's best mountain climbers, for they can travel, heavily laden, over Himalayan terrain at a rate of more than forty miles per day. One observer noted, "They can scale an almost perpendicular rock with break-neck speed and without fear. They can clamber up the sheerest precipice with the utmost calm."[8]

In the mountaineering world, the Hunzans are known not only for their vigor and physical stamina, but also for possessing buoyant spirits and remaining positive under even the most trying circumstances. In an issue of the *Journal of the Royal Geographical Society*, the head of one expedition wrote:

> The Hunzan men were with us two months, continuously on the move, over what is probably some of the worst country in the world for laden men. Always ready to turn their hand to anything, they were the most cheerful and willing set of men with whom we have ever traveled.[9]

Another mountaineer described a situation when a horse had broken free and run away. His Hunzan porter went after the horse, keeping up the high mountainous pursuit in bare feet in drenching rain for nearly two days, finally catching the horse and bringing it back.[10]

Over and over again the leaders of the most difficult mountaineering expeditions describe the Hunzans as a people who seem never to suffer from fatigue. One said it was commonplace to see them walk twenty miles in a day, heavily laden, over irregular mountainsides, and then dance far into the night. And then to do the same the following day, and the next.[11]

Another said that he saw a Hunzan, in midwinter, make two holes in an ice pond, then repeatedly dive into one and come out at the other, apparently finding the near-freezing water invigorating, as comfortable as a polar bear.[12]

## AN OPTOMETRIST STUDIES THEIR EYES

In the 1960s, the emcee of the famed U.S. television program *People Are Funny*, Art Linkletter, funded a visit to Hunza by Dr. Allen E.

Banik, a Nebraska optometrist with a long interest in health, aging, and longevity.

Dr. Banik paid particular attention to the Hunzans' eyes and vision. In the West, he well knew, most people experience a gradual loss of flexibility in their vision beginning in their forties and fifties, a condition called presbyopia. As presbyopia develops, people need to hold books, magazines, newspapers, menus, and other reading material at arm's length in order to focus properly. When they perform near work, such as embroidery or handwriting, they may get headaches or eyestrain. The prevailing belief among modern optometrists is that there is no getting around it—presbyopia happens to everyone at some point in life, even those who have never had a vision problem before.

Yet Dr. Banik found that even the most elderly of the Hunzans did not suffer from presbyopia or any of the other diseases and weaknesses of eyesight to which elder Americans are prone. "In all respects," he observed,

> the Hunzans' eyes were notable. I found them unusually clear; there were few signs of astigmatism. Even the oldest men had excellent far- and near-vision—an indication that their crystalline lenses had retained elasticity.[13]

Dr. Banik (along with his co-author, Renee Taylor) went on to describe his findings in his book titled *Hunza Land: The Fabulous Health and Youth Wonderland of the World*. He was enraptured with these people, and wrote:

> This race, which has survived through centuries, is remarkable for its vigor and vitality. . . . In 2,000 years of almost complete isolation, the Hunzans seem to have evolved a way of living, eating, thinking and exercising that has substantially lengthened their life span. They have no money, no poverty, no disease. . . . It is a land where the people enjoy not only purity of body but also mutual trust and integrity. . . .
>
> The Hunzans are a hardy, disease-free people unique in their enjoyment of an unparalleled life span. . . . It amazed me to see

the number of older citizens going about their work and showing none of the signs of decrepitude that are so often evident in the United States. . . .[14]

Dr. Banik concluded that the health and longevity of the Hunzan people begins in their childhood. Moved by the happiness of the children, he reflected, "They laugh readily and seem to have a kindly feeling toward everyone. There is no juvenile delinquency in Hunza."[15]

## A PEOPLE WHO CELEBRATE LIFE

Almost everyone who has visited Hunza has described the atmosphere of peace and the resilient and seemingly always good-natured attitude of the people. When Illinois senator Charles Percy, a member of the U.S. Senate Special Committee on Aging, visited Hunza, he remarked on the

> general air of goodwill that permeated our visit. Wherever we walked, the villagers saluted us and clasped our hands between theirs. Men greeted men, women greeted women. Children ran into the orchards to gather the fresh, sweet apricots for us or offered wild flowers and apples.[16]

Others have spoken of their amazement at the degree of freedom enjoyed by Hunzan women, especially in a Muslim country. They go unveiled, work in the fields in trousers, and inherit property. Divorce is legally as easy for women as it is for men, although it is not common. Women are not abused or overworked. They typically have only two or three children at widely spaced intervals. There is tremendous respect for breast feeding. Babies are breast fed for up to three years, and even longer in some instances.

When the American Geriatrics Society's Dr. Jay Hoffman returned from Hunza, he summed up the picture effusively:

> The Hunzans appear to be happiest people in all the world. They are happy because they are truly alive. . . .[17]

## SECRETS OF THE SOIL

Today, Rodale Press is the largest independent book publisher in the United States, and publishes magazines (including *Prevention, Men's Health, Runner's World, Organic Gardening, Backpacker, Bicycling,* and *Mountain Bike*) in forty-two countries. And the Rodale Institute is the world's preeminent advocate for organic farming and gardening.

Both Rodale Press and the Rodale Institute were started by Jerome Irving Rodale. J.I., as his friends called him, had a lifelong interest in health and well-being, and through his success as a publisher, he popularized the organic movement in America. A 1971 cover story by *The New York Times Magazine,* describing his efforts to promote organic gardening and a healthful lifestyle, called him the "guru of the organic food cult." (That organic food was then called a "cult" shows you how far we've come in the past few decades. Today, *Organic Gardening* is the most widely read gardening publication in the world.)

J. I. Rodale believed deeply in organic food. He felt that the health of a people depends on the quality of food they consume, and the quality of their food depends on the health of the soil in which that food is grown. Nothing, in his eyes, could be more fundamental, nor more important, than the health of the soil.

What does all this have to do with the Hunzans?

Everything. J. I. Rodale was a dedicated student of the Hunzan way of life, and it was from studying the Hunzans that he developed many of his seminal ideas about organic agriculture. He believed that the legendary health and vitality of the Hunzan people grew directly out of Hunzan soil, and that the vitality of their soil derived from their agricultural practices, which he considered to be the finest in the world. In his view, Hunzan agriculture was the pinnacle of the organic way of life and the ideal model for humanity to follow.

Two years before he published the first issue of *Prevention,* J. I. Rodale authored a book titled *The Healthy Hunzas.*[18] In this book, Rodale detailed how, over a period of two thousand years, the hard and continuous labor of the Hunzans had produced a spectacular series of fertile terraces throughout the valley, with brilliantly designed irrigation systems that divert water periodically from the mountain streams and rivers to the terraces.

If Rodale was effusive in extolling the sophistication and scope of the Hunzan agricultural terraces and irrigation systems, the American Geriatrics Society's Dr. Jay Hoffman was downright ecstatic after seeing them:

> The thing that impressed us most was the terraces that stretched far out into the distance through the valley and up the mountainsides. . . . Even the best engineers who have visited Hunza cannot understand how the originators of these terraces were able to erect thousands of them, each irrigated in the greatest engineering feat ever witnessed. . . . Though they are not listed as such, I like to think of them as one of the seven wonders of the world [due to] the magnificence, engineering skill, and scientific competence built into these terraces.[19]

When I first heard Dr. Hoffman likening the Hunzan agricultural terraces to the seven wonders of the world, I felt certain he was exaggerating. But as I've learned more about the terraces and how they work, I've come to feel that his enthusiasm was warranted.

There are thousands of terraced fields in Hunza, creating a sweeping staircase of extraordinary beauty up the entire length of the valley. The soil they are filled with has been brought up the steep mountain slopes in baskets from the river thousands of feet below. Each of them is diked so that the edges are a few inches higher than the ground. This enables the terraced fields to be flooded with the rich mineral waters that come down from the surrounding mountains through more than sixty miles of channels and aqueducts that have been arduously carved and hacked into the cliffs over the centuries. The heavily silt-laden waters carry a finely ground rock powder made by the pulverizing action of the glaciers which dominate the Hunzan landscape. The waters thus not only irrigate the Hunzan crops but also deposit a thin film of precious minerals over the already fertile soil.

As this process has been repeated endlessly over the centuries, it has constantly conditioned and enriched the soil with essential minerals. Rodale was convinced that this had everything to do with the marvelous well-being of the Hunzans:

> The magnificent health of the Hunzans is due to . . . the way in which their food is raised. . . . I am sure that the powdered rock dust which flows onto the Hunzan land is a significant factor in the outstanding results obtained by the Hunzans.[20]

Over the many centuries, Hunzan agriculture was entirely organic, of course, because no fertilizers or pesticides were available. But in the recent past there was one year in which the Pakistani government warned the Hunzans that a major infestation of insects was expected, threatening their crops. The Pakistanis offered pesticides as protection, but the Hunzan leadership decided against their use. Instead, the people collected the wood ashes from their cooking fires and placed them on the soil around the plants where the invading insects would have liked to land. The presence of the highly alkaline wood ashes repelled the insects. Then, as the ashes broke down into the soil, they enriched it with their high mineral content. In this way, the Hunzans protected their crops without doing any damage to the soil, and in the process even adding to its fertility.

On a different occasion, though, the Hunzans were persuaded to try a synthetic fertilizer by a salesman who convinced them that their crop yields would be increased. The farmers soon discovered that more water was needed to grow the fertilized crops, and that though the harvest was larger, the quality of the grains that grew was inferior. So they returned to their organic methods, and from that point on they prohibited the use of synthetic fertilizers.

Highly aware of both the agricultural value and the microbial dangers inherent in human waste, Rodale was deeply impressed that without the aid of modern technology the Hunzans had developed methods to compost human waste so that it could be safely used to augment their soil. He wrote:

> In every phase of their agricultural operations, the Hunzans show a sagacity that is uncanny. One ponders over the amazing fact

that it took the civilized world so long to learn the simple facts of water and sewage hygiene, and yet the Hunzans, in their primitive hideaway, applied it effectively a thousand years ago. . . . The Hunzan is downright uncanny in his methods of coaxing food out of the soil. . . . His finger is on the pulse of the land. Soil erosion is at a minimum because he is intelligent and understands the danger of soil loss. He has the time and the energy to farm in a manner that conserves the soil.[21]

Rodale understood what the erosion of the soil base can do to a culture. Soil erosion has played a determining role in the decline and demise of many great civilizations, including those of the ancient Egyptians, Greeks, and Mayans. In *Topsoil and Civilization*, Vernon Carter and Tom Dale point out that wherever soil erosion has destroyed the fertility base on which civilizations have been built, these civilizations have perished.[22]

Topsoil is the dark, nutrient-rich soil that holds moisture and feeds us by feeding our plants. It is one of the basic foundations of our sustenance upon this earth. Two hundred years ago, most of America's cropland had at least twenty-one inches of topsoil. But today, most of it is down to around six inches of topsoil, and the rate of topsoil loss is accelerating. The United States has already lost 75 percent of one of its most precious natural resources. It takes nature, unassisted, five hundred years to build an inch of topsoil. Currently, the United States loses another inch of topsoil every sixteen years.

Rodale, who was among the first to awaken modern society to the importance of soil health, saw the significance of the fact that the Hunzans had fed their entire society for thousands of years from their little valley without any topsoil loss whatsoever. It was for him an epiphany that their soil has only grown richer over the years, and that they have actually created fertile soil in places that were once little more than bare rock.

How have the Hunzans managed such a feat? They put everything that can possibly enhance the soil to use, wasting nothing. When their goats and sheep climb high up the mountainsides in the

summer, the children make a game out of going up to find the drop-
pings, then bringing them down to be added to the compost piles.
Every solitary thing that can serve as food for fruit trees and vegetables is diligently collected, including dead leaves, rotting wood, and
any animal waste they can find. These are all composted in carefully
designed sunken compost pits, then carefully distributed over every
square foot of the thousands of terraces.

Theirs has been the most magnificent, most enduring, most unremitting agriculture in the earth's history. While we in the United
States have decimated our soil in only two hundred years, the Hunzans have depended on theirs for two thousand and made it steadily
more fertile in the process.

## THE FOOD THEY EAT

What kinds of foods do the Hunzans grow on the fertile terraces that
have been called one of the great wonders of the world? They grow a
wide variety of fruit, including apricots, peaches, pears, apples,
plums, grapes, cherries, mulberries, figs, and many types of melons.
They enjoy all of these plus a multitude of wild berries, both fresh
and sun-dried. Their apples are huge, weighing more than a pound
each. But of all their fruits, the ones they eat by far the most are their
celebrated apricots. The Hunzans have developed more than twenty
varieties of apricots whose flavor and nutrient value are worlds beyond the types commonly grown in the West today. Their apricots
have been described as among the most luscious fruits on earth.

Apricot orchards are everywhere in Hunza, and nearly every family has apricot trees under cultivation. To view the Hunzan valley in
late summer is to see thousands of brilliant orange roofs shimmering
in the sun, for the roof of every building is literally covered with drying apricots. Every flat rock surface is also covered with them, split
open to receive the sun's drying rays. The fruits are eaten fresh in the
summer, and then throughout the winter and spring they are eaten as
dried fruit and also used extensively in cooking and baking. A typical
breakfast in Hunza in the winter is a porridge made from dried apricots and millet, upon which freshly ground flaxseeds are sprinkled.

## THE TRADITIONAL DIETS OF THESE LONG-LIVED
## CULTURES ARE REMARKABLY SIMILAR[23]

|  | Abkhasia | Vilcabamba | Hunza |
|---|---|---|---|
| Percent of calories from carbohydrates: | 65% | 74% | 73% |
| Percent of calories from fat: | 20% | 15% | 17% |
| Percent of calories from protein: | 15% | 11% | 10% |
| Overall daily calories (adult males): | 1,900 | 1,800 | 1,900 |
| Percentage of diet from plant foods: | 90% | 99% | 99% |
| Percentage of diet from animal foods: | 10% | 1% | 1% |
| Salt consumption | low | low | low |
| Sugar consumption: | 0 | 0 | 0 |
| Processed food consumption: | 0 | 0 | 0 |
| Incidence of obesity: | 0 | 0 | 0 |

The Hunzans have minimal pastureland, which makes animal husbandry nearly impossible. So like the Vilcabambans and Abkhasians, they eat very little meat. On certain rare feast days they eat goat or sheep meat, and on other days they consume a fermented milk product made from goat or sheep milk. But according to Leaf, meat and dairy products together constitute only 1 percent of their total diet.

It is actually quite intriguing how similar the traditional Hunzan diet is to the traditional diets of the Vilcabambans and Abkhasians. Though they live in very different parts of the world, the traditional diets of all three of these extraordinarily healthy societies are very low in calories by modern standards. In all three cases, protein and fat are almost entirely of vegetable origin. And all three depend entirely on natural foods rather than processed and manufactured ones.

People in each of these cultures eat substantial amounts of whole grains. In Hunza, the primary grains are wheat, barley, millet, buckwheat, and the hard, pearly seeds of a grass called Job's tears.

Vegetables also play a prominent role in the Hunzan diet, particularly greens, including mustard greens, spinach and lettuce, root vegetables such as carrots, turnips, potatoes, and radishes, an assortment of beans, chickpeas (garbanzo beans), lentils, and other sprouted legumes, plus many kinds of pumpkins and other squashes. They cultivate many kinds of herbs for both culinary and medicinal purposes, including mint and thyme. They grow flaxseeds, and rare is the meal that does not contain freshly ground flaxmeal in one form or another.

In Hunza, a large part of the diet is eaten uncooked. In the summer, as much as 80 percent of the food is eaten in its natural state. Vegetables in season are picked just prior to consumption and almost always eaten raw. Fresh corn on the cob, for example, is never cooked. In the winter, the Hunzans soak lentils, beans, and peas in water for several days, then lay them out on wet cloths in the sun. They are eaten raw when they begin to sprout.

When vegetables are cooked, they are typically lightly steamed using a minimal amount of water. And the water used to cook them is always consumed along with the vegetables themselves, thus utilizing the food value that has become concentrated in the cooking water.

By eating much of their food uncooked and cooking the rest of their food only lightly, the Hunzans accomplish a couple of things. They keep to a minimum the fuel needed for cooking, an ecological imperative in Hunza where fuel sources are none too abundant. And at the same time they conserve the nutrient value of the vegetables.

## A NOTE OF SOBRIETY

The Hunzans may be among the healthiest of any peoples on earth. Their many disease-free and clear-seeing elders are nourished by a cuisine rich in nutrients and by an environment of extraordinary beauty, with healthy air, water, and soil. Hunza has long been a remarkable place, and we have much to learn from it.

At the same time, though, it makes sense to be cautious when evaluating claims about a distant land that many of us may never so much as visit. Some researchers have become so enamored with the Hunzan way of life as to lose their objectivity.

One starry-eyed researcher who studied Hunzan health and wrote a book on the subject said that men and women work in the fields at 120 years of age or older until their time comes to die. He said they then eat supper with the rest of the group and go to bed. In the morning when the family arises, they discover that the oldster has quietly died in his or her sleep. "What a wonderful way to live and to die," he reflected, "without suffering the pangs and misery of disease that eventually end in death for most people on earth. The awful suffering that usually precedes death is not known in Hunza land."[24]

While I'm sure that the downward slide of chronic disease and deterioration that often lasts for years in the lives of elders in the modern Western world is far shorter in Hunza, I believe this author's comments are fanciful and romanticized. No doubt some fortunate individuals in Hunza have died as he described, and many in Hunza have undoubtedly continued in good health until perhaps only a few weeks or even days before their death. But we have no solid evidence that anyone in Hunza has ever lived to the age of 120, and more important, nothing is served by describing the lives and deaths of the Hunzans as totally free of suffering.

I suspect that some of the researchers who have studied life in Hunza have at times become caught up in their zeal to describe a land they perceive to be a paradise on earth. Some, unable to speak the native language, have seen only what the Hunzan rulers have wanted them to see. Others have visited only in the summer, and so have never seen how difficult the cold winters in the mountains can be.

And there is yet another factor that could distort their perceptions. Writers and scientists with already established ideas about healthful lifestyles can tend to look for that which validates their views. People can become gullible when they want to hear what they've already made up their minds to believe. It is certainly possible that some of those who have been most fervently enthusiastic

about life in Hunza have to some degree been guilty of making the
Hunzans out to be something they are not.[25] Unfortunately, this is not
an easy matter today to appraise definitively, as the social and political challenges of contemporary Pakistan are beginning now to invade
even this isolated and pristine land (a development I'll discuss more
fully later on).

But whatever the failings and exaggerations of some researchers
might have been, it remains an indisputable fact that in Hunza, as in
Abkhasia and Vilcabamba, a large proportion of elder citizens have
retained their faculties, remained vigorous, and enjoyed life right up
until only weeks or months before their deaths. It is an established
fact that the elderly in each of these regions have had extremely low
rates of heart disease, cancer, obesity, arthritis, asthma, dementia,
and the other degenerative infirmities that plague so many older people in the West. It is a fact that they have remained for the most part
remarkably fit and active as they age.

## RESPONDING TO ADVERSITY

What is the Hunzans' secret? Part of it, I believe, is that when faced
with hardship and privation, they have responded with courage and
creativity. In countless ways, these resourceful people have turned
around what would seem to be disadvantages.

They have a shortage of fuel, so they eat much of their food raw,
thus enhancing its nutritive value. They have no refrigeration, so they
harvest their food just before eating, once again gaining a nutritional
advantage. They have no electric lighting, so in the long winters they
sleep longer hours, thus conserving their energy at a time when the
sun's radiance is at its lowest ebb. Living in an extremely rocky and
steep area with almost no flat land on which to grow crops, they have
built the most ingenious terraces in the history of the world. Faced
with a serious lack of soil, they have wasted nothing and carefully
put back into their gardens anything that could nourish the earth,
over time producing gardens of extraordinary fertility. Situated in a
rocky environment that provides almost no pastureland, they have
adopted a healthy vegetarian diet. Lacking the many laborsaving devices of the modern world, they are extraordinarily active, thus gen-

erating a vitality and level of fitness almost incomprehensible to those of us accustomed to modern conveniences.

How is this relevant to life in the modern world? I'm certainly not suggesting that everything about the Hunzan way of life is worthy of (or possible for) our emulation. But we can learn from these people. While we have developed a mass consumption lifestyle and a throw-away culture that are doing terrible harm to the earth, they seem to have created a balanced and healthy life with the limited resources at their disposal. While the modern world seems to require excessive and unsustainable levels of resource consumption, the Hunzans have, of necessity, come to understand the role of moderation and restraint in leading balanced and healthy lives. They have learned to waste nothing and to find a use for everything.

What makes these people remarkable to me is not that they have known no suffering, but that they have found ways to use their obstacles and challenges to become stronger as a people. What I love about them is not that their lives are perfect, but that in their responses to adversity they have discovered their powers. They remind me of Friedrich Nietzsche's maxim "What does not kill me makes me stronger."

It has always been a mystery to me why some of life's deepest insights and larger truths are ushered into our lives by limitations and sorrow. As a child, I often wondered why God didn't put more vitamins in ice cream, which tasted so sweet and delicious, but instead put them in vegetables, which to me at the time did not. But as I've grown I've learned something that the Hunzans seem as a people to grasp. There is no such thing as a problem that isn't somehow also a gift. Very often it is in our hardships and trials that we are strengthened. Suffering can be a form, as the spiritual teacher Ram Dass puts it, of "fierce grace."

Certainly all of us have our share of suffering in this life. In a world of great diversity, this is one thing we all have in common. The Reverend Dale Turner reminds us that

> each of us has a handicap of one kind or another. For some, it is
> a physical, mental or emotional infirmity; others suffer estrange-
> ments within the family circle; and there are others who struggle

through a lifetime with feelings of inferiority or timidity. There
are millions who suffer the handicaps that accompany economic
privation. . . . One has this handicap, and one that. The race of
life is run in fetters.[26]

## WHEN YOU GET A LEMON, MAKE LEMONADE

No, I don't want to live entirely as the Hunzans do. But I am inspired
and heartened by the courage and creativity with which they deal
with their difficulties, turning challenges into opportunities. There is
something about the modern world, on the other hand, that leads
people to respond to problems and suffering with distraction and
consumption. When we respond in this way, something precious is
lost.

I have known too many older people in the modern Western
world who have gotten into the habit of shrinking from challenges.
They try to avoid all discomforts. They aren't handicapped or disabled, but they might as well be. Disappointed in themselves and in
life, they have bit by bit abandoned their visions and hopes. Somehow they have become so discouraged and disheartened that their
passion for life has been replaced by an obsession with convenience
and security. They are perfectly healthy, yet use their age as an excuse
not to pursue their dreams.

In their resourcefulness and perseverance, the Hunzans stand for
another possibility entirely. And this is what makes their example so
pertinent to life in the modern world.

In spite of your best efforts, the process of aging may bring with it
the loss of certain abilities. These may be abilities you have possessed
for almost all of your life, abilities you have relied upon and taken for
granted. But you do not have to allow this loss to undermine your
spirit, to stop you from contributing your unique gifts to this world
and those you love, or to blind you to the opportunities and choices
that still exist in each moment.

I do not believe that by following a healthful lifestyle you can
guarantee that you will never fall ill. The longer I've lived and the
more of life I've seen, the more I've come to the conclusion that in the

course of our lives each one of us will encounter more than our share of hardship and misfortune. No one—the Hunzans, the Abkhasians, and the Vilcabambans included—is immune from suffering and sorrow. But the examples of these cultures suggests that there are indeed steps you can take that will greatly lessen the suffering in your life and make you more capable of responding consciously and creatively to whatever adversities may come your way. These are steps that will make you healthier, stronger, less prone to illness, and more aligned with the powers of healing and joy. The more I've learned about these remarkable people, the more I've understood that—at every age—you can respond to whatever life brings you with the power of your aliveness and the beauty within your heart.

I'm thinking now of Samuel Ullman. He lived most of his life (1840–1924) in Natchez, Mississippi, and Birmingham, Alabama, where as a white businessman and lay rabbi he devoted his life to securing educational benefits for black children similar to those provided for whites. Today, his life and commitment to social justice are enshrined in the Samuel Ullman Museum at the University of Alabama in Birmingham. Though he became totally deaf as he grew older, he did not let that stifle his creativity or his passion. Instead, he continued to express himself and to work on behalf of others. Long after becoming deaf, he wrote a poetic essay titled "Youth" that has touched people all over the world with its eloquence:

> Youth is not a time of life; it is a state of mind. It is not a matter of rosy cheeks, red lips and supple knees; it is a matter of the will, a quality of the imagination, a vigor of the emotions; it is the freshness of the deep springs of life.
>
> Youth means a temperamental predominance of courage over timidity, of the appetite for adventure over the love of ease. This often exists in an adult of 60 more than a child of 20. Nobody grows old merely by a number of years. We grow old by deserting our ideals.
>
> Years may wrinkle the skin, but to give up enthusiasm wrinkles the soul. Worry, fear, self-distrust bows the heart and turns the spirit back to dust. Whether 60 or 16, there is in every human

being's heart the lure of wonder, the unfailing childlike appetite of what's next.

In the center of your heart and my heart there is a wireless station. So long as it receives messages of beauty, hope, cheer, courage and power from people and from the infinite, so long are you young.

# The Centenarians of Okinawa

*Of all the self-fulfilling prophecies in our culture, the assumption
that aging means decline and poor health is probably the deadliest.*
—Marilyn Ferguson

From our look at a few of the cultures in which elders have led extraordinarily healthy and long lives—the Abkhasians, Vilcabambans, and Hunzans—we know they have each traditionally eaten a low-calorie, plant-based, whole-foods diet. We also know of the respect for elders and the other social and environmental realities that have helped them to live with such vitality and vibrancy. But the lack of reliable age verification data for these societies has been a problem. Unfortunately, none of the elders in any of these societies have been studied with rigorous scientific methodology. Additionally, these regions have become less pristine in recent years, making it that much harder to understand their traditions and health realities.

What would be ideal for our effort to comprehend the factors that influence the health and longevity of human beings would be to find a present-day culture where people live extraordinarily long and healthy lives, where infant and childhood mortality are low, and where the diseases that plague our society are rare. In order to be ideal for our purposes, such a fabulously healthy and long-lived society would also be part of our modern world. Thus, its example would be directly relevant to our lives, and it would be sufficiently accessible that it could be methodically studied by teams of trained scientists.

In the best of all worlds, scientific researchers with impeccable credentials would already have been investigating and assessing these long-lived, healthy people for decades, subjecting them and their medical data to many different kinds of tests and analysis. We would have the data—complete medical files, comprehensive biochemical test results, dementia screens, Activities of Daily Living (ADL) surveys, nutrition surveys, age verification documents. Ideally, this data would give us incontrovertible proof that the people in this culture have far less heart disease, breast cancer, colon cancer, prostate cancer, diabetes, obesity, osteoporosis, and dementia than is the norm in the Western world. We would have at hand thorough and irrefutable documentation on the lives, ages, and health of a society where an inordinately large number of individuals have reached more than 100 years of age in vibrant health and enjoyment of life.

If there were such a present-day society and we had that kind of data on its members, we'd have a major clue to knowing how to live as long as possible and how to have the good health to enjoy it.

Remarkably, such a society does exist, and its members have indeed been the subject of thirty years of scientific investigation of the highest credibility. We've found quite likely the nearest thing to a modern Shangri-la, and we've got the documentation to prove it.

## OKINAWA

The southernmost Japanese prefecture (state) of Okinawa is made up of 161 beautiful islands that are the dwelling place of 1.4 million people. Adorned with palm trees and blessed with an abundance of flora, fauna, and pristine rain forest, these subtropical islands form an archipelago stretching for eight hundred miles between the main Japanese islands and Taiwan. Okinawa is often called "Japan's Hawaii" because the weather is so pleasant, with an average temperature of 82 degrees Fahrenheit in July and 61 in January.

To most North Americans, Okinawa is known for being home to

the largest American military presence in the Far East as well as for having been the site of the longest and bloodiest battle of World War II. Some of us recall that more people were killed during the Battle of Okinawa than were killed by the atomic bombings of Hiroshima and Nagasaki combined. The war memorial built by the Okinawans at Itoman at the southern tip of the main island is reminiscent of the Vietnam memorial in Washington. But it is much larger, and it is the only such memorial on earth that lists the names of all the people killed, civilian and military, on both sides of the battle.

More recently, Okinawa has become known for something quite opposite to the death and destruction of war. Its new renown began to emerge in 1975, when the Japan Ministry of Health and Welfare began to fund the Okinawa Centenarian Study—a study that continues to this day. The purpose of the study has been to assess whether there is any validity to the numerous reports of extraordinary health and longevity in Okinawa.

After three decades of study, the results have exceeded the expectations of even the most optimistic researchers. The Japanese prefecture of Okinawa has now been scientifically established to be the home of the longest lived and healthiest people ever thoroughly studied. These results have been published in many scientific papers, and were popularized in a bestselling 2001 book titled *The Okinawa Program.*[1]

The most important evidence needed for any study of longevity and health is reliable age verification data. This has unfortunately been lacking in Abkhasia, Vilcabamba, and Hunza. In Okinawa, however, this problem is solved. In Okinawa, every city, town, and village has a family register system that has scrupulously recorded births, marriages, and deaths since 1879.[2] Thanks to the meticulous keeping of birth and health records, there is no doubt about the claims to longevity. The data, in this case, are reliable. *Okinawa is home to the world's healthiest documented elders, to the world's longest recorded life expectancies, and to the highest concentrations of verified centenarians in the world.*[3]

The word "centenarian" refers to someone who has lived to the age of 100 years or more. Scientists consider centenarians particularly important to study because they are usually living examples of successful aging. Many studies, including the New England Centenarian Study as well as the Okinawa Centenarian Study, have found that people who make it to 100 and beyond have often been remarkably healthy for most of their lives.[4] In medical terms, they typically experience a rapid terminal decline very late in life, resulting in a compression of morbidity to their final years. This means that any health problems they might experience tend to take place at the very end of their very long and otherwise very healthy lives. *Studies of centenarians have found that 95 percent of those who make it to 100 have been free of major diseases into their nineties.*[5]

When it comes to authenticated supercentenarians (those who have lived to 110 and beyond), Okinawa is in a class by itself. Okinawa today accounts for 15 percent of the world's documented supercentenarians, despite being the home of only 0.0002 percent of the world's population.[6]

The authors and principal investigators of the Okinawa Centenarian Study have impressive credentials:

- Makoto Suzuki, M.D., Ph.D., is a cardiologist and geriatrician, professor emeritus and former director of the Department of Community Medicine at the University of the Ryukyus in Okinawa. Currently he is the chair of the Division of Gerontology at Okinawa International University. He has written more than two hundred peer-reviewed scientific publications.
- Bradley Willcox, M.D., is physician-investigator in geriatrics at the Pacific Health Research Institute and clinical assistant professor in the Department of Geriatrics, John A. Burns School of Medicine, University of Hawaii. He is also the principal investigator of the U.S. National Institutes of Health–funded study "Genetics of Exceptional Longevity in Okinawan Centenarians."
- D. Craig Willcox, Ph.D., is a medical anthropologist and gerontologist. A professor at Okinawa Prefectural University, he is also a research associate with Harvard University's New England Centenarian Study.

I emphasize the credentials of the Okinawa Centenarian Study's authors in order to make the point that the people who have developed the extraordinary body of information we have about health and longevity in Okinawa are a group of well-respected clinicians and scientists. Science is not, however, the only valid way of obtaining knowledge, nor must people have credentials to be wise. Many of the world's most outstanding people have had only limited schooling. Winston Churchill, for example, as well as Will Rogers, Irving Berlin, Walt Disney, Frank Lloyd Wright, Pablo Picasso, and Henry Ford never went beyond high school.

Sometimes an overabundance of education can turn people into walking encyclopedias who forget that there are vast realities that cannot be measured or analyzed. I find it deeply meaningful, though, when a group of highly educated scientists use their specialized skills and knowledge for the greater good of all. And this is what the researchers who have conducted the Okinawa Centenarian Study have done, bringing both scientific expertise and human understanding to their investigation of wellness and longevity in Okinawa.

Along with their research teams, they have visited and studied more than six hundred centenarians and thousands of other elders in their eighties and nineties. Their vans have been loaded with equipment to collect vital information for complete geriatric assessments. They've taken syringes for drawing blood for biochemical and genetic analyses, reflex hammers for assessing the health of the nervous system, electrocardiographs for measuring the health of the heart, questionnaires and surveys for assessing mental status, and cutting-edge heel-bone densitometers (portable machines that measure bone health and osteoporosis risk).[7]

Having meticulously studied the elders in Okinawa, these researchers tell us that it is an everyday occurrence in Okinawa to find "energetic great-grandparents living in their own homes, tending their own gardens, and on weekends being visited by grandchildren who, in the West, would qualify for senior citizen pensions."[8] They say it is commonplace for people in Okinawa to live past the age of 100 and remain active, healthy, and youthful looking. Pointing out that the word "retirement" does not exist in the traditional Okinawan dialect, they add:

By 1990, Okinawan life expectancy figures had even *surpassed* the absolute limits of population life expectancy assumed by the Japan Population Research Institute. Limits had to be revised *upwards* simply to account for the phenomenal longevity of the Okinawans.[9]

After more than thirty years of ongoing study, the medical research team reports that among the elders of Okinawa, heart disease is minimal, and breast cancer is so rare that screening mammography is not needed. The three leading killers in the West—coronary heart disease, stroke, and cancer—occur in elderly Okinawans with the lowest frequency of any elder population ever thoroughly studied by modern science.[10] The medical research team states:

> Our study found the elders to have incredibly young arteries, low risk for heart disease and stroke, low risk for hormone-dependent cancers (healthy breasts, ovaries, prostates and colons), strong bones, sharp minds, slim bodies, natural menopause, healthy levels of sex hormones, low stress levels, and excellent psycho-spiritual health. . . . If North Americans lived more like the elder Okinawans, we would have to close eighty percent of the coronary care units and one-third of the cancer wards in the United States, and a lot of nursing homes would also be out of business.[11]

There is something deeply poignant about the contrast between the health and longevity enjoyed by the elders in Okinawa and the experience of aging that is common among elders in the United States and other Western countries today. If you visit most nursing homes in North America, you'll see a less than pretty picture. You'll find elders in various states of decrepitude, helplessness, and, all too often, despair.

And it's not just in the last years of life that the difference is dramatic. In Okinawa, elders tend to stay remarkably fit and healthy until the last year or two of life, but in the modern Western world, the prevailing lifestyle takes a toll far earlier in life. In the United States and similar countries today, most of us hit our peak between twenty and thirty and gradually decline after that. By the age of seventy, most of us have lost 60 percent of our maximal breathing capacity, 40 percent of our kidney and liver functions, 15 to 30 percent of our bone mass, and 30 percent of our strength.[12]

It's far different in Okinawa, where many elders are still in good health, completely independent, and still doing active physical work such as farming even a century or more after their birth. In a typical case, a very elderly man being interviewed in the Okinawa Centenarian Study said he was in perfect health. After completing a full geriatric assessment including an electrocardiogram, the researchers concluded that he was correct. Try as they might, they could find nothing wrong with his body. Even at the age of 100, he was utterly healthy.

Was this man a rare case? Far from it. The researchers studying the elderly in Okinawa kept finding people like him, people perfectly healthy at 100.[13]

## IS THERE HEART DISEASE IN OKINAWA?

The human heart doesn't actually look very much like a valentine, but it is nevertheless a wondrous and beautiful muscle. About the size of a large pear, it begins to beat only a few weeks after conception, and then proceeds to pump forth the rhythm of our lives through every moment of our uterine and earthly existence. Only at the moment of our death does it cease.

This beating has a definite purpose: to pump blood to all parts of the body. The life of our very cells depends on the oxygen and nutrition brought to them by the flow of our blood. If for some reason any muscle did not receive a fresh flow of blood, it would quickly die.

Since the heart is also a muscle, it, too, must continuously receive fresh blood. You might think that receiving a blood supply would never be a problem for the heart, since its chambers are always full of blood. But the heart is not able to directly utilize any of the blood contained within its pumping chambers. Instead, the heart muscle feeds from the blood supplied to it through two specific vessels, called the coronary arteries.

In a healthy person, the blood flows freely and easily through the coronary arteries, and the well-supplied heart keeps pumping away as it should. But if one of the coronary arteries, or one of its branches, should become blocked and thus unable to furnish the heart with blood, then even though the heart's chambers are full of blood, that part of the heart dependent on the blocked-off artery will die.

In medical terms, this is called a "myocardial infarction." Most of us know it by another name—a heart attack. Heart attacks are the single largest cause of death in the United States today, for both men and women. Every 25 seconds, another person is stricken. Every 45 seconds, another life is lost.

Though heart attacks strike suddenly, and often without fore-warning, they do not "just happen." They are actually the final step of a slow and lengthy process that takes place in our arteries, called "atherosclerosis."

Atherosclerosis is the process by which arteries gradually accumulate fatty and waxy deposits on the inner walls, thus reducing the size of the openings through which the blood can flow. The foreign deposits which adhere to the inner walls of the arteries are called "atheromas" or "plaques."

When these plaques become advanced enough, the fatty contents of the deposits will rupture into the artery and form a clot. These clots may clog up the already reduced arterial opening, and thus entirely prevent the flow of blood through the artery. If a clot forms in one of the two coronary arteries that supply the heart with its only source of life-giving blood, and the coronary artery becomes blocked by the clot, the heart is deprived of its supply of blood, and the result is a heart attack.

You may know that most men in North America today die from diseased coronary arteries that lead to fatal heart attacks. But it's not only men. If you are a woman in North America, you have nearly a 50 percent chance of dying from heart disease—ten times your risk of dying from breast cancer. We take arteriosclerotic heart disease so for granted today that we may not realize it is one of the greatest epidemics mankind has ever faced, carrying off a larger percentage of the population than did the Black Death in the Middle Ages.

This is why it is so significant that according to the Okinawa Centenarian Study, elder Okinawans have only 20 percent as many heart attacks as North Americans do.[14] According to the medical researchers who have conducted the study, even in old age the Okinawans have very healthy blood vessels. Their coronary arteries are amazingly young, supple, and clean.[15]

Furthermore, if Okinawans do suffer a heart attack, they are more than twice as likely as North Americans to survive.[16] But there's still more to it than that. Coronary heart disease dramatically lowers quality of life. The arterial disease that leads to heart attacks not only damages the vessels leading to the heart but also damages the rest of the circulatory system, causing premature aging of the whole body.

I have been deeply moved by the reality that if North Americans were to live and eat the way the elderly Okinawans do, there is every likelihood that we, too, would greatly reduce premature aging, enhance the quality of our lives, and reduce our risk of heart disease by 80 percent.

Can you imagine what would happen if a pharmaceutical company developed a drug that could accomplish these benefits and risk reduction? It would be marketed and sold in a manner that would make the sales efforts for Viagra look modest in comparison. It would be trumpeted in practically every magazine, newspaper, and television health report in the world. And it would make tens if not hundreds of billions of dollars for its manufacturer. But since there is comparatively little profit to be made from encouraging lifestyle changes, the wider public has little idea of the extraordinary benefits such changes can bring.

## CANCER

Yes, you might be saying, but what about cancer? What good would it do me to avoid heart disease as I age, only to succumb to the terrors of cancer?

If you think that way, you are not alone. Many people live in dread of developing cancer. And they have reason. More than thirty years have elapsed since the war on cancer was officially declared by U.S. president Nixon. And despite the enormous effort expended in terms of manpower, resources, and money, we actually appear no closer to winning the war than we were on the day it was declared. New drugs are constantly being approved, many of which can cause a temporary shrinkage in tumor size. But very few have yet been found that can eradicate any kind of cancer permanently.

On March 22, 2004, a cover story appeared in *Fortune* magazine with the discouraging title "Why We're Losing the War on Cancer." The author was Clifton Leaf, the magazine's executive editor and a survivor of adolescent Hodgkin's disease. Feeling extraordinarily lucky to have survived, he nevertheless had the courage to ask, "Why have we made so little progress in the war on cancer?" His article revealed how poorly things are going in the world of cancer treatment today:

- More Americans will die of cancer in the next fourteen months than have died from all the wars the United States has fought combined.
- Even adjusting for age, the percentage of Americans dying from cancer has not improved since the war on cancer began.
- The much-vaunted improvement in survival from cancer is largely a myth. "Survival gains for the more common forms of cancer are measured in additional months of life," wrote Leaf, "not years."
- Most of the improvement in longevity of cancer patients can be attributed to early detection, not treatment. Patients now often die at the same stage in their cancer's development as they once did, but since they knew earlier that they had cancer, it can appear that they "survived" longer with the disease.
- The few dramatic breakthroughs (such as in Hodgkin's disease) occurred mainly in the early days of the war on cancer. There has been little substantial progress in recent decades, despite the claims to the contrary.

This lack of progress in the world of cancer treatment is largely hidden from the public. Physicians don't like to talk about their failures, and drug companies are always hyping the newest drug. This can give the false impression that progress has been made when it hasn't. But recognizing that the war on cancer has thus far been largely a disappointment doesn't mean you have to lose hope. It can help you turn your attention to where there are solid grounds for real hope—*prevention.*

If we are going to get serious about cancer prevention, there is much to be learned from the elder Okinawans. Why? Because when it comes to cancer, the medical data for these fortunate people are nothing short of amazing. Despite living to such extremely old ages compared to North Americans, their cancer rates are orders of magnitude better than those found in the West. *Compared to someone in the United States, an Okinawan elder is 85 percent less likely to die from breast cancer, 88 percent less likely to die from prostate cancer, 70 percent less likely to die from ovarian cancer, and 70 percent less likely to die from colon cancer.*

These are staggering statistics. And behind these numbers is the unrelenting reality of how many people in the West are suffering and dying needlessly.

While prostate cancer is the most common cancer in males in North America and Europe, and the second leading cause of death from cancer among males in the modern industrialized world, it is extremely rare in Okinawa. When researchers in the Department of Urology at Ryukyus university conducted a study on prostate cancer in Okinawa, they found so few cases that they never bothered to publish the results.[17] Most Okinawan men have never even heard of the disease.

## WHAT ABOUT BREAST CANCER?

Breast cancer kills forty-six thousand women in the United States each year. On average, each of these women has her life cut short by twenty years. But these numbers tell us nothing of the personal anguish and suffering, the immense financial burdens, the motherless children, and the shattered families that result.

Just about every adult in the Western industrialized world knows someone who has breast cancer or who will get it. It is so common that if one of your sisters doesn't develop it, one of your daughters or cousins probably will. In contrast, the Okinawan medical research team tells us:

> If you are an Okinawan woman, the chances are that no one you know has breast cancer or will develop it. You may have heard of it but never seen it—it is that rare. . . . You have to put 100,000 Okinawan women in a room to find six who will die from it.[18]

This is a stunning finding for a fully industrialized society. You might imagine that if such low breast cancer rates were to be found anywhere, it would be some place like Hunza or Vilcabamba, places so pristine that their residents have remained unexposed to the carcinogenic chemicals that permeate our environment today. Or perhaps such a low breast cancer rate would be found in a society where people do not live long enough to get cancer.

But the extremely low rate of breast cancer among the elders in Okinawa cannot be explained by a lack of chemicals or pollution, nor by shortened life spans. Three of Okinawa's rivers now rank among the five most polluted rivers in Japan.[19] And life spans among women in Okinawa are the longest ever fully documented for any nation or region in world history.

## OSTEOPOROSIS

Another of the afflictions that cause a great deal of suffering among older people in the United States, particularly among postmenopausal women, is osteoporosis. You can probably guess what I'm going to say next. Yes, Okinawans are immensely favored here, too. The Okinawans have much stronger bones, and less than half as many hip fractures as North Americans.[20]

In the West, postmenopausal women have often been told to take estrogen replacement therapy to protect their bones and their hearts and to reduce menopausal symptoms. They've been told that if they don't take estrogens, their risk for heart disease and osteoporosis will skyrocket. For years, Premarin was the best-selling pharmaceutical drug in the United States—even though we now know it had the unfortunate side effect of elevating breast cancer rates.

In Okinawa, however, aging women have not sought help from drug companies. For them old age is typically a time of vitality, peace, and opportunity. While millions of women in the West have taken estrogen replacement therapy, virtually no elderly Okinawan women have done so.

One of the reasons is that you don't have to replace what you haven't lost. According to the Okinawa Centenarian Study, the average 100-year-old Okinawan woman has about the same estrogen level as the average woman in the United States who is thirty years her junior.[21] This is a remarkable finding, because estrogen levels in women naturally decrease as they age, and very low estrogen levels are often a marker for advanced aging. And it helps explain why—without taking drugs—menopausal and postmenopausal women in Okinawa have far fewer hot flashes, less than half the hip fractures, and 80 percent less heart disease than do women in the United States.


## TESTOSTERONE

While postmenopausal estrogen decline in women has received a great deal of press, there is a parallel problem in men. In the United States and other modern Western nations, testosterone levels peak in most men during their thirties and decline after that at a rate of between 1 and 2 percent per year. It is increasingly recognized that this decline can have serious health implications in older men, particularly when it is severe.[22] Classic signs of testosterone deficiency include thinning hair, decreasing libido, increasing body fat, declining muscle mass, memory problems, decreasing vitality, and higher rates of depression.

The Massachusetts Male Aging Study is one of many studies to confirm that good health among older men correlates with higher levels of testosterone. This study and others have found higher levels of bioavailable testosterone to be associated with greater bone density, decreased risk for hip fractures, increases in muscle strength, and better heart health.

Men who maintain higher testosterone levels as they age have significantly less heart disease and fewer symptoms of mental senility when compared to men with low levels of testosterone.[23] Higher testosterone levels are also correlated with improved erectile capability in men. Not surprisingly, an ever-increasing number of older men in the West today are beginning to experiment with testosterone products, hoping to attain the benefits of the levels they enjoyed when they were younger. In Okinawa, however, this is not necessary.

The Okinawa Centenarian Study found that elder Okinawan men have testosterone levels nearly identical to those found in American men thirty years younger.[24] Hence the following story:

A very elderly gentleman was sitting on an Okinawan bus. The bus was crowded, and people were standing in the aisles. The elder noticed a pretty girl standing in front of him. Chivalrously, he offered her his seat. "I know I'm an old man, but I would be pleased if you would take my seat."

"Thank you," she said with a smile, "but I don't mind standing."

The bus continued along its jerky way, until it stopped abruptly, throwing the standees about, with the young woman landing on top of the elder gentleman. As they disentangled, the man offered again. "I don't want to see you tossed about. If you won't take my seat, why don't you just sit on my lap so there won't be so much crowding?"

She smiled and perched herself on his lap. The bus bumped its way along its route.

After a minute or so, the elder Okinawan gentleman tapped the young lady on the shoulder. "Young lady," he said, "I think you had better stand up again, because I am not as old as I thought I was."

## HOW DO THEY DO IT?

What could account for the many marvelous health advantages enjoyed by the elder Okinawans? As in Abkhasia, Vilcabamba, and

Hunza, there is in Okinawan culture a tremendous respect for the elderly, and also a profound sense of sharing and caring for others at all stages of life. And as is true in these other societies, Okinawans have always had a great deal of physical exercise built into the daily practices of their lives. One difference, though, is that instead of living at a high elevation with thin, pure air and a lot of uphill exercise, most Okinawans live at or near sea level.

If you ask the elder Okinawans themselves for the key to their legendary health and longevity, they most often point to the simple, nutritious, and wholesome food they eat.

In the West, we often look to food for entertainment, amusement, distraction, and compensation for emotional and sensory deprivation in other areas of our lives. But in Okinawa, people think about food in an entirely different way. Many of the traditional Okinawan proverbs about eating sound like phrases you might find on the wall of a health food store in the West. One such proverb translates as "Food should nourish life—this is the best medicine." And another: "One who eats whole food will be strong and healthy."

What does modern science say about all this? According to the researchers who conducted the Okinawa Centenarian Study, the elders' diet has indeed played a profound role in the health they have attained. Thanks to these researchers' meticulous investigations, we have an extraordinarily detailed picture of the foods the elders have eaten. And we can see that the diets of the world's exceptionally healthy and long lived peoples have a great deal in common:

- They are all low (by Western standards) in overall calories.
- They are all high in good carbohydrates, including plenty of whole grains, vegetables, and fruits.
- They are all "whole-foods" diets, with very little (if any) processed or refined foods, sugar, corn syrup, preservatives, artificial flavors, or other chemicals.
- They all depend on fresh foods, eating primarily what is in season and locally grown rather than relying on canned foods or foods shipped long distances.
- They are all low (though not super-low) in fat, and the fats

come from natural sources, including seeds, nuts, and in some cases fish, rather than from bottled oils, margarines, or saturated animal fats.

- They all derive their protein primarily from plant sources, including beans, peas, whole grains, seeds, and nuts.

## EAT LESS, LIVE LONGER

One of the most telling of all the differences between the traditional diets in Abkhasia, Vilcabamba, Hunza, and Okinawa and the modern American diet is that they are all much lower in overall calories. Even with their very active lifestyles, the average man in these regions consumes only around 1,900 calories a day. In the United States, in contrast, where lifestyles are far more sedentary, the average man consumes 2,650 calories a day.

And many Americans eat far more than that. In the documentary *Super Size Me,* filmmaker Morgan Spurlock ate all his meals at McDonald's for a month, easily consuming more than 5,000 calories a day. Of course, it's not just McDonald's. A single order of fries and a Thickburger at a Hardee's restaurant add up to more than 2,000 calories. On the dessert front, a single slice of Cheesecake Factory's carrot cake has more than 1,560 calories. And Americans typically eat huge desserts *after* consuming fatty, high-calorie meals.

From the point of view of people in the longest living cultures, however, they aren't eating a "low-calorie diet." From their perspective, the food *we* eat is *high* in calories. And they have a point in seeing our caloric standards as extravagant rather than seeing their intake as restricted. While we are busy consuming greasy burgers, sugar, white flour, and other high-calorie, low-nutrition foods, these societies have attained extraordinary health and longevity on diets that provide far more essential nutrients than standard American fare while remaining far lower in overall calories.

The Okinawans almost never overeat, because they like to leave some room in their bellies at the end of each meal. They don't like feeling "stuffed." This actually makes quite a bit of sense, because of an interesting quirk in human physiology. You may have noticed that you sometimes feel more full about twenty minutes after you stop eating than you did while you were still eating. This is because it takes the stretch receptors in your stomach about twenty minutes to tell your brain (via the hormone cholecystokinin) how full you really are. If you eat until you experience yourself to be 100 percent full, you actually go about 20 percent over capacity with every meal. And if you do that regularly, your stomach will stretch a little bit each time to accommodate the extra food. Then you have to eat more next time to get the same feeling of fullness.[25]

This is one of the reasons it is more satisfying and healthful to eat slowly. When you aren't rushing, your stomach has time to signal to the appetite centers of your brain that food has arrived, and you experience greater pleasure and contentment.

The elder Okinawans say they stop eating when they are 80 percent full. They say they "eat less in order to live longer." For them, this is just common sense and the way of their traditions. But everything we are learning from the latest medical research on successful aging confirms the wisdom of their principles.

When Dr. Richard Weindruch and Dr. Rajinder Sohal, world leaders in studies of low-calorie diets, wrote about the Okinawans in *The New England Journal of Medicine* in 1997, they pointed to the low (by American standards) caloric intake of the elder Okinawans as a key factor in their outstanding health and life expectancy.[26] Similarly, Professor Yasuo Kagawa of Jichi Medical School, who has studied the Okinawans, attributes their longevity and health primarily to the relatively low amount of overall calories they consume.[27]

These researchers have good reason for thinking this way. One of the most remarkable findings of modern scientific research is that no intervention, including the elimination of smoking, has been found to be as important in overall life extension as cutting back on calories while maximizing dietary nutrients.

Many researchers have contributed to the development of this understanding, but few more than Roy Walford, M.D., who has long been recognized internationally as one of the top experts in the field of gerontology. His research at UCLA was funded for more than thirty-five years by the National Institutes of Health, and he published more than 350 articles on aging and health in medical journals. He writes:

> We can with an order of probability bordering on certainty extend maximum human life span by means of a calorically restricted optimal nutrition diet. . . . There is now abundant hard evidence—not testimonial evidence, not clinical anecdote, not based on plausibility arguments, and not even correlational evidence, although all these exist in plenitude—but hard, well-controlled and steadfastly confirmed experimental evidence that a low calorie diet that provides optimum nutrition will greatly extend average and maximum life spans, postpone the onset and decrease the frequencies of most or all of the "diseases of aging," maintain biomarkers at levels younger than chronological age, maintain sexual potency, general vitality, and ability to engage in sports into advanced age, and delay deterioration of the brain.[28]

It is true that in many underdeveloped countries where overall caloric consumption is low, life spans are often painfully short. But these underfed populations are also malnourished. Their diets are not only restricted in calories—they are also deficient in many vitamins, minerals, protein, and other essential nutrients.

Similarly, there is no medical benefit to anorexia nervosa—a psychological disorder in which people (usually young women) experience a compulsive urge to eat little or no food in a fixation on reducing their weight. They literally starve themselves slowly, sometimes even to death, as did the popular singer Karen Carpenter in late 1982.

The point is not that any low-calorie diet is helpful. The point is that a low-calorie diet that also provides optimal nutrition is most advantageous for health and longevity. There is no advantage—and there is real danger—to reducing calories below the body's legitimate needs. This is particularly true for children and for pregnant women, whose caloric needs are especially high. But the evidence is overwhelmingly clear that for people at every stage of life the best diets are those in which every calorie comes packed with nutrients.

Prior to 2006, most calorie restriction studies had been done using rats and other small animals. When animals are fed spartan diets with optimal nutrition, they typically live 30 percent or more longer than their amply fed littermates, and have far less heart disease and cancer. But such studies have been difficult to do with humans. In 2006, however, researchers published a remarkable study in the *Journal of the American College of Cardiology*.[29] The study of twenty-five members of the Calorie Restriction Society, a group of people who follow Dr. Walford's ideas and who consume a nutrient-rich, low-calorie diet, found that people who eat low-calorie diets that are sound and well balanced have extraordinarily healthy hearts that retain youthful vigor for many years after they would have been expected to show signs of aging.

The twenty-five calorie-restricted participants had been voluntarily eating a nutritionally balanced diet providing at least 100 percent of the recommended daily intake for each nutrient, but averaging only 1,671 calories a day, for periods ranging from three to fifteen years. (People eating a typical Western diet consume between 2,000 and 3,000 calories a day.)

Luigi Fontana, M.D., Ph.D., of Washington University in St. Louis, the study's principal investigator, said the members of the Calorie Restriction Society had hearts that seemed fifteen years younger than would have otherwise been expected. They had signficantly lower blood pressure, less inflammation, and less myocardial fibrosis. Their hearts were able to relax between beats in a way similar to hearts in much younger people. They had substantially lower levels of inflammatory markers, including C-reactive protein, tumor necrosis factor–alpha, and transforming growth factor–beta 1. And those in the calorie-restricted group had significantly more elastic ventricles than controls, and better diastolic function. "Diastolic function declines in most people as they get older," said Fontana. "But in this study we found that diastolic function in calorie-restricted people resembled diastolic function in individuals about 15 years younger."

And Fontana pointed out something else. The participants eating a calorie-restricted, optimal-nutrition diet had been doing so for an average of only six years, but their hearts appeared fifteen years younger. That could mean that the diet reverses aging.

According to John O. Holloszy, M.D., a co-author of the study, "It's very clear that calorie restriction has a powerful, protective effect against diseases associated with aging. We don't know how long each individual will end up living, but they certainly have a longer life expectancy than average because they're most likely not going to die from a heart attack, stroke or diabetes. And if, in fact [as the study indicates] their hearts are aging more slowly, it's conceivable they'll live for a very long time."[30]

While this was the first study to look in medical depth at humans who have deliberately maintained a low-calorie, high-nutrient diet over the course of years, many other studies have shown that diets that provide optimal nutrition while remaining low in calories improve blood sugar control, produce younger-appearing and leaner bodies, and increase mental sharpness. As well, diets super-high in nutritive quality but relatively low in calories have been shown to retard the basic rate of aging in humans, to greatly extend the period of youth and middle age, to greatly reduce the risk for such late-life diseases as heart disease, diabetes, and cancer, and even to lower the overall susceptibility to disease at any age.

I love food, and I doubt that I will ever deliberately adopt as restrictive a diet as that of the Calorie Restriction Society members. But I think it's important to recognize that if you want to live a long and healthy life, this is one of the keys: Avoid processed foods and empty calories, and instead eat a diet low in calories and high in nutrients. Your susceptibility to cancer, heart disease, stroke, diabetes, autoimmune disease, and many other ailments will be only a tiny fraction of what it would be otherwise. Plus, such a diet will give you, according to Dr. Walford (who hitchhiked and riverboated across Central America for his fifty-eighth birthday),

> better eyesight and hearing at every age; a sharper, more alert problem-solving mind; an increased feeling of well-being; enhanced sexuality and fertility at a more advanced age.[31]

Roy Walford's description of the kind of health that typically ensues from a low-calorie, highly nutritious diet may seem too good to be true, particularly when we are accustomed to seeing the examples of unhealthy aging that abound in the modern Western world. But he is not indulging in wishful thinking; he is engaged in clear-eyed and dispassionate scientific observation and analysis. His description accurately depicts the healthy aging of the Okinawans, the Abkhasians, the Vilcabambans, and the Hunzans, all of them peoples whose diets have indeed been very low (by Western standards) in overall calories while abundant in nutrients. The marvelous health Dr. Walford predicts for those who follow a highly nutritive low-calorie diet is no pipe dream. It has consistently been shown to be the reality of the healthiest and longest lived peoples on earth.

# PART

# 2

# OUR FOOD,
# OUR LIVES

# 5

## Eat Well, Live Long

*It's not just a matter of playing the genetic cards you're dealt. We have the power to shape our own lives. The reality is a much more optimistic scenario than if it were just a matter of picking the right parents.*

—John Rowe, M.D., Professor of Geriatrics at Harvard
Medical School and Chair, MacArthur Foundation
Research Network on Successful Aging

The question of the optimum diet for humans has been debated endlessly in recent years. Authors have sold millions of copies of books advocating all kinds of approaches. Some, including Dean Ornish, M.D., say the way to go is low-fat, high-carbohydrate; others, such as Robert Atkins, M.D., advocate lots of fat and protein and very low carbohydrates. Advocates of these and other approaches can, and no doubt will, continue to argue back and forth for years to come. But what, I ask, can we learn from our elders? What can we learn from those cultures where people have actually lived spectacularly long and healthy lives?

According to the authors of the Okinawan Centenarian Study, the elder Okinawans who have attained the most phenomenal health and longevity statistics ever fully documented eat an average of seven servings of vegetables a day, seven servings of whole grains per day,

## COMPARING THE DIETS OF AMERICANS AND OKINAWAN ELDERS[1]

|                     | Americans    | Okinawan Elders |
|---------------------|--------------|-----------------|
| Meat/poultry/eggs   | 29 percent   | 3 percent       |
| Dairy products      | 23 percent   | 2 percent       |
| Fruit               | 20 percent   | 6 percent       |
| Vegetables          | 16 percent   | 34 percent      |
| Grains              | 11 percent   | 32 percent      |
| Soy foods           | 0.5 percent  | 12 percent      |
| Fish                | 0.5 percent  | 11 percent      |

Percentages are by weight. For the sake of this comparison, we are leaving aside for the moment the immense quantities of sugar, corn syrup, and added fats eaten by Americans and avoided almost entirely by the elder Okinawans.

and two servings of soy products per day. They eat fish two or three times a week. Their consumption of dairy products and meat is nearly nonexistent. And they eat very little sugar or added fats.[2]

If you look at the chart above, you'll notice certain things right away. You'll see that the Okinawan elders eat a great deal less meat, poultry, eggs, dairy products, and fruit than Americans. And that they eat far more vegetables, grains, soy foods, and fish. (The elder Okinawans may very well have the highest soy consumption of any people in the world.)

There are several things that the chart does not illustrate, however, which are also quite important. For one, the Okinawan elders do not eat margarines or any other hydrogenated oils or trans-fat foods. And although the chart reveals that the elder Okinawans eat far more grains, there are also crucial differences between the types of grains eaten. The Okinawan elders eat primarily whole, unrefined grains. In the West, however, most of us have taken a different path.

## THE WHITER THE BREAD, THE SOONER YOU'RE DEAD

White flour is what you get when you strip away the fiber-rich bran and the nutrient-rich germ from the wheat, leaving only the nutrient-depleted starch. Wheat is the primary grain consumed in the modern Western world, and most of it is eaten as white flour. *In the United States, 98 percent of the wheat eaten today is eaten in the form of white flour.*

The reason wheat was originally refined and processed into white flour was to extend shelf life. This provided certain advantages to commerce, but the consequences to human health that have followed from the shift from whole wheat to white flour have been painful indeed.

Here is a table showing the percentage of nutrients lost when whole wheat flour is refined into white flour:

| | |
|---|---|
| Protein: | 25 percent lost |
| Fiber: | 95 percent lost |
| Calcium: | 56 percent lost |
| Copper: | 62 percent lost |
| Iron: | 84 percent lost |
| Manganese: | 82 percent lost |
| Phosphorus: | 69 percent lost |
| Potassium: | 74 percent lost |
| Selenium: | 52 percent lost |
| Zinc: | 76 percent lost |
| Vitamin $B_1$: | 73 percent lost |
| Vitamin $B_2$: | 81 percent lost |
| Vitamin $B_3$: | 80 percent lost |
| Vitamin $B_5$: | 56 percent lost |
| Vitamin $B_6$: | 87 percent lost |
| Folate: | 59 percent lost |
| Vitamin E: | 95 percent lost |

Many people think that when white flour is "enriched" with added vitamins, the nutritional value is restored. But this is far from true. Of the twenty-five nutrients that are removed when whole wheat flour is milled into white flour, only five nutrients are chemically replaced when the white flour is enriched.

The importance of whole grains in cancer prevention was vividly illustrated in a 2001 report published in the *Journal of the American Dietetic Association.*[3] The authors conducted a "meta-analysis," reviewing the entire body of available scientific literature on whole grains and cancer risk. Here's what they found: Of forty-five studies on whole grains and cancer, forty-three showed whole-grain intake to provide significant protection from several cancers. Specifically, a protective association was seen in 9 of 10 mentions of studies on colorectal cancers and polyps, 7 of 7 mentions of gastric cancer, 6 of 6 mentions of other digestive tract cancers, 7 of 7 mentions of hormone-related cancers (breast, prostate, ovarian, and uterine cancer), 4 of 4 mentions of pancreatic cancer, and 10 of 11 mentions of other cancers.

Whole grains clearly protect against cancer. But that's far from all. Reporting on the Iowa Women's Health Study in the *American Journal of Public Health,* researchers found that women who ate at least one serving a day of whole grain foods had "substantially lower risk of mortality, including mortality from cancer, cardiovascular disease, and other causes" compared to those who ate less.[4] That's from just one serving of whole grains a day. Sadly, though, most Americans don't get even that. Whole grains make up less than 1 percent of the average American's diet.

It's important to understand that while both whole and refined grains are high in carbohydrates, they do not act the same way in the body. Whole grains, you may recall, include all parts of the plant kernel, including the fiber-rich bran and the nutrient-rich germ. Refined grains, on the other hand, have had these nutritious components stripped away during milling. White flour, white rice, and other refined grain products are absorbed rapidly into the bloodstream, causing rapid fluctuations in blood sugar levels. The fiber found in whole grains slows these fluctuations, helps lower cholesterol levels, keeps the digestive tract healthy, and provides many other advantages. Plus, whole grains also provide important nutrients, including B vitamins, vitamin E, and many other health-promoting substances.

Do you know why they call it Wonder Bread? Because if you eat it, it's a wonder you're still alive.

## SUGAR TIME

The diets that have enabled the world's longest-lived peoples to live such healthy lives are very high in whole grains and other healthful carbohydrates. In this way they could hardly differ more from the low-carb regimen advocated by Robert Atkins, M.D., and similar authors. But there is a very real problem the low-carb diets are seeking to correct. The problem is that Western diets include far too many refined carbohydrates. The elder Okinawans and other members of the world's healthiest peoples rarely if ever eat such foods.

When it comes to eating unwholesome carbs, Americans quite literally take the cake. It's incredible how many Krispy Kreme doughnuts, Dunkin' Donuts, and Hostess Twinkies and Ding Dongs Americans manage to down each year. The number is in the tens of billions. Nearly a third of all calories in the average American diet today come from refined sugar and corn syrup.

Food manufacturers put such massive amounts of refined sugars in foods for a simple reason—to stimulate appetite. People whose appetites are stimulated eat more food. This is good for sales, but it is also why excess sugar consumption is so strongly linked to obesity. People eating highly refined and processed foods typically consume 25 percent more calories than those on a more natural diet.

I've known that the the amount of sugar consumed by children and adults in the industrialized Western world today is entirely out of hand. But I hadn't realized how bad it's gotten. At present, the average American consumes a staggering total of 53 teaspoons of sugar each day. This amounts to a five-pound bag of sugar every ten days for each man, woman, and child.

Thanks to the roughly $4 billion a year in federal subsidies handed to corn growers in the United States, high-fructose corn syrup has become so cheap that it can now be found in almost every processed food, even ones like soups and salad dressings that didn't used to be sweetened. Some studies indicate that corn syrup is even worse than cane sugar. Though that remains to be settled, some things are beyond doubt. A single 12-ounce can of soda pop has about 13 teaspoons of sugar in the form of high-fructose corn syrup. Today, the average American drinks about 55 gallons of soda pop a year.[5] Ten to 15 percent of all calories consumed by America's teenage girls come from soft drinks.[6] Many U.S. schools today actually have more soft drink machines than water fountains.

What's so bad about sugar and corn syrup? A lot, if you eat too much. Excess sugar consumption is linked not only to obesity, but also to kidney stones, osteoporosis, heart disease, and dental cavities. Sugar and corn syrup are also addictive—the more you eat, the more you want. Plus, the more sugar and other empty calories you eat, the more other calories you have to eat just to get your minimum daily requirement of vitamins and other nutritional factors.

The result isn't pretty. We've got a lot of overfed and overweight people who are always hungry and are actually undernourished. Despite the excessive number of calories they are eating, their cells are not getting the nutrients they need.

Furthermore, sugar (like white flour) is low in fiber, so not only do you get a lot of calories that provide almost no nutrients, but also, because such carbs are absorbed quickly, you get a blood-sugar spike and an insulin surge, which causes you to gain weight.

And then there are your teeth. Naturally occurring bacteria in your mouth feed on sugar. Within a few minutes of your eating foods high in sugar, bacteria in your mouth produce by-products that bathe your teeth in an acid that eats away at your tooth enamel, leading to cavities and decay.

So essentially, if you want to become malnourished, obese, and toothless, foods high in sugar and corn syrup are your ticket.

Although I'm not a big fan of the low-carb diets, I do recognize that they've done good in reducing the amount of refined carbohydrates people eat. As a result of the widespread popularity of these diets, Interstate Bakeries was forced in 2004 to file for Chapter 11 bankruptcy protection.[7] The company's foremost products? Twinkies and Wonder Bread.

## THE MAN WHO HAD EVERYTHING

Sometimes, we don't realize how valuable our health is until we've lost it. This was brought home to me a few years ago when I met a neighbor of my parents', a man named Marvin Davis. As my dad and I were walking over to Marvin's house where we had been invited for dinner, my dad mentioned that Marvin was one of the richest men in the world. I later found out that *Forbes* magazine estimated his worth to be $5.8 billion. The oil tycoon was known for buying and selling things like the Twentieth Century–Fox studio, the Pebble Beach golf course, and the Beverly Hills Hotel.

His home, as you might expect, was palatial. One of the first things I noticed was that all the doors, even the doors to the bathrooms, seemed to be double-width. I wondered why . . . until I met our host. The poor man—poor, obviously, not in wealth, but in health—must have weighed four hundred pounds. He was so large that he apparently could not fit through a normal door, even an oversized one. I couldn't help but be moved by the pathos of his situation. Here was a man who was so rich he could buy almost anything in the world, yet he was so hugely overweight that he could not go to the bathroom without several attendants to help him.

I don't think I can adequately describe the feelings I had that evening as I watched Marvin eat multiple servings of steak, lobster, and caviar. As I spoke with him and watched him interact with others, he seemed distracted, burdened, and unhappy. Some might have envied his immense financial fortune, but I found myself feeling sorry for him. I kept remembering something Maurice Sendak said: "There must be more to life than having everything."

It was hard not to notice the dramatic contrast with the peoples of Abkhasia, Vilcabamba, Hunza, and Okinawa. Lean, light, and happy, they walk with a spring in their step and speak with a lilt in their voice. They eat slowly, give thanks for what they have, never overeat, and are remarkably content. They laugh and joke a lot, and their eyes sparkle with joy and peace. Though most have little in the way of material possessions, they rarely hoard resources beyond their needs. Instead, they are eager to share what they have with others. In their cultures, it is not the person who accumulates wealth who is esteemed. It is the love in people's hearts and the wisdom in their lives that counts. It is not how much you have that matters, but how much you give of yourself to others.

No, I did not envy Marvin Davis. Perhaps I was being unfair to him, but to me he seemed to embody something that has gone terribly amiss in modern society. If we can afford it, we buy it; if it tastes good, we eat it. We are very big on consumption.

There is a deep problem with this. If we continue to pursue short-term gratification without regard for the long-term consequences, the results can only be disastrous. Insatiable is not sustainable.

When Marvin Davis died in 2004, the *Los Angeles Times* featured a lengthy front-page article about his life, saying he had been the richest man in Southern California for several decades.[8] The article spoke of his buying and selling professional football, basketball, and baseball teams and mentioned some of the other ways he spent and used his billions. Perhaps out of respect, it did not use the word "obesity."

## THE GIRTH OF A NATION

Human beings come in all shapes and sizes, and this diversity is part of our beauty. Yet modern society can be very cruel to people whose bodies do not fit the cultural ideal. I certainly do not want to add to the suffering that larger people often have to endure in modern culture as a result of their size. No one should ever be ostracized or put down for their weight.

But we need to start talking about the dire health consequences of obesity. The number of Americans who die prematurely each year as a result of being overweight is now rapidly approaching the number who die prematurely from cigarette smoking.[9] *Obesity now contributes more to chronic illness and healthcare costs than does smoking.*[10] The Rand Institute equates being obese with aging prematurely by twenty years.[11]

When researchers at the Fred Hutchinson Cancer Research Center in Seattle studied 73,000 adults aged 50 to 76, they found that obesity was correlated with forty-one different adverse health conditions.[12] Some of these conditions are life-threatening, such as heart failure. Others, like high blood pressure, increase the risk of more serious diseases. Still others, including insomnia and chronic fatigue, reduce the quality of life.

Obesity is a serious disease, and it's becoming an epidemic in modern society. Liposuction is now the leading form of cosmetic surgery in the United States, with nearly half a million operations performed per year. More than half of U.S. physicians are themselves overweight.[13]

A few weeks ago, when I accompanied a friend to a doctor's appointment, I found it unnerving that the receptionist must have weighed at least three hundred pounds. Then she sent us in to see the physician. Compared to him, the receptionist was slim.

In 2001, the U.S. surgeon general declared obesity to be an epidemic, noting that the percentage of American children who are overweight had tripled in the previous twenty-five years. In 2006, the *International Journal of Pediatric Obesity* announced that nearly half the children in the western hemisphere will be obese by 2010. According to James Hill, director of the Center for Human Nutrition at the University of Colorado Health Sciences Center, "If these trends continue, within a few generations every American will be overweight."[14]

Already, almost two-thirds of all Americans are overweight or obese.[15] And the problem is not just an American one. Obesity is increasing today in every country in the world.[16]

It's increasing in Alaskan Eskimos, in the Evenki (reindeer herders in Siberia), and in the Walpiri (Australian Aborigines). More than 25 percent of children in Egypt, Chile, Peru, Germany, and Mexico are now obese. Nearly 20 percent of four-year-olds are obese in Zambia and Morocco.[17] In Mexico, the average family of five drinks six gallons of Coca-Cola a week, and 65 percent of the population is overweight or obese.[18]

Dr. Stephan Roessner, president of the International Association for the Study of Obesity, is alarmed. "There is no country in the world," he says, "where obesity is not increasing. Even in [developing] countries we thought were immune, the epidemic is coming on very fast."[19]

In England, childhood obesity has tripled in the last twenty years. In 2004, a British parliamentary committee examining the obesity epidemic highlighted the death of a three-year-old girl from heart failure brought on by her excess weight. One expert quoted in the report by the House of Commons Health Committee told of children who require ventilator assistance at home for respiratory conditions because of their obesity. The children were "choking on their own fat," said Sheila McKenzie, M.D.[20]

## ARE ATKINS AND SOUTH BEACH THE ANSWER?

The books written by Robert Atkins, M.D., have sold more than twenty million copies in more than twenty languages. When the Atkins diet was at its peak in the first six months of 2004, no fewer than 1,864 new "low-carb" products were launched in the United States, including low-carb pasta and low-carb gummy bears.[21] Every sector of the food industry, from Heinz ketchup to Michelob beer, was jumping on the low-carb bandwagon. Kraft brought forth low-carb Oreo cookies. Round Table Pizza presented a low-carb pizza crust. Even W. Atlee Burpee & Co., the seed seller, was ranking their vegetable seeds according to carbohydrate content in order to help customers choose which seeds to plant in order to grow "low-carb" foods in their home gardens. One 2004 survey found that half the U.S. population was either on a low-carb diet, had tried a low-carb diet, or planned to try a low-carb diet in the future.[22]

People can be desperate to lose weight, and many have looked to low-carb diets to accomplish this ardently longed-for result. When people do lose weight on these diets, it's largely because they are consuming fewer calories, owing primarily to reduced consumption of unhealthful refined carbohydrates. In the short term, these diets can actually cause more weight loss for the same number of calories consumed than most other low-calorie diets. Proponents of these diets call this "the metabolic advantage" of a low-carb diet. On a severely carbohydrate-restricted diet, the human body has to expend energy (burn calories) to manufacture carbohydrate for tissues that absolutely require glucose, like the brain and the red blood cells. Thus, extra calories are expended without exercise.

Unfortunately, the weight lost in this manner doesn't usually stay off. The "metabolic advantage" doesn't last. In 2004, the British medical journal *The Lancet* published a study finding that any weight loss advantage Atkins and other low-carb diets may have is gone within a year.[23] The report also noted that side effects experienced by those on carb-restricted diets include constipation, headaches, bad breath, diarrhea, muscle weakness, and cramps.

These kinds of side effects are actually quite common on very low-carb diets. In another study, this one funded by Atkins himself, 70 percent of patients on an Atkins diet for six months were constipated, 65 percent had halitosis (bad breath), 54 percent reported headaches, and 10 percent were losing hair.[24]

Still, the battle of the diets has continued. In 2005, *The Journal of the American Medical Association* published the results of a head-to-head comparison of four popular diets, including Atkins and Ornish.[25] Tufts University researchers randomly assigned each of 160 overweight people to one of the four diets, gave them an instruction book and four educational sessions, and tracked their weight over the next year. At the one-year mark, those following the Ornish diet had the greatest weight loss, while those following Atkins had the least weight loss. Moreover, those following the Ornish program had the greatest reduction in LDL ("bad") cholesterol, while those following Atkins had the least reduction. Those following the other two diets, Weight Watchers and The Zone, fell between Ornish and Atkins in both weight loss and LDL reduction. Among the participants who completed the study, those on the Ornish diet lost an average of 14.5 pounds and reduced their cholesterol by 21.5 mg/dl—the best results of all the diets tested.

Unlike the other diets tested, Ornish's low-fat, plant-based diet has been scientifically proven to reverse atherosclerosis, decrease angina (chest pains), bring about permanent weight loss (five years or longer), and dramatically reduce cardiac events such as heart attacks. Studies finding these benefits have been published in the most respected peer-reviewed medical journals. These studies have found

that even people with advanced heart disease can avoid coronary bypass surgery and angioplasty by following the Ornish diet and making the other lifestyle changes in his program. On the other hand,
there is significant research pointing to dangers for the low-carb approach. In 2000, for example, the journal *Angiology* published a
study that found a worsening of blood flow to the heart on the Atkins
diet.[26]

A central tenet underlying the low-carb diets is that carbohydrates
raise blood insulin levels, causing our bodies to store more fat. A
chapter in Atkins's book is titled "Insulin—The Hormone That
Makes You Fat."

In 2003, the researchers who put people on the Atkins diet, the
Zone diet, the Weight Watchers program, and the Ornish diet presented their findings to the American Heart Association convention.
Of the four diets, Ornish's was the only one to lower insulin significantly, even though that's what the Atkins and Zone diets are designed to do.

## ARE LOW-CARB DIETS SAFE?

When Atkins's book was originally published, the medical community did not exactly applaud. The chair of the Nutrition Department
at Harvard University warned physicians that recommending the
Atkins diet "borders on malpractice."[27] The president of the American College of Nutrition said, "Of all the bizarre diets that have been
proposed in the last 50 years, this is the most dangerous to the public if followed for any length of time."[28]

The chief health officer for the state of Maryland was asked,
"What's wrong with the Atkins diet?" He replied:

> What's wrong with . . . taking an overdose of sleeping pills? You
> are placing your body in jeopardy. . . . Although you can lose
> weight on these nutritionally unsound diets, you do so at the risk
> of your health and even your life.[29]

More recently, when the American Dietetic Association called the
Atkins diet "a nightmare diet," Robert Atkins attempted to dismiss

such criticism as "dietitian talk."[30] "My English sheepdog," he snorted, "will figure out nutrition before the dietitians do."[31]

Unfortunately for Atkins and his sheepdog, however, almost every reputable health science organization in the world has issued statements strongly warning against his diet. The list includes the American Heart Association, the National Academy of Sciences, the American Cancer Society, the American Institute for Cancer Research, the American Kidney Fund, the American College of Sports Medicine, and the National Institutes of Health.

In 2002, the American Heart Association published an advisory in the leading medical journal *Circulation* warning the public about the perils of such diets. "They put people at risk for heart disease, and we're really concerned about this," said Robert H. Eckel, M.D., senior author of the paper and chairman of the American Heart Association's Nutrition Committee. "These diets will raise the . . . bad cholesterol and increase the risk for cardiovascular disease, particularly heart attacks."[32]

Eckel, who is professor of medicine at the University of Colorado Health Sciences Center, was commenting specifically on the Atkins, Zone, Protein Power, Sugar Busters, and Stillman diets.

Eckel noted that people often temporarily lose weight on these diets, and as they shed pounds, their overall cholesterol levels may temporarily drop. "But what I see after people have lost weight on such a diet, then their weight stabilizes for a period of weeks or months and often the cholesterol, particularly the bad cholesterol, now becomes more elevated. . . . Many people's LDL cholesterol [the bad cholesterol] goes up if they remain on the diet."[33]

I was a featured guest on Dr. Atkins's radio show several times, and I spoke with him on a number of other occasions as well. I am sure that he believed he was helping people to enjoy healthier lives. Similarly, I have no doubt that the people currently advocating other low-carb diets believe in what they are doing. But these diets are deeply misguided in blaming carbs alone for the Western world's obesity epidemic. They have gotten people to eat fewer refined carbohydrates like sugar and white flour, which is a positive step. But even with that, they have regrettably caused significant harm to some of their followers.

In 2004, Jody Gorran, a fifty-three-year-old man from Delray Beach, Florida, sued the estate of Dr. Robert Atkins and the company that promotes his diet. While he was following the Atkins diet, his cholesterol shot from 146, well within the normal range, to 230, considered in the hazardous range. Before he started the diet, medical tests showed that his arteries were clear, but within two years of following the Atkins approach, he had three episodes of chest pain, and doctors found a 99 percent blockage in a major artery. They needed to perform angioplasty and insert a stent to keep it open.

In 2003, the South Beach diet became the latest low-carb diet to become wildly popular. Like the Atkins diet, South Beach begins with a two-week initiation phase which drastically restricts carbohydrates. Later, the diet differs from Atkins in that it does not encourage saturated fats like butter and sausage, and allows more fibers and whole grains. Although no fruit or whole grains are allowed in the first two weeks of the plan, small amounts are allowed afterward.

South Beach is certainly an improvement over Atkins, but it's hard for me to be enthusiastic about any diet that looks askance on natural foods like apples, apricots, berries, beets, carrots, and whole-grain bread. Somehow the idea of eating bacon and eggs for breakfast and then taking cholesterol-lowering drugs doesn't strike me as a healthy approach. But that is what the author of the South Beach diet, cardiologist Arthur Agatston, does, and that is what he recommends.[34]

While in the White House, U.S. president Bill Clinton consulted with Dr. Dean Ornish, who advised him to stay away from high-fat animal products. The president, however, loved burgers, and chose instead to follow the South Beach diet. After the former president underwent emergency quadruple coronary artery bypass surgery to relieve clogged arteries in 2004, he said he wished he had never gone on a low-carb regimen of steaks and cheeseburgers, but had instead followed the advice he had received from Dr. Dean Ornish.

He probably would have been better off if he had. The healthy and long-lived people of Okinawa, Abkhasia, Vilcabamba, and Hunza eat a diet very much like the Ornish diet—a low-fat, whole-foods, plant-based diet made up entirely of natural foods and rich in complex carbohydrates. And they are among the leanest people on earth.

## THE LOW-CARB CRAZE BEGINS TO FADE

The low-carb diet craze reached its peak in 2004, with far fewer people following diets like Atkins and South Beach in subsequent years. On August 1, 2005, Atkins Nutritionals, Inc., the company that promoted low-carb eating into an international diet craze, filed for bankruptcy court protection. The company had $300 million in debts it could not pay.[35]

Though this was a sad day for the company and the people who depended on it, it was good news for public health, because it signaled that more and more people were beginning to understand that you do not have to eschew healthy carbs to lose weight. If you are going to heed the example of the world's longest living cultures, the answer is not to stop eating carbohydrates entirely, but to stop eating refined carbohydrates, and instead eat healthier, unprocessed carbs like whole grains, vegetables, and fruits, along with seeds, nuts, and legumes, as the basic building blocks of your diet.

The evidence is consistent. People who eat plant-based diets centered on whole grains, vegetables, nuts, seeds, and legumes tend to be dramatically slimmer than those whose diets incorporate significant amounts of animal products. In 2004, for example, an intensive four-nation study involving more than four thousand men and women aged 40 to 59 revealed that the thinnest people eat the most healthful carbs. The study's lead author, Linda Van Horn, Ph.D., professor of preventive medicine at Northwestern University, presented the findings at the 44th American Heart Association Annual Conference. "Without exception, a high-complex-carbohydrate . . . diet is associated with low body mass," she said. "Desirable carbohydrates are complex, high-fiber carbohydrates: whole grains, fruits and vegetables."[36]

How do the medical researchers who have conducted the Okinawa Centenarian Study feel about the low-carb diets? Having meticulously analyzed the diets and health of many of the world's longest lived people, these researchers write:

> Never in the history of nutrition research has the evidence been more clear and consistent: a high [unrefined] carbohydrate, low calorie, plant based diet is the best for long-term health. There's no doubt about it anymore, despite what you might have read in books advocating low-carb, high-protein diets.[37]

## SIMPLE PLEASURES

The lifestyles of the elder Okinawans, like those of the Abkhasians, Vilcabambans, and Hunzans may seem spartan compared to the modern world, where we consume so much sugar and other tasty high-calorie, low-nutrient foods. But these long-lived peoples are most certainly not life deniers. They take pleasure in their senses and excel at having a good time. They are life-affirming folks who enjoy the simple delights and transformative joys of the world around them. They rarely consume foods like candy, chips, ice cream, or hot dogs, but they are brimming with life. They smile a lot. They laugh out loud. They sing and dance.

In fact, when I look at our overworked, under-slept, fast-food modern world, I think it may be we who are sensually deprived and they who are the true celebrants.

Take alcohol, for example. I am sure you know how much damage arises in the modern world from the excessive consumption of alcohol. People in each of the long-living cultures enjoy alcoholic beverages. But rather than indulging to excess, they savor their pleasures, drink only in moderation, and have no concept of alcoholism. In fact, they enjoy life far too much to want to escape from it by becoming inebriated.

In their enjoyment and appreciation of moderate amounts of alcohol, these cultures are fully congruent with the modern research that has found substantial heart and other health benefits to *moderate* consumption of red wine. (These benefits, needless to say, disappear when people drink excessively.)

## THE ROLE OF GENES

There are people who believe that your health is not greatly affected by what you eat, how you live, or whether you enjoy your life. They believe the only way to ensure a long and healthy life is to be blessed with favorable genes. Are they right?

Not according to one of the foremost experts on the relative importance of lifestyle choices and genetics, John W. Rowe, M.D., president of the Mount Sinai School of Medicine and the Mount Sinai Hospital in New York City. Since its inception, he has chaired the MacArthur Foundation Research Network on Successful Aging, which conducted a major study of both identical and nonidentical twins who were raised apart. Dr. Rowe explains:

> The bottom line is very clear: with rare exceptions, only about 30 percent of physical aging can be blamed on genes . . . and as we grow older, genetics becomes less important. . . . These findings shatter the myth that our course in old age is predetermined. MacArthur research provides very strong evidence that we are, in large part, responsible for our own old age.[38]

There are of course some diseases (such as hemophilia, cystic fibrosis, ichthyosis, sickle cell anemia, hemochromatosis, Tay-Sachs disease, and Huntington's disease) that are strongly or entirely determined by genetics. I do not wish to minimize the importance of knowing all we can about how genes affect health. But we now know that even when there is a genetic predisposition for cancer, heart disease, hypertension, rheumatoid arthritis, and many other conditions, a healthful diet and regular exercise can at the very least substantially delay, and more often completely prevent, the emergence of the disease.

The Study of Adult Development at Harvard University is arguably the longest study of aging in the world. It is a prospective study, meaning that it has not depended on people's memory of what took place in the past. Instead, nearly a thousand people have been followed by researchers for more than sixty years. It is also a rarity in medicine, for it has studied the lives of the healthy rather than only those who are ill.

Looking back in 2002 over what had been learned in more than six decades, the study's director, George E. Vaillant, M.D., concluded that in most cases genes are not the preeminent factor that many have believed:

> To many it seems as if heart attacks and cancer are visitations from malicious gods and that much of the pain of old age is in the hands of cruel fate, or at least of cruel genes. The whole process of aging sometimes feels completely out of our control. But blessed with prospectively gathered data, I was astonished at how much of . . . healthy aging or lack of it is predicted by factors . . . that are more or less controllable.[39]

What about the Okinawans? Might the underlying reason for their fabulous health and longevity be some kind of special genetic status? Might they be blessed with favorable genes that enable them to remain healthy when others would fall ill?

These questions have been thoroughly studied. Migration studies have found that when Okinawans move elsewhere and adopt the diets of their new locations, they get the same diseases at the same rates, and die at the same ages, as the people whose customs they embrace. The life expectancy for Okinawans who move to Brazil, for example, drops seventeen years.[40]

The U.S. National Institutes of Health funded a study called "Genetics of Exceptional Longevity in Okinawan Centenarians." The study found that most of the Okinawans' advantage stems not from genetics, but from the way they live and the food they eat.

By far the most dramatic evidence that genetics is not the primary reason for the blessings of Okinawan health can be seen today in the lifestyles and health of the younger Okinawans, who of course share the same genes as their elders. It is a sad and sobering reality that the health practices and way of life that have produced such outstanding results for the elders for so long are today being abandoned by younger generations.[41]

How has this happened? At the end of World War II, without

Okinawans' having any voice in the matter, the American military seized massive amounts of Okinawan property in order to build numerous military bases and housing estates for American military families. The Americans did not requisition or pay for this land. They simply seized it, often at bayonet point, and then bulldozed the houses on it so they could use the land however they wanted.

In 1951, Okinawa legally became a possession of the United States, and the U.S. military occupation of Okinawa lasted until 1972, twenty years longer than the Allied occupation of mainland Japan. Even after Okinawa reverted to Japanese sovereignty in 1972, the United States has maintained an enormous military presence in Okinawa.

Today, there are still more than fifty thousand U.S. military personnel and thirty-nine U.S. military bases in Okinawa, occupying about one-sixth of the land mass of the prefecture. This massive presence has had a mammoth impact on the culture and lifestyle in Okinawa. With the soldiers have come American fast-food restaurants. McDonald's, KFC, A&W, Burger King, and Baskin-Robbins have become commonplace. Okinawa now has more hamburger restaurants than anywhere else in Japan.

In addition, in the 1960s the Japanese government noticed that young people in Okinawa weighed less and ate fewer calories than young people in the rest of Japan. Mistakenly thinking this was a problem, the government proclaimed the young Okinawans underweight and began to institute a school lunch program designed to rectify the "problem." Full-fat milk and refined white bread replaced a low-calorie plant-based diet centered on vegetables, whole grains, soy foods, and fish.

As a result of these influences, younger Okinawans today are eating a much more Western diet than their elders have ever eaten. They are consuming far more calories, far more fat, far more processed food, far more meat, sugar, and corn syrup. Relying ever more on convenience foods and eating many of their meals in American fast-food restaurants, they are becoming less physically active and less involved in their communities.

The contrast could hardly be more striking. The elders are still eating their traditional diets filled with sweet potatoes, fresh vegetables, and tofu. But the younger residents of Okinawa, heavily influenced by the tens of thousands of U.S. troops based there, now spend three times more money per capita on processed meat and nearly five times more on canned foods than do the residents of any other Japanese prefecture.

The elder Okinawans, whose health and longevity have been so thoroughly documented, eat a diet that—like those of the Abkhasians, Vilcabambans, and Hunzans—is plant-based and low-calorie and contains very little sugar or processed food. But when members of the younger generation buy food at markets, their shopping carts are filled with bacon, jelly rolls, sausage, and soda pop. The younger Okinawans today have actually become the world's largest per capita consumers of Spam and other canned and processed meats.[42]

As you might expect, there have been health consequences to abandoning the ancestral Okinawan ways. They are serious, and I find them to be terribly sad. Younger Okinawans today have the highest level of obesity in Japan, the worst cardiovascular risk profile, the highest risk of coronary heart disease, and the highest risk for premature death. What a stark and painful contrast this presents to their elders, who are the healthiest and most long-lived people ever thoroughly studied by modern science.

Today, Okinawans in their forties and fifties are increasingly overweight, and are more likely to die of heart attacks and cancer than their elders who are in their nineties and beyond. Newspapers publish an increasing number of obituaries of people who have died in what might otherwise have been the middle of their lives. Most of those deaths are from diabetes, cancers, strokes, and heart disease—diet-related diseases rarely seen in the older generations. One of the saddest parts of life for Okinawan elders today is how often they must attend the funerals of their grandchildren.

The rapid and nearly total shift in dietary habits and in health between the generations in Okinawa is a source of deep sorrow to anyone who sees the calamity that is taking place. It is tragic to witness such a wholesome way of life being discarded in favor of one so harmful. And yet, at the same time as we mourn what is being lost, we can also realize that we are being offered an opportunity to learn something important. In Okinawa today we can see both an ultimate example of healthful living and its opposite—both within the same gene pool, and both taking place at a time when they can be studied carefully by scientific investigators.

The researchers have done their job. They have made clear what the factors are that have produced the vastly different health outcomes among different generations in Okinawa. It's up to each of us what we do with what we have learned.

# 6

## Nutrition and the Health of Humanity

*You are not old until regret replaces your dreams.*
—Anonymous

The distressing contrast between the eating habits and health of the elder and younger Okinawans is a sad reenactment of a pattern that has taken place in many indigenous cultures as they have become colonized by Western influences and processed foods. Beginning in the nineteenth century and becoming nearly unstoppable in the twentieth, it is a pattern that has devastated the cultural traditions of native peoples in nearly every corner of the globe. And it began to be thoroughly documented in the 1930s.

The 1930s were an interesting time in the evolution of modern civilization. Photographic equipment was just becoming relatively inexpensive and portable, and yet there were still many cultures and tribes of people worldwide who had not yet been exposed to the growing influence of Western culture. And it was in the 1930s that an American dentist named Weston A. Price traveled to nearly every corner of the world, camera in hand, seeking to understand the relationship between the food people were eating and the health they were experiencing.

As he trekked around the globe, Price specifically sought out people who were still eating their native foods. He asked about their dietary habits, then examined and photographed their teeth. At the same time, he undertook similar studies and took similar photos of people from the same cultures who had become exposed to Western foods and who had begun to substitute foods like white flour, white sugar, marmalade, and canned goods for their native diets.

The differences, as shown by the many photographs in Price's 1939 book *Nutrition and Physical Degeneration,* were startling.[1] Time and again, Price found that those people who were still eating their native diets had very little if any dental caries (decay or crumbling of teeth) and appeared to be in radiant health, while their counterparts who were now eating refined and processed foods from the West were exhibiting massive tooth decay and malformation of their dental arches as well as suffering from a growing cascade of illnesses and dysfunctions. Price came to believe that dental decay was caused primarily by nutritional deficiencies, and that the same conditions that promote tooth decay also promote disease elsewhere in the body.

For nearly a decade, Weston Price and his wife, Monica, traveled each summer to different parts of the world. Their investigations took them to isolated Swiss villages and to an island off the coast of Scotland. They studied Aborigines in Australia, Maoris in New Zealand, traditional Eskimos in Alaska, indigenous tribes in Canada and the Florida Everglades, Peruvian and Amazonian natives, South Sea islanders, and tribespeople in Africa.

All told, Price found fourteen different tribes whose diets, though radically different from one another, seemed to provide not only nearly complete immunity from tooth decay, but also extraordinary resistance to illness. And in every case, he also found that when members of these tribes began to eat what Price called "the displacing foods of modern commerce," the results were uniformly disastrous. While eating their native foods, they enjoyed robust, vibrant, and nearly disease-free health, but when they began eating imported white flour, sugar, jams, jellies, cookies, condensed milk, canned vegetables, margarine, vegetable oils, confections, and other refined foods, their health rapidly deteriorated.

Price was a dentist, and his principal concern was the teeth and dental arches of the people he encountered. He found that as long as these people consumed their native diet, their mouths and jaws developed so that they never experienced crowded teeth, overbites, underbites, or tooth decay. When their wisdom teeth came in, they always had plenty of room. But as his photographs poignantly show, once they abandoned the wisdom of eating their native foods for eating "civilized" foods, the results were ruinous. Now all kinds of dental problems that had been previously unknown became rampant.

And it wasn't just dental problems. Price found that as people shifted to refined foods, birth defects increased, and people became more susceptible both to infection and to chronic disease. As people ate ever more refined and devitalized foods, he said, they and their offspring became increasingly weaker and more prone to all kinds of diseases.

## THE DAMAGE DONE BY PROCESSED FOODS

Before eating such foods, Price said, native peoples enjoyed magnificent health and exhibited superb physical traits. He wrote of their eyesight with awe, pointing out that they could see many stars that are visible to those of us in the modern world only with the aid of telescopes. The Maori of New Zealand, he said, could see the moons of Jupiter with their naked eyes. The proof was that they could describe the moons to someone looking through a telescope, and their descriptions were accurate.

He wrote of the Aborigines of Australia, who could see animals moving a mile in the distance, and whose skill in tracking was so uncanny that it was as though they possessed a sixth sense.[2] Over and over again he found indigenous people who had for countless generations built superbly functioning bodies which they maintained in excellent health as long as they ate only their traditional native foods.

But, Price warned ominously, once modern Western foods became part of native peoples' diets, the destruction developed rapidly. He wrote:

[Indigenous peoples like] the Aborigines of Australia have reproduced for generation after generation through many centuries—no one knows for how many thousands of years—without the development of a conspicuous number of irregularities of the dental arches. Yet in the next generation after these people adopt the foods of the white man, a large percentage of the children developed irregularities of the dental arches with conspicuous facial deformities.[3]

Again and again, Price warned of the menace of processed foods. To his eyes, their incorporation into the human diet represented a dire threat to human health and quality of life. "If a scale were extended a mile long," he said,

and the decades measured by inches, there would apparently be more degeneration in the last few inches than in the preceding mile. This gives some idea of the virulence of the blight contributed by our modern civilization. . . .[4] It should be a matter not only of concern but deep alarm that human beings can degenerate physically so rapidly by the use of a certain type of nutrition, particularly the dietary products used so generally by modern civilization.[5]

Price saw this tragedy occurring among all the indigenous peoples he visited. The peoples he studied were diverse. They were of widely different cultures and ethnicities, and they lived at different altitudes, latitudes, and climates. Yet in writing about culture after culture, Price speaks of the radiant health that was theirs before the advent of processed and refined foods, and the inevitable deterioration that ensued after such foods became part of their diets. It is not just his words that account for the power of Price's message. Some of the photographs he took are inspiring depictions of the health enjoyed by native peoples in all corners of the globe while they continued to eat the foods that were natural to their environment. Others of his photos are graphic and haunting illustrations of what happened when these ancestral ways were discarded in favor of "civilized foods."

To Price, the conclusion was obvious: The consumption of sugar, refined flour products, sweetened foods, canned foods, polished (white) rice, and other processed foods brought the white man's diseases to native populations. If people were to remain healthy, it was imperative that they resist dietary colonization and return to their ancestral wisdom and native diets.

## IMMENSE VARIETY IN THE TRADITIONAL DIETS OF NATIVE PEOPLES

Remarkably, Price saw that these native diets upon which indigenous people had long thrived differed greatly from one another. They were, in fact, as varied as the environments in which the people lived. Tribes who made their homes near rivers, lakes, or the ocean typically based their diets on fish and other marine life. Those who lived in cold northern climates where plant life was sparse tended to base theirs on wild game. Yet others, living in more temperate areas, were mostly vegetarian, eating primarily whole grains, fruits, and vegetables, much like the Abkhasians, Vilcabambans, Hunzans, and Okinawans (none of whom Price ever met or studied). Some were essentially lacto-vegetarian in that their diet consisted mostly of plant foods such as seeds, nuts, whole grains, vegetables, and fruits, but also included dairy products. A number of others ate a diet that could best be called "pesco-vegan," in that it did not include significant amounts of meat, dairy products, or eggs, but was rich in a wide variety of plant foods and in fish. Some, like the African Masai, ate primarily the blood, milk, and meat of their cattle. Others, like the Kikuyu tribe just to the northwest of the Masai, ate mainly sweet potatoes, corn, millet, beans, and bananas.

The diversity was endless. In some cultures, most of the food was cooked. In others, much of it was eaten raw. Some cultures ate liberally of dairy products from pastured cows, goats, or camels, while others lived "in isolation so great that [they] had never seen milk in any larger quantity than drops."[6] Some of these native peoples lived in ecosystems so inhospitable that they were forced to depend on only a few varieties of plant foods, while others enjoyed a great multitude of fruits, vegetables, grains, and legumes. In some tribes, whole grains were the staples of the diet, and were considered sacred. In others, grains played little or no role, and other foods, including sometimes the livers of certain wild animals, were the ones held sacred.

As diverse as these diets were, they did, to Price's eyes, have certain things in common. Most notably, none contained any refined or devitalized foods such as white flour, sugar, canned foods, pasteurized or skimmed milk, or refined and hydrogenated vegetable oils. And they all tended to be low (compared to modern diets) in calories. Price also noticed that all contained at least a small measure of animal food, even if only insects, fish, or milk. How interesting that the common features he found among the diets of all the healthy native peoples he studied are found also in the diets of the elder Okinawans, Abkhasians, Vilcabambans, and Hunzans.

## A MAN AHEAD OF HIS TIME

At a time when many in the West looked upon native people as savages in need of the civilizing influence of Western culture, Weston Price saw the ignorance, the arrogance, and the destructiveness of this attitude. At a time when indigenous cultures were everywhere being destroyed by westernization, he wrote with immense respect for the ancestral wisdom of native tribes. I am sure that if his voice had been heeded, the cultures and the health of more indigenous peoples would have survived.

Moreover, Price was one of the earliest and most outspoken voices against the increasing tide of refined and processed foods. In this, he was something of a grandfather to the natural-foods movement of today. There is no telling how much suffering and disease would have been avoided if his message had been heard, and the shift to ever more processed and refined foods had been averted.

Though writing in the 1930s, much of what Weston Price said has withstood the test of time and has been corroborated by subsequent research. He was one of the first to observe that many of the common diseases in our culture—including cancer, heart disease, diabetes, asthma, arthritis, tooth decay, and obesity—were rare among indigenous peoples throughout the world whose diet was made of natural, fresh, unprocessed foods, grown in their environment. And he saw that when these peoples began to eat denatured and devitalized food, when sugar and white flour and canned foods made their way into their mouths and stomachs, the incidence of these diseases began to skyrocket. He was not exaggerating when he reported that many traditional peoples, often living a hand-to-mouth existence, maintained vibrant health, lived long, and enjoyed youthful vitality. It is a fact that in some cultures, most modern diseases were unknown, women had fast and comparatively painless childbirths, and men could run all day without fatigue. All this we know not only from Price, but also from many other researchers who have corroborated these views.

Author and cancer expert Ralph Moss has described what took place in the mid-nineteenth century, when well-trained medical personnel began to travel and even to live among indigenous peoples.[7] The news they brought back was startling. These diverse populations, many of whom had little in the way of material possessions, were generally much healthier than their Western counterparts. True, some had high infant mortality rates, and they easily succumbed to infectious diseases they had never before encountered, such as measles, smallpox, and tuberculosis. But they had far less asthma, allergies, indigestion, heart disease, and cancer.

The almost total nonexistence of cancer was particularly striking, because it was at this very time that cancer rates in the West were beginning to skyrocket. This led the French surgeon Stanislas Tanchou, M.D., to formulate what became known as "Tanchou's Doctrine"— the theory that the incidence of cancer increases in direct proportion to the "civilization" of a people.[8] This doctrine came to be embraced by John Le Conte, M.D., an influential physician who became the first president of the University of California.[9] Le Conte's enthusiasm led to a host of medical missionaries, anthropologists, and others searching avidly for cancer among the native peoples of the world. But the result was always the same. For seventy-five years, not a single case of cancer was documented among the tens of thousands of native people studied by competent medical examiners. A Harvard-trained anthropologist named Vilhjalmur Steffansson, for example, lived for eleven years among the Eskimo and never saw a case. In later life, he wrote a book titled *Cancer: A Disease of Civilization?*[10]

Unfortunately, whatever protection these native populations had against cancer began to be lost when many began to adopt Western ways in the 1920s. From then on, the rates of cancer among native peoples began a steady rise, eventually nearly reaching those of white populations.

## PAINTING THE WHOLE PICTURE

Clearly, Weston Price was on to something profoundly important. There is no doubt that there are aspects of modern Western civilization that are toxic, disease-causing, and carcinogenic. Overall, he did a remarkable job, particularly given that he lived and wrote when nutritional science was in its infancy. His work began long before Casimir Funk coined the word "vitamin."

However, it is also important to recognize the limitations of his views. In most cases, Price spent only a brief amount of time with each of the cultures he photographed and wrote about. He traveled primarily in the summertime, which gave him a partial picture of the peoples and the lands he visited. In most cases, he never saw the hardships of winter, nor the diseases and other difficulties that would come with the cold. Considering his intense interest in the health of the people he visited, it is regrettable that there are in his writings hardly any comments about infant mortality.

He did not speak the languages of his hosts, and typically lived with them for only a matter of days, or at most a few weeks—hardly enough time to gain a deep understanding of a culture that is different from one's own. If the peoples he visited wanted to keep anything hidden from his Western eyes, they would have had little difficulty doing so.

Further, Price was not trained in cultural anthropology and had not undertaken the discipline of learning to identify and detach from his own cultural biases. The fact that everywhere Price went he saw the same pattern could be interpreted as evidence that he discovered a law of great significance. But it could as easily be taken as an indication that he had certain predilections that he took with him wherever he went and which influenced what he saw and did not see. If everywhere you go you see the same thing, perhaps that says as much about the eyes with which you are looking as it does about the places you are visiting.

Price wrote extensively and movingly about the demise of indigenous people's health. As he describes it, the cause was always the white flour, sugar, jams, jellies, cookies, condensed milk, canned vegetables, margarine, vegetable oils, confections, and other refined foods they began to eat once they were exposed to Western ways. While I am certain that eating large quantities of such foods caused these people immense harm, and I applaud Price for illuminating this truth, it is important to remember that other developments were occurring at the same time that also contributed to the degeneration of native health that he so vividly catalogued and photographed. He barely mentions, for example, the role of unfamiliar germs for which indigenous peoples had no resistance, the health consequences stemming from the breakdown of social networks and kinship groups, the health implications of shifting to a more sedentary life, and the abuse of alcohol, which often became available to indigenous people through the same channels as processed food.

## BEYOND IDEALIZING NATIVE PEOPLES

Unfortunately, in Weston Price's zeal to show the damage done by processed foods, he portrayed all indigenous peoples prior to their exposure to such foods as essentially exemplary. In the more than five hundred pages of his book, for example, there is not a single negative reference to any feature of the lifestyles or the health statuses of any of the peoples he visited who were still eating their native food.

Indigenous peoples, like people everywhere, come in all shapes, sizes, and kinds. Some cultures have embodied great wisdom and compassion, while others have not. Most have found ways of living that have endured over time, though not all have developed lifestyles and customs that are worthy of emulation. There have been some indigenous peoples, for example, who have engaged in ritual human sacrifice, slavery, and the brutal oppression of women.

While some present-day hunter-gatherer communities such as the Pygmies and Bushmen in Africa are exquisitely cooperative and non-violent peoples who embody a marvelous respect for life, other tribes have developed habits that are not so life-affirming. The Ache people, for example, are a small indigenous population who live in the rain forest of eastern Paraguay. They were studied between 1978 and 1995 by anthropologists Kim Hill and Magdalena Hurtado from the University of New Mexico and their colleagues.[11] The Ache are indigenous hunter-gatherers who were relatively uninfluenced by the outside world until the 1970s. They are a strong and vigorous people who until very recently ate only their native foods. Price never visited them, but he would have found them splendid and impressive.

However, 40 percent of newborn Ache females do not live to see their first birthday. And it is the Ache custom to kill children whose parents die so that the tribe will have no orphans. Hill and Hurtado tell of interviewing an Ache man who had killed a thirteen-year-old girl who had been beautiful, healthy, and happy, simply because her mother had died in an epidemic.

To give another example of the heights (or depths) of decadence reached in some peoples long before the coming of refined and processed foods: When the Spaniard Hernán Cortés first entered the Aztec capital in Mexico in 1519, he found a thriving society in which twenty thousand people per year were being sacrificed by the Aztec royalty. Captives were taken to the top of pyramids where, upon a flat stone ritual table, they had their hearts ripped out. Then the limbs were removed, cooked, and eaten by the royalty.

Though we can learn wonderful things about health and the positive possibilities of human culture from many traditional ways of life, there are very real dangers in romanticizing indigenous people. We need to be discerning.

Today, many of Weston Price's followers consume a great deal of meat and milk and zealously push others to do the same, citing his admiration for the health of the Masai, whose diet consisted primarily of the blood, milk, and meat of their cattle.[12] In Price's eyes, the ability of the Masai to dominate their neighbors proved the superiority of their diet. He wrote,

> In every instance these cattle people dominated the surrounding tribes. They were characterized by superb physical development, great bravery, and a mental acumen that made it possible for them to dominate. . . . The Masai until checked carried on a re-

lentless warfare, consisting largely of raids, in which they slaughtered the men and carried off the women and children and drove
away the cattle or goats.[13]

Although Price saw such warlike and aggressive behavior as evidence of strength and health, another view would see it as blood-
thirsty and cruel. Our needs today, in an ever more connected world,
are not for a diet that enables us to raid and dominate our neighbors,
but for one that enables us to live healthy lives in harmony with one
another and the rest of creation. Our needs are not for a diet that
makes us more aggressive and warlike, but for a diet that enables us
to live fruitful lives, strong in well-being within ourselves and the
ability to live in peace with others.

In his glorification of native peoples, Weston Price urged us
back—back to a simpler time, back to a less technological time, back
to a time before modernity contaminated our lives and polluted our
environment, back to the diets of our ancestors.

But we no longer live in the world of our ancestors. What is available to us is different. Just as each of the intact native peoples Price
visited in the 1930s was finely attuned to the foods in their surround-
ings and had learned to live in harmony with the world in which they
lived, we must now learn how to live healthy lives and to eat wisely
from the foods that exist in our environment. Certainly his work
speaks compellingly to anyone willing to listen about the dangers of
white flour, sugar, candy, canned foods, and the other processed
foods that caused these people so much harm. It is of great consequence for us to listen, because the majority of the packaged foods
screaming at us to buy them from the aisles of our supermarkets, and
most of the foods sold in our fast-food chains, are refined, devitalized, and adulterated foods. We must hear what he had to say because 30 percent of the calories in the modern Western diet today
come from sugar, and 98 percent of the wheat eaten today in the
West is eaten in the form of white flour. The harm done by the movement away from natural whole foods is literally incalculable.

But very few of us can go back to the diets of the ancients. The
world has changed irrevocably. Living off wild plants and caribou is
not practical in New York City.

We cannot all depend on fish as some native peoples have done, because most of the world's fisheries are now depleted or in steep decline, and because our oceans and lakes are polluted and many of today's fish are high in mercury and other toxic contaminants. We cannot all depend on wild game because there is not nearly enough of it, and many species are nearing extinction. We cannot all eat grass-fed beef because there is not nearly enough rangeland to feed our growing numbers. And if we eat commercial beef today we may well be contributing to the destruction of the rain forests and to the extinction of the few indigenous peoples who remain intact.

Like it or not, we cannot go back. Our task is to use our intelligence and discernment to determine the optimal way of life for ourselves, our families, and our societies here and now.

The direction now is not back to a past that can never be again. Our direction is forward. Forward to creating agricultural systems and diets that permit us to live long, vibrant, healthy lives along with the other six billion of us on the planet. Forward to using our wisdom to become better stewards of the planet, to living more lightly on the earth, to reducing our ecological footprint.

Our task is not to return to what Price called "the glory and power of the people who lived proudly in past centuries."[14] Our task is to honor the past, learn from it, and move on toward a healthy and sustainable future.

We must treasure tradition, but we must also embrace change.

# The Most Comprehensive Study of Nutrition Ever Conducted

*Life is not measured by the number of breaths you take, but by the moments that take your breath away.*

—Anonymous

Things are changing everywhere in the world today, and with astonishing speed. It may be that we see more change in a year today than our distant ancestors saw in a millennium.

Perhaps the place on earth where today's changes are most pronounced and taking place most rapidly is the nation where there are the most human beings—China. Only twenty-five years ago, for example, private car ownership was prohibited by the Chinese government. But now China is nearly the world's largest car importer, and every major car and truck manufacturer in the world is rushing to China to set up production lines. The number of cars in China increased a staggering 130-fold between 1980 and 2001.

Not long ago, China had an annual per capita income of only about $200, but now a consumer economy is arising with phenomenal speed. In 1996, China had 7 million cell phones and the United States had 44 million. Only seven years later, China had rocketed to 269 million versus 159 million here.

The largest shopping mall in the United States is the widely heralded "Mall of America" in Bloomington, Minnesota. But in the last few years four malls have been built in China that are bigger than the Mall of America, and the South China Mall in Dongguan City is three times its size.[1]

China is not alone. A great many of the world's peoples seem eager to adopt modernity and become mass consumers as fast as possible. But China is the country where the pell-mell pursuit of consumption is happening fastest, and where the environmental implications are being felt most intensely. China is now dealing with massive and uncontrolled air and water pollution. From the dismal air quality in its cities to the spreading deserts in its northwest, China is a nation with enormous environmental problems.

When so much is changing in our world, and at such a mind-boggling pace, some of us easily forget that the needs of our bodies for fresh air, clean water, exercise, a healthy environment, and wholesome natural food remain essentially the same as they have been for tens of thousands of years. Remarkably, it is a study that took place in China, just as the world's most populous nation began its recent massive changes, that may hold a key to our understanding how to live the longest and healthiest lives we can. I'm referring to the extraordinary China Study, which *The New York Times* called "the most comprehensive large study ever undertaken of the relationship between diet and the risk of developing disease."[2]

How did it happen that in a nation about to embark on such a massive economic and social transformation, the diet and health of an extremely large number of people were studied with a level of depth that is unmatched anywhere in world medical history? It's an intriguing story.

## THE CHINA STUDY

In the early 1970s, the premier of China, Chou En-lai, was dying of cancer. In the grip of this terminal disease, Premier Chou initiated a nationwide survey to collect information about the extent and location of cancer in China. The result was the most ambitious biomedical research project ever undertaken, involving more than

650,000 workers. The cancer survey was truly monumental. It catalogued the death rates for twelve different kinds of cancer in more
than twenty-four hundred Chinese counties, accounting for 880 million Chinese citizens—96 percent of China's population.[3]

The survey found that cancers were vastly more common in some
parts of China than in others. This was of compelling interest for two
reasons: first, because the difference in cancer rates between some
Chinese *counties* was actually far greater than the difference between
many of the world's *nations;* and second, because these differences
were occurring in a country where 87 percent of the population belong to the same ethnic group (the Han people) and are genetically
quite similar.

The difference in cancer rates between counties was staggering.
Some counties, for example, had death rates from colon cancer that
were twenty times greater than those of other counties. Similar differences were found for breast cancer, lung cancer, liver cancer, and
many other forms of cancer. The counties with the highest rates of
some cancers had rates that were more than a hundred times greater
than were found in the counties with the lowest rates of these cancers.[4]

These are truly remarkable figures. To put them into perspective,
consider the great interest in why Long Island has an increased rate
of breast cancer. Many tens of millions of dollars have been spent and
countless person-years of labor have gone into investigating why two
counties on Long Island have rates of breast cancer that are 10 to
20 percent higher than the New York state average. In China, by
comparison, the survey found that some counties have breast cancer
rates twenty times (2,000 percent) higher than others.

The world medical community wanted to know what was going
on in China. Why was there such massive variation in cancer rates
among different Chinese counties? What could account for such phenomenal variation in cancer rates among genetically similar people?
What could explain the fact that men in one part of China die from
cancer of the esophagus 435 times more frequently than men in another part? And why was overall cancer so much less common in
China than in the United States and other Western nations?

Medical authorities throughout the world understood that the answers to these questions, if they could be determined, would not only be of great value to the Chinese people. They would be of tremendous value to the entire world.

In 1983, seven years after Premier Chou died of liver cancer, and as a direct extension of the nationwide cancer survey he had instigated, the China Study was begun. It was to become the most ambitious international scientific inquiry undertaken in medical history dealing with lifestyle factors and human health.

The China Study was in every way an international endeavor. It was a collaborative effort between Cornell University in the United States, the Chinese Academy of Preventive Medicine, the Chinese Academy of Medical Sciences, and Oxford University in England. And it was headed jointly by Dr. Junshi Chen, deputy director of the most significant government diet and health research laboratory in all of China; Dr. Junyao Li, one of the authors of the Chinese nationwide Cancer Atlas Survey and a key scientist in China's Academy of Medical Sciences; Professor Sir Richard Peto of Oxford University, considered one of the premier epidemiologists in the world; and Dr. T. Colin Campbell, co-author of the landmark U.S. National Academy of Sciences report "Diet, Nutrition, and Cancer."

Dr. Campbell was chosen to be the project director. His credentials were impressive: As well as being co-author of the National Academy of Sciences report, he was author of more than three hundred scientific papers, and he was the senior science advisor to the American Institute of Cancer Research / World Research Fund.

Funding for this massive enterprise was shared by the nations involved. Much of the initial funding came from the U.S. National Cancer Institute and the National Institutes of Health. The Chinese Ministry of Health pitched in by paying the salaries of more than 350 health workers who, armed with computers and faxes (the China Study introduced the first fax machine into China in 1985), proceeded to generate the most comprehensive data base ever compiled on the multiple causes of disease.

## AN AMAZING OPPORTUNITY

The world medical community realized that the China Study represented a once-in-the-history-of–humanity opportunity. In the 1980s,
China was a perfect "living laboratory" for studying diet and disease
patterns, unparalleled anywhere else in the world. This was because
the Chinese still tended to spend their entire lives in the same area.

China was perhaps the last place in the world where such a study
could be undertaken. In the Western world, many of us move frequently, and our food comes from all over the world. But China in
the 1980s still offered the possibility of studying vast numbers of
people who had lived in only one area for their entire lives. At that
time, more than 90 percent of the adults in the counties studied still
lived in the area where they were born.

Furthermore, these people had eaten food from the same area
their whole lives. And the differences in diets between even neighboring regions in China was great. If your only experience of Chinese
food comes from Chinese restaurants in the West, you might not realize how greatly diets in China vary from one region to another.
Villagers on the mountainous north bank of the Yangtze River,
for example, have for many generations relied mainly on steamed
breads and sweet potatoes. Only fifty miles away, however, on the
rich farmlands to the south, villagers have long depended primarily
on rice.

The China Study sought to discover whether the varying diets
in different parts of China would correlate to the widely varying
death rates from cancer and other diseases. To find out, researchers
launched the most widespread and massive international scientific investigation ever devised.

Researchers went into sixty-five counties across China, adminis-
tering diet and lifestyle questionnaires and collecting urine and blood
samples from tens of thousands of people. They recorded everything
families ate over a three-day period and analyzed food samples from
marketplaces around the country.

The counties that were studied stretched across the entire Chinese
land mass, from the far northwest to the southern coastal region to
Taiwan. Researchers traveled for days across rough terrain in order

to reach nomads on the Soviet border and villagers in an oasis near the Gobi desert.

Altogether, twenty-four provinces (out of twenty-seven in all of China) were selected for the China Study, representing a vast range of climates and topographies. Some were in the semitropical coastal areas of southeast China. Others were in the frigid areas in the northeast part of the country near Siberia. Some were located in the arid regions near the northern steppes. Still others were in high mountainous areas in the Himalayas.

The counties chosen also had widely varying population densities. One remote county near the Gobi desert had only twenty thousand nomadic residents. Another county, on the outskirts of Shanghai, was home to 1.3 million people.

The number of skilled person-hours put in by health professionals involved in this study was immense. To attempt anything remotely resembling the China Study in the West would have been prohibitively expensive.

When the China Study was at last finished, researchers had a study that was utterly unmatched in its quality and comprehensiveness. They had what *The New York Times* described as "the Grand Prix of epidemiology."[5]

## DISEASES OF POVERTY / DISEASES OF AFFLUENCE

One of the first findings to emerge from the China Study data was that certain groups of diseases often occur in similar economic settings. Scientists have long spoken of two classes of disease: "diseases of poverty" and "diseases of affluence."

"Diseases of poverty" include infectious diseases like pneumonia, tuberculosis, diarrhea, respiratory illnesses, and measles. Diarrheal diseases are seldom fatal in industrial countries, but they claim the lives of millions of children in the developing world. Among well-nourished children, measles is rarely fatal, yet this disease kills some 800,000 children annually, nearly all of them already weakened by hunger. Respiratory illnesses are usually a minor problem in a healthy population, but they take a heavy toll among malnourished people with weakened immune systems.

The China Study made clear that the underlying causes of "diseases of poverty" are actually nutritional inadequacy and poor sanitation. In fact, since it is not poverty itself that causes these diseases, but the lack of clean water and adequate food, it would be more precise to call them "diseases of nutritional inadequacy and poor sanitation."

Similarly, the China Study demonstrated that the underlying cause of most "diseases of affluence"— including diabetes, coronary heart disease, obesity, and many forms of cancer—is not affluence itself, but rather the nutritional excess that typically accompanies affluence. In fact, so tightly are "diseases of affluence" linked in the China Study data to eating habits that Dr. T. Colin Campbell, the project's director, has said that it would be more accurate to cease referring to "diseases of affluence" and instead adopt the term "diseases of nutritional extravagance."[6]

Noting that the more wealthy and urban Chinese have begun to eat diets higher in oils and animal products, Dr. Campbell explains:

> In Shanghai and Beijing eating meat has acquired a certain social cachet. Unfortunately, this gastronomic form of social climbing is just the diet that we now know causes so many of the diseases we suffer from in the West—cancer, heart disease, and diabetes.[7]

After examining a multitude of possible factors, the scientists undertaking the China Study found that diseases of nutritional extravagance were most markedly associated with high blood cholesterol. *You may already know that high cholesterol is a widely recognized risk factor for heart disease. But the China Study found that higher blood cholesterol levels were also consistently associated with diabetes and many cancers.*

This dramatic correlation between higher cholesterol levels and what have been known as "Western lifestyle diseases" was found to be consistent even though cholesterol levels in China tend to be lower than are commonly found in the West. In fact, vastly lower cholesterol levels were one of the chief reasons that, at the outset of the China Study, death from heart disease was a stunning 17 times less frequent in China than in the West. The China Study found that in some parts of China, particularly the southwestern Chinese provinces of Sichuan and Guizhou, heart disease was virtually nonexistent. During a three-year observation period, not a single person died of coronary heart disease before the age of sixty-four among 246,000 people in a Guizhou county and 181,000 in a Sichuan county.[8] According to Richard Peto of Oxford University, one of the China Study's principal investigators, "the Chinese experience shows that most Western coronary heart disease is unnecessary."[9]

The primary foods that cause blood cholesterol levels to rise are well known today. They are saturated fats (found mostly in animal products) and hydrogenated fats (found mostly in pastries, cookies, margarines, and other processed foods). And increasingly, as Dr. Campbell makes clear in his outstanding 2005 book titled *The China Study*, animal protein is also being seen as a major cause of high cholesterol.[10]

Meanwhile, the foods that decrease cholesterol levels are also well known. They are soy products, whole grains, vegetables, and fruits. In general, the higher the intake of fiber (found in unprocessed plant foods but not in any animal products) and legumes (peas and beans) in your diet, the lower the level of cholesterol you will have in your blood.

As a result of the vast amount of information gathered in the China Study, Dr. Campbell came to believe that the scientific evidence indicates a diet based on plant foods with a minimal amount of foods derived from animals as the ideal diet for human beings. In fact, his book *The China Study* is one of the strongest scientific arguments ever amassed for such a way of eating. The China Study itself, remember, had begun in the attempt to understand the reason for the vast differences in cancer rates among Chinese counties. According to Dr. Campbell, the primary answer turned out to be the differences in animal food consumption:

> One of the most dramatic findings of the China Project was the strong association between foods of animal origin and cancer. . . . We found that one of the strongest predictors of Western diseases

was blood cholesterol. . . . Lower blood cholesterol levels were linked to lower rates of heart disease, cancer and other Western diseases. . . . As blood cholesterol levels decreased from 170 mg/dL to 90 mg/dL, cancers of the liver, rectum, colon, lung, breast, stomach, esophagus, brain (in both adults and children), and leukemia (in both adults and children) decreased. . . . It's not enough simply to make a few small dietary changes to prevent cancer. A major shift towards plant-based foods and away from animal foods is likely to produce much greater benefits.[11]

## CANCER AND ANIMAL FOODS

If the correlation between cancer and animal food consumption is indeed as powerful as the China Study found, you would expect other studies to find the same thing. It turns out that many have. A study of 122,000 female American nurses, for example, found that those women who ate meat daily were two and a half times more likely to get colon cancer than those women who ate meat less than once a month. In 2001, a comprehensive Harvard review of the research on dairy products and prostate cancer found that those who had over the course of their lives consumed the most dairy products had *double* the rate of advanced prostate cancer and *four times* the rate of metastatic prostate cancer. A high intake of fruits and vegetables, on the other hand, was associated with a lower risk of advanced prostate cancer.[12]

Other studies, including the famous Physicians' Health Study, have also confirmed a link between dairy product consumption and prostate cancer. And a study of more than twelve thousand Seventh-Day Adventist men found that those who drank soy milk regularly rather than cow's milk had a whopping 70 percent reduction in their risk of prostate cancer.[13]

Today, men in China who are still eating their traditional whole-foods, plant-based diet without any dairy products have one of the lowest rates of advanced prostate cancer in the world. And no one can say these low rates are due to a genetic advantage, because Chinese American men living in the United States and eating the standard American diet have been shown to have rates ten times as high as their genetic counterparts still eating in the traditional way in China.

Just how important it is to eat a plant-based diet to prevent cancer was confirmed in 1997, when the American Institute for Cancer Research issued a major international report, *Food, Nutrition and the Prevention of Cancer: A Global Perspective.*[14] This report analyzed more than 4,500 research studies dealing with diet and cancer, and its production involved the participation of more than 120 contributors and peer reviewers, including participants from the World Health Organization, the Food and Agriculture Organization of the United Nations, the International Agency on Research in Cancer, and the U.S. National Cancer Institute.

Included in the report was a study by a panel of fifteen of the world's leading researchers in diet and cancer who reviewed more than two hundred case-controlled studies on the link between fruits and vegetables and cancer. An astounding 78 percent of these studies found fruits and vegetables to have a statistically protective effect in regard to one or more kinds of cancer. Only 22 percent showed no significant link. None showed an increase of cancer with consumption of these foods.

The overall report's number one dietary recommendation?

Choose predominantly plant-based diets rich in a variety of vegetables and fruits, legumes, and minimally processed starchy staple foods.[15]

As both the project director of the China Study and the senior scientific advisor to the American Institute for Cancer Research who organized the landmark international report, Dr. T. Colin Campbell knows these studies intimately. As a result of what he has learned, he has become outspoken on the diet-disease connection. He says,

The vast majority of all cancers, cardiovascular diseases, and other forms of degenerative illness can be prevented simply by adopting a plant-based diet.

There is a certain irony in Dr. Campbell's becoming one of the most outspoken scientific proponents of a plant-based diet. He was raised on a dairy farm and grew up eating lots of meat and eggs. He wrote his Ph.D. dissertation on the ways animal protein could be produced more efficiently so we could eat more animal-based foods. But as he describes in *The China Study,* his remarkable career doing nutritional research at the highest levels convinced him that a diet as low as possible in animal-based products is the healthiest choice. He says he was just paying attention to what the scientific evidence was showing him.

His diet now is 99 percent vegetarian. He and his wife, Karen, have raised five children on a plant-based diet.

## CHINA TODAY

The China Study was undertaken just as China was beginning to move from centuries of grinding poverty into a newfound affluence. The study made it clear that there would be immense benefits to this nation of more than a billion people if it would use its new wealth to solve the problems of malnutrition and poor sanitation while retaining respect for a whole-foods, natural, plant-based diet. Such an approach would go a long way toward eliminating the "diseases of poverty" without generating the "diseases of affluence."

This would have been the wisest approach, but regrettably, it is not what has taken place. Many Chinese today—still carrying memories of food rationing, food lines, and empty, grumbling bellies—are eager to dispense with traditional staples like whole grains and fresh vegetables in favor of the cookies, chocolates, potato chips, jellies, pudding, fried chicken, and burgers that they associate with a more Western and affluent lifestyle. Having for the most part only recently been exposed to such foods, they are easy prey for the advertising and other marketing tactics of the mostly U.S.-based junk food companies, who make it all seem so modern and terrific, and who never seem to get around to mentioning the inevitable health consequences.

Sadly, the Chinese government and people are today not heeding the lessons of the China Study. The nation that spawned the largest study of diet and health in the history of the world is ignoring its findings. Hundreds of millions of Chinese are abandoning traditional diets rich in fiber and whole grains in favor of diets far higher in sugar and animal fat. The small farms that have long supplied open-air markets are being replaced by vast agribusiness conglomerates that feed ever-larger supermarket chains and fast-food restaurants.

The people of China now have more money, more "stuff," and more problems. They are increasingly being poisoned by the air they breathe, the water they drink—and the food they eat.

China has traditionally been a vegetarian culture, while hamburgers have long been a defining feature of the U.S. lifestyle. As recently as 1974, the United States consumed close to fifty times more meat than China. But by 2005, the Chinese diet was becoming increasingly similar to the standard U.S. diet, and China was consuming nearly twice as much meat as the United States. In the thirty years between 1974 and 2004, meat consumption in China increased an astonishing 12,700 percent.[16]

In 1989, Kentucky Fried Chicken became the first foreign fast-food franchise to set up shop in China. McDonald's and others soon followed. By 2004 there were more than twelve hundred KFC outlets in China—the company was opening nearly one a day—and the CEO of Yum Brands, which owns KFC, was telling *Fortune* magazine that KFC "makes almost as much money in China today as it makes in the U.S."[17]

The dietary changes are enormous. While TV commercials starring pop heartthrobs are persuading millions of Chinese teens to drink Pepsi, China's children are now weaned on cheeseburgers from McDonald's, pizza from Pizza Hut, and fried chicken from KFC.

While these changes are fattening the bottom lines of multinational corporations, they are also fattening the bottoms of the Chinese. As recently as 1995, only one in ten Chinese was overweight. But today, according to one study, almost a third of all Chinese adults are overweight.[18]

Amazingly, according to this study, *the number of Chinese who have become overweight in the last decade is greater than the entire population of the United States.*

Meanwhile, the number of obese (extremely overweight) and morbidly obese people is increasing, too, and not just among adults. As late as 1995, childhood obesity was virtually nonexistent in China. But a 2000 study by the Shanghai Children's Health Care Institute found that nearly 10 percent of Chinese children between three and six years old were obese.[19]

Recent studies are also finding a sharp rise in levels of blood cholesterol throughout China in the last decade, and in the incidence of high blood pressure and diabetes in both children and adults.[20] Urban areas in particular are already seeing a dramatic increase in heart disease and cancer.

It is unsettling to reflect on what these changes portend for the future health of the Chinese people. Already, cardiovascular disease and cancer have become the leading causes of death among Chinese adults. Like all Asians, the Chinese are acutely susceptible to diabetes and develop the disease at far lower weights than people of other races. Asians, particularly those from Far Eastern nations like China, Korea, and Japan, are 60 percent more likely to become diabetic than whites of the same weight.[21] Sadly, we are only seeing the first glimpses of the long-term damage likely to occur. The health impacts of China's shift away from traditional diets and lifestyles have only just begun to manifest themselves.

There is a sad and eerie resemblance between the food choices increasingly being made in China today and those now being made by the younger generation in Okinawa. In each case, people are eager to consume the high-fat, high-sugar diet symbolized worldwide by U.S.-based companies like McDonald's, KFC, and Coca-Cola. And in each case, they do so seemingly ignorant of the health implications of the direction they are taking. It is a tragedy of epic proportions that the knowledge and wisdom painstakingly garnered by the China Study, the Okinawa Centenarian Study, and many similar undertakings is not shaping the public policies of these nations, and not entering into the consciousness and affecting the choices of their people.

Americans like to think that because they spend considerably more on healthcare than any other nation in the world, their health is exemplary. But such is far from the case. In fact, the Centers for

Disease Control and Prevention released a report in 2006 showing that recent immigrants to the United States are far healthier than their U.S.-born counterparts, despite having no health insurance and little access to health care. The study found that when people of African, Asian, and Hispanic descent move to the United States they become progressively less healthy the longer they stay in the country. With each passing year, they become more likely to suffer from high blood pressure, obesity, and cardiovascular disease. The reason? The diets and lifestyles in the United States are far less healthy than those in many other countries.

As an American, I find it deeply disturbing that a diet that in many ways emanates from my country is causing so many problems, and is spreading around the world. I take heart, though, from the fact that as we work for policy changes that will someday help societies everywhere benefit from the discoveries of the China Study and the Okinawa Centenarian Study, we can as individuals already make use of this vast wealth of information.

When you heed the lessons of the China Study and the Okinawa Centenarian Study, and follow in the footsteps of the world's healthiest and longest lived peoples, you are taking a major step toward a healthier and more satisfying existence. But your choices don't affect only your life. You are also joining with the energies of millions of other people who are seeking a healthier way of life, creating a counterforce that can and will alter the course of history.

Most of us, of course, don't think of ourselves as agents of social change. Few of us dare imagine that by the way we live our lives we can affect the greater stream of events. But each of us does create an impact by how we act, and in the sum of all our actions will be written the story of our time.

Every time anyone challenges the culture of fast food and consumerism that is running amok in our world, a ripple of hope goes forth. As these ripples come together from a million different locations, they create a current that becomes increasingly powerful. When we make a statement by how we live, we set an example that radiates outward, an example that by its authenticity inspires others and helps realign the world.

When you ask that your food be natural, nourishing, and consistent with the wellness of your body and the wholeness of your spirit, you are taking an important step toward a long and healthy life, but you are doing something more, too. In rebelling against the McDonaldization of the world, you are helping to create a healthier future for all who are yet to come.

# 8

## The Road to Health and Healing

*And still you may protest, "But what about the person who drinks like a fish, smokes like a furnace, eats like a hog, and is nonetheless 85 years old?" By the same analogy, you may once in a while drive from San Francisco to Los Angeles at 120 miles an hour and still get there—but don't bet on it. Maybe suicide doesn't work the first time around, but try again. The odds get better.*
—Walter Bortz, M.D., Co-Chair, AMA-ANA Task Force
on Aging and President, American Geriatrics Society

In concluding that there are dramatic health benefits to a plant-based diet, the China Study's Dr. Colin Campbell helps us understand one of the keys to the good health of the world's longest-lived peoples. And he is in good company. Consider, for example, the extraordinary accomplishments of Dean Ornish, M.D.

Dr. Ornish has been instrumental in bringing diet to the forefront of medical thought. A graduate of Harvard Medical School, he has seen his work featured prominently in popular media, including on the covers of *Newsweek, Time,* and *U.S. News & World Report.* Dr. Ornish has succeeded in having his heart disease treatment program covered by more than forty insurance carriers, and his numerous *New York Times* bestselling books have helped millions of people to take charge of their health and improve their lives.

Dr. Ornish's best-known research is the Lifestyle Heart Trial, in which he treated patients with advanced heart disease not with drugs, but with lifestyle changes alone.[1] He put a group of patients on a very low fat plant-based diet for a year, and asked them to stop smoking, to get regular moderate exercise, to spend a half hour a day stretching, meditating, relaxing, or doing some other form of stress reduction, and to participate in weekly psychological and social support groups. Meanwhile, a control group was treated with the standard American Heart Association heart disease program, which includes a significant amount of low-fat animal products and utilizes cholesterol-lowering drugs.

The results revolutionized the treatment of heart disease worldwide. Those patients who completed Dr. Ornish's experimental program achieved medically unprecedented improvements in health and vitality. On average, their total cholesterol dropped from 227 mg/dL to 172 mg/dL, and their LDL ("bad") cholesterol dropped even more dramatically—from 152 mg/dL to 95 mg/dL. Furthermore, the frequency, duration, and severity of their chest pain plummeted. The more closely the patients adhered to the lifestyle recommendations, the more their hearts healed. Nearly all of the patients in Ornish's program not only arrested the development of their heart disease but actually experienced marked improvement. Things not only stopped getting worse; they got dramatically better—something that had never been seen before in the history of heart disease treatment.

And what about the control group who followed the American Heart Association program? They did not fare nearly as well. Their chest pain became worse in frequency, duration, and severity. While Ornish's experimental group experienced a 91 percent reduction in the frequency of chest pain, the control group had a 165 percent rise. Further, their bad-cholesterol levels were significantly higher than in Ornish's experimental group, while the blockages in their arteries also increased.

More than two thousand patients have now completed the Ornish program in hospitals throughout the United States. Most have been able to avoid coronary bypass surgery and angioplasty by making lifestyle changes, thus saving enormous amounts of both suffering and money. Highmark Blue Cross/Blue Shield cut their costs in half in the first year, and Mutual of Omaha saved $30,000 per patient in the first year.

The bottom line, and the reason why more than forty U.S. insurance companies now cover all or part of the Ornish program, is that only one out of every six patients on the American Heart Association program can expect to achieve discernible heart disease reversal, while on the Ornish program, with its very low fat and plant-based diet, three out of every four patients can expect such life-changing results.

A common misconception about Dean Ornish's work is that he recommends a very low fat diet for everyone. Actually, his studies have shown that a whole-foods plant-based extremely low fat diet (along with other lifestyle modifications) works miracles for reversing heart disease (and also prostate cancer). However, if your goal is simply to lose a few pounds or drop your cholesterol, then it's not necessary to cut your fat that low. Besides, simply focusing on how much fat you eat and trying to get it as low as possible can lead you astray, because the type of fat you eat is every bit as important as the amount.

In February 2006, massive media attention focused on the results of the Women's Health Initiative dietary modification study. If you believed the headlines, you would have thought low fat diets had been found to bestow no advantages at all. But if you read past the headlines, you'd have learned things were not that simple.

For one thing, the study didn't distinguish between fats that are beneficial and those that are harmful. For another, the study participants who were eating a "low fat diet" didn't reduce their consumption of fat very much. Twenty-nine percent of their diet was comprised of fat, not the study's goal of 20 percent. And even this may have been an overestimation, since people often say they are following a healthier diet than they really are. Remarkably, the comparison group reduced its consumption of fat nearly as much.

It was deeply unfortunate that many people got the impression from the headlines that dietary and other lifestyle changes don't actually matter that much, when in fact they matter greatly. In 2005, for example, the landmark INTERHEART study of more than 29,000 men and women in 52 countries found that nine factors related to diet and lifestyle accounted for 94 percent of the risk of a heart attack in women and 90 percent of the risk of a heart attack in men. This was seen in all geographic regions and in every racial and ethnic group worldwide.

## HOW TO BE HEART DISEASE PROOF

Less well known than Dr. Ornish, but equally convinced of the health advantages of a plant-based diet, is Cleveland Clinic general surgeon and researcher Dr. Caldwell B. Esselstyn, Jr. Writing in *The American Journal of Cardiology,* Dr. Esselstyn describes his twelve-year study in which, as he puts it, "patients became virtually heart-disease proof" while eating a diet with almost no animal products.[2]

All of the patients in Esselstyn's study had severe heart disease at the outset, yet after twelve years on his program, 95 percent of them were alive and well. How sick were they to begin with? The eighteen patients in Esselstyn's study had experienced forty-eight serious cardiac events between them in the eight years before they joined the study. But in the twelve years of the study, the seventeen patients who stayed with the program experienced a grand total of zero cardiac events.

Is a diet with very few animal products too extreme for most people to follow? Esselstyn doesn't think so. He writes:

> Some criticize the plant-based diet as extreme or draconian. Webster's dictionary defines draconian as "inhumanly cruel." A closer look reveals that "extreme" or "inhumanly cruel" describes not plant-based nutrition, but the consequences of our present Western diet. Having a sternum divided for bypass surgery or a stroke that renders one an aphasic invalid can be construed as extreme; and having a breast, prostate, colon or rectum removed to treat cancer may seem inhumanly cruel. These diseases are rarely seen in populations consuming a plant-based diet.[3]

Similarly, Dr. Dean Ornish reflects,

I don't understand why asking people to eat a well-balanced vegetarian diet is considered drastic, while it's medically conservative
to cut people open or put them on powerful cholesterol-lowering
drugs for the rest of their lives.[4]

In November 2005, *National Geographic* published a cover story
that echoed its influential articles of the 1970s. Titled "The Secrets of
Living Longer," the lead article featured three contemporary groups
of long-living people, those from Okinawa, Japan, Sardinia, Italy,
and Loma Linda, California, all of whom eat a plant-based diet. At
the conclusion of the issue, *National Geographic* summarized the
"secrets of long life" in two words: "Go vegetarian."[5]

Similarly, the researchers who conducted the 25-year Okinawa
Centenarian Study strongly advise, "Minimize your animal food consumption."[6] As Dr. Ornish explains, "Animal products are the main
culprit in what is killing us. We can absolutely live better lives without them."

In suggesting that animal-based foods should to a large degree be
replaced by plant-based foods, doctors like T. Colin Campbell, Dean
Ornish, and Caldwell Esselstyn may seem to be on the margins of
current Western society, particularly in a day when so many have
been drawn to the short-term promises of the Atkins diet and its low-
carb relatives. But unlike Dr. Atkins, these doctors and their ideas are
fully supported by the medical literature, and what they propose has
been demonstrated to work over the long term.

I've had the privilege of knowing each of these doctors (Ornish,
Esselstyn, and Campbell) as a personal friend, and I know that each
of them is lean and thriving on the plant-based whole-foods diets they
espouse—diets which are strikingly similar to those on which the
elder Okinawans, the Abkhasians, the Vilcabambans, and the Hunzans have long thrived. I also know that each of these doctors consumes at least occasional small amounts of wild fish. In this, they are
in accord with traditional wisdom, for no society has ever, to my
knowledge, sustained itself for long exclusively on plant foods. There

may have been some traditional cultures whose only animal product consumption consisted of grasshoppers, beetles, grubs, or other insects, but all have partaken of at least a minimal amount of animal foods.

For the Hunzans, it's occasional goat or sheep milk, and on rare feast days goat or sheep meat. For the Vilcabambans, it's a few free-range eggs, and once in a great while, some wild game. For the Abkhasians, it's regular helpings of a fermented dairy drink called *matzoni,* and occasional grass-fed beef. And for the Okinawan elders, it's regular consumption of wild fish.

In this way these cultures, which of course have evolved without the benefit of vitamin pills or other supplements, obtain nutrients that might be lacking or deficient on an exclusively vegan diet, such as vitamin $B_{12}$. And they have also helped to assure themselves of an adequate supply of another nutrient that we all need for health and healing: omega-3 fatty acids.

## A CRITICAL NUTRIENT

The benefits of getting an adequate supply of omega-3s are many and vast. Getting enough omega-3s is crucial to optimum physical and mental health in all stages of life. They have been shown to help reverse heart disease, boost immune function, fight degenerative disease, enhance fertility, improve mental health, and promote healthy skin. An adequate supply makes you less vulnerable to inflammatory and autoimmune diseases, less likely to have asthma, and less prone to many mental and emotional disorders including depression and Alzheimer's disease.

In times past, people got ample omega-3s from eating a variety of wild plants or from wild game. But today, people eat few wild plants, and modern meats, dairy products, and eggs contain greatly reduced levels. As a result, most people in the modern industrialized world are woefully deficient in these critical nutrients. The dietary availability of omega-3 fatty acids has declined in the United States today to only 20 percent of the level found in American diets a century ago.

Where, then, can you get them? Omega-3s are plentiful in flaxseeds and in flaxseed oil and in fatty wild fish such as salmon, herring, mackerel, and sardines, and can be found in lesser amounts in walnuts, hemp seeds, green leafy vegetables, and canola and soy oil.

Flaxseeds have long been a staple part of the diet in Hunza and Abkhasia and are widely eaten in Europe, though they have only recently started to become popular in the United States. As a source of omega-3s, they have some distinct advantages over fish. Unlike fish, they are packed with nutrients called *lignans* that lower cholesterol, reduce the risk of heart disease, and lower the risk of breast cancer, colon cancer, and prostate cancer. Thanks to their high lignan content, flaxseeds have also been shown to be tremendously valuable both in reducing PMS in premenopausal women and in reducing unpleasant symptoms of menopause. How high in lignans are flaxseeds? When researchers at the University of Toronto examined sixty-eight different foods, searching for those highest in lignans, they found that flaxseed contains between 75 and 800 times more lignans than any other food.[7]

Moreover, flaxseeds contain none of the pollutants and heavy metals such as mercury that are unfortunately increasingly common in today's fish.[8]

On the other hand, wild fatty fish such as salmon have some advantages over flaxseeds and flaxseed oil. Most notably, they are far better sources of the long-chain omega-3s DHA (docosahexaenoic acid) and EPA (eicosapentaenoic acid), which are necessary for healthy functioning and development. Both DHA and EPA are important for the heart, and DHA is especially critical for the brain development of fetuses and newborns.[9] DHA makes up 15 to 20 percent of the cerebral cortex and 30 to 60 percent of the retina, so it is essential for the healthy development of the fetus and baby and all growing children. Plus, omega-3s from wild fish may help prevent prostate cancer, while the same apparently cannot be said of omega-3s from plants. The Okinawan elders, who have one of the lowest rates of prostate cancer in the world, get their abundant omega-3s from wild fish.

With the exception of single-celled ocean plants and some seaweeds, no plant, including flax, provides any significant long-chain fatty acids. While the human body can convert the shorter-chain omega-3s found in flaxseeds and flaxseed oil into DHA and EPA, there seems to be a great deal of variation in how efficiently different people's bodies can accomplish this conversion.

The widely touted value of fish as a health food is primarily due to the extremely high concentrations of long-chain omega-3 fatty acids found in wild salmon and other wild fatty fish. No salmon, or any other fish or animal for that matter, manufactures omega-3s, but wild salmon get them by eating certain algae that make these important nutrients, which are then concentrated and stored in the salmon's body fat. Wild salmon are plentiful sources of omega-3s. Farmed fish, however, have far fewer of these essential nutrients.

## FARMED AND DANGEROUS[10]

The salmon and other fish that people are eating today are increasingly the product of fish farms. In 1990, only 6 percent of the salmon consumed in the world came from fish farms. Only eight years later, though, half were farmed, and the percentage has continued to rise since then.[11] Today, virtually all the catfish and rainbow trout, and most of the shrimp and salmon, eaten in the United States are raised by fish farmers. Alaska salmon is always wild, but all the Atlantic salmon currently available in supermarkets or restaurants is farmed. Canned salmon may be either fresh or farmed (though if it's Atlantic salmon, it's farmed). If it doesn't say whether it's wild or farmed, it's usually farmed.

Are there reasons to avoid farmed fish? Yes, and very good ones. Wild salmon have long captured the imaginations of human beings largely because they spend part of their lives in freshwater streams and part in the salty sea, using a sense of smell a thousand times more acute than that of dogs to migrate for thousands of miles and return to their birthplace to spawn. With farmed salmon, however, it's a far drearier story. With up to fifty thousand salmon confined in each underwater cage, the water they breathe and drink rapidly becomes putrid with their accumulated wastes. They must, as a consequence, be routinely administered a plethora of drugs, hormones, antibiotics, and vaccines to keep them alive under these conditions.

Wild salmon develop their characteristic pinky-orange color from eating krill. The flesh of farmed salmon, on the other hand, is a dull grayish color which would be unattractive to consumers, so chemically synthesized astaxanthin is added to their food to create the desired color.

Many studies have found farmed fish to be far higher than wild fish in toxic chemicals and other pollutants that affect the central nervous system and the immune system and can cause cancers and birth defects.[12] The farmed salmon industry insists that the studies have been too small to be significant. But in 2004, after two years and almost two million dollars, a study was released which contained an exhaustive analysis of salmon from around the world. The study was performed by some of the world's leading experts on industrial pollution, from Cornell and elsewhere, and was published in the journal *Science*.[13]

The study found that the levels of PCBs, dioxins, and banned insecticides such as toxaphene in farmed fish were so high that, based on U.S. Environmental Protection Agency (EPA) guidelines, no one should be eating farmed salmon more than once a month. Farmed fillets bought in supermarkets in Boston and San Francisco were so heavily contaminated that even half a serving a month might be too much. Since these recommendations take into account only the increased cancer risk, the researchers warned that women and girls should be eating even less than that, noting that pregnant women can pass these contaminants on to their fetuses, impairing mental development and immune system function.

The Association of Salmon and Trout Producers called the new study "dangerous, alarmist and a shot in the dark." George Lucier, a former director of the U.S. Department of Health toxicological program and the author of more than two hundred studies on toxic chemicals, disagreed. Backed by other independent U.S. experts, he called the results "undeniable."

## THE HAZARDS OF MERCURY

Many of today's fish are unfortunately contaminated with methyl mercury.[14] This is a serious problem, because methyl mercury attacks the brain and the entire nervous system and causes behavioral problems and loss of intelligence in children. Many recent studies link mercury exposure to impairments of immune and reproductive systems and to cardiovascular disease. Chronic low-level exposure in utero or in the early years of life delays development and hampers performance in tests of attention, fine motor skills, language, visual spatial skills, and verbal memory. At high concentrations, mercury causes not only mental retardation but cerebral palsy, deafness, blindness, and death.

Humans are exposed to methyl mercury primarily through eating fish. So widespread has this problem become that one out of every six women of childbearing age in the United States today has blood mercury concentrations high enough to damage a developing fetus. This means that 630,000 of the four million babies born in the United States each year are likely to experience some level of neurological damage because of exposure to hazardous mercury levels in the womb.

In 2002, a study of affluent residents of the San Francisco Bay Area found that those eating swordfish, sea bass, halibut, and ahi tuna steaks had dangerous concentrations of mercury in their blood.[15] The study, the first to look at mercury levels among middle- and upper-income people who eat fish for their health, was conducted by Dr. Jane Hightower, a doctor of internal medicine at the California Pacific Medical Center in San Francisco. Dr. Hightower explained, "We found that when people eat fish, their mercury goes up. They stop eating the fish, their mercury goes down. It's that simple."[16]

One child in the study had a blood mercury level that was triple the level allowed by the EPA and the U.S. National Academy of Sciences. She was lethargic, was losing verbal skills, and could no longer tie her shoes. She was eating two cans of tuna a week.

Dr. Hightower instructed her ill and high-mercury patients to give up fish for six months, or eat fish that doesn't accumulate mercury, such as wild salmon, sardines, sole, tilapia, or small shellfish. When they followed her advice, their mercury levels fell dramatically, though sometimes it took many months for improvement to occur.

Unfortunately, mercury contamination of fish is far more widespread than is commonly recognized. In 2005, the *Chicago Tribune* conducted one of the most comprehensive studies of mercury in com-

mercial fish ever undertaken, and came to some disturbing conclusions. In a series of articles fully deserving of a Pulitzer Prize for investigative journalism, the newspaper described

> a decades-long pattern of the U.S. government knowingly allow-
> ing millions of Americans to eat seafood with unsafe levels of
> mercury. Regulators have downplayed the hazards, failed to take
> basic steps to protect the public health and misled consumers
> about the true dangers.[17]

For years, the U.S. government has been telling the public that
canned light tuna is a safe low-mercury choice. But the *Chicago Tribune* investigation found that

> U.S. tuna companies often package and sell a high-mercury tuna
> species as canned light tuna—a product the government specifi-
> cally recommends as a low-mercury choice. The consequence is
> that eating canned tuna—one of the nation's most popular
> foods—is far more hazardous than what the government and in-
> dustry have led consumers to believe.[18]

## WHAT TO DO?

Fish are the most plentiful food source for the critical long-chain
omega-3 fatty acids DHA and EPA, but they are also the most plentiful food source for PCBs, DDT, and dioxins, in addition to mercury
and other heavy metals. And the extent to which overfishing is
wreaking havoc on fish populations is hard to exaggerate. We have
so depleted our oceans, lakes, and rivers that more than one-third of
all fish species are now known to be vulnerable to, or in immediate
threat of, extinction. In the past fifty years, the populations of every
single species of large wild fish have fallen by 90 percent or more.[19]

If you do eat fish, don't make the mistake of going overboard, because this is one situation where more is not better. When researchers
studied the eating habits and health outcomes of more than 23,000
postmenopausal women for five years, they found that those eating
the most fish had a fifty percent greater risk of developing breast can-

cer than those eating little or none. Publishing their results in the November 2003 *Journal of Nutrition,* the researchers found the increased risk of breast cancer from high fish consumption held true even after controlling for a multitude of other risk factors, including alcohol, obesity, hormone use, and more.[20] Another study, published in *Circulation,* a journal of the American Heart Association, found that the half of the population eating the most fish had over twice the risk of dying from a heart attack.[21]

What explains the higher rates of breast cancer and heart disease in fish eaters? The problem seems to stem from the pollutants, particularly mercury. "Fish is not merely a source of omega-3 fatty acids," the investigators warned, "but also of methyl mercury."[22]

One option is to take fish oil capsules. According to Dr. Alexander Leaf, who in recent years has become one of the world's leading experts on fish oils, three grams a day of fish oil provides one gram of DHA and EPA, which is all you need. More than that, he says, is just extra fat. Several brands (including Arctic Pure, Nordic Naturals, and Xtend-Life) use oil from fish caught in the cleanest and coldest waters, and their products have been molecularly distilled, removing any mercury or other heavy metals, dioxins, PCBs, and other contaminants.

If you prefer not to consume fish in any form, it's important to include ample amounts of ground flaxseeds or flaxseed oil (one to two tablespoons a day) in your diet. In my household, we grind flaxseeds in a designated electric coffee grinder every few days, keep the ground flaxmeal in the fridge, and sprinkle it on all kinds of dishes.[23] You also might want to consider taking supplementary DHA. Algae-derived DHA is presently available commercially as Omega-Zen-3 or Neuromins DHA.

It's also important to keep your consumption of omega-6 fatty acids from being too high, because excessive omega-6s compete with the omega-3s found in flax and other plant foods, making them less available to your body. The ideal dietary ratio of omega-6s to omega-3s is about two to one, but people eating the standard American diet today typically have a ratio of more like fifteen to one.

How can you make sure your omega-6 intake isn't excessive?

- Get most of your fat from whole plant foods such as nuts, seeds, and avocados.
- Use extra-virgin olive oil or canola oil rather than oils high in omega-6s such as sunflower, safflower, or corn oil.
- Limit your consumption of processed and fried foods, and avoid anything even partially hydrogenated, for these are often made with high-omega-6 oils.

## IRONING OUT THE TRUTH

Besides DHA and EPA, are there any other nutrients that people in the industrialized world who are eating healthful plant-based diets need to be concerned about? Yes, there are, including vitamin $B_{12}$ (which all vegans should take regularly), vitamin D, iodine, and carnosine. Unless you live in a southern climate and are outdoors a great deal year-round, you probably need either to take supplementary vitamin D or to eat foods to which the vitamin has been added. Both cow's milk and many brands of soy milk are regularly fortified with this vitamin in the United States and Europe today.

It's also a good idea to include iodized salt or seaweeds in your diet, or take supplementary iodine. Vegetarians may benefit from taking supplemental carnosine, a nutrient that tends to be low in plant-centered diets and that helps prevent glycation reactions in the human body. (Glycation, also known as the Maillard reaction, is recognized as a major contributor to premature aging.) Of course, the best supplement is a diet that includes a wide variety of green vegetables, beans, whole grains, nuts, and seeds.

Many people believe they need to eat meat to get enough iron. The beef industry has certainly given that impression in its ads. But those ads are misleading.

Iron is a mineral that forms part of the hemoglobin of your red blood cells and helps carry oxygen to your body's cells. When your iron stores are low or depleted, you can't get enough oxygen to your cells. A form of anemia results, and you may feel tired.

Contrary to meat industry insinuations, however, vegetarians are not more prone to iron deficiency than are meat-eaters. Iron deficiency anemia is one of the most common nutritional deficiencies around the world, but most of it occurs in developing countries rather than in affluent countries, and the cause is more likely to be parasites than diet.

The form of iron found in plant foods is called *nonheme iron*. The kind found in meat (including poultry and fish) is called *heme iron*. Heme iron is far more easily absorbed by the body than iron obtained from plant sources. The beef industry tries to make this seem like an advantage for heme iron, but in fact it is a disadvantage with very real drawbacks.

Hemochromatosis is the most common genetic disorder known to occur in humans, with 24 million people worldwide at risk for this serious disease. People with this condition store an excessive amount of iron in their bodies, which is in turn associated with increased rates of coronary artery disease and liver cancer. The fact that heme iron from meat is so readily absorbed presents a risk to people with hemochromatosis, but excess iron also poses dangers for people who do not have this genetic problem.

Antioxidants are deservedly recognized for their role in sustaining health and helping to prevent cancer, heart disease, and other forms of chronic illness. Iron, on the other hand, is the opposite of an antioxidant. It is a potent *oxidant*. Excess iron in the body causes the production of free radicals which in turn can damage cells, leading to many kinds of disease and causing premature aging. For example, when sufficient quantities of heme iron are present, as is likely to happen when diets contain appreciable quantities of beef, cholesterol is oxidized into a form that is more readily absorbed by the arteries. This leads to increased rates of heart disease.

With nonheme iron—the kind found in plants—it's a totally different story. Your body absorbs only what it needs. When your iron needs are higher, your body absorbs more; when they are lower, it absorbs less. And in this case, the wisdom of the body has profound implications for health and longevity.

It is widely recognized that women consistently outlive men almost everywhere in the world. Many of the world's leading experts in longevity, including Thomas T. Perls, M.D. (Assistant Professor of Medicine at Harvard Medical School, and founder and director of the New England Centenarian Study), believe the reason is women's menstruation. With the monthly shedding of the uterine lining, women during their menstruating years have significantly lower iron levels in their bodies than men. Since iron generates the formation of free radicals, Dr. Perls says, a lower iron burden leads to a slower rate of aging, reduced cardiovascular disease, and decreased susceptibility to other age-related diseases in which free radicals play a role.

Physicians have traditionally prescribed iron supplements and even transfusions for premenopausal women with "iron-poor blood." However, says Dr. Perls, iron supplementation for premenopausal women may actually be damaging: "It's possible that higher iron levels, which may have been considered 'normal' only because they are common in males, actually speed the aging process."[24]

Many studies have shown that males who make frequent blood donations have lowered iron levels and heightened resistance to the oxidation of LDL cholesterol, and thus are far less likely to develop atherosclerosis and heart disease. Regular blood donation in both men and menopausal women seems actually to improve the chances of longevity by lowering the amount of iron in the body and thus reducing the rate of oxidative damage.

According to Dr. Perls, lower iron levels in adults (up to a point, of course) are an advantage:·

> Although dietary iron is of great importance in children to ensure adequate red blood cell production, it may turn out that adults, and perhaps even adolescents, are speeding up their aging clocks by maintaining iron levels that are now considered "normal," but may in fact be excessive.[25]

With heme iron (the kind found in meat), your body absorbs virtually all the iron in the food, regardless of whether it is health-supporting to do so. With nonheme iron (the kind found in plants), however, you absorb only as much as you need. Many researchers now believe this is one of the reasons people eating vegetarian and other plant-based diets characteristically live healthier and longer lives than those who eat significant amounts of meat. Plant foods rich in nonheme iron include whole-grain breads and cereals, legumes, nuts and seeds, and dark green leafy vegetables. Some dried fruits are also good sources, particularly raisins, apricots, and dates.

## CHOOSING WISELY

The debate about how much, if any, animal foods are optimum to include in one's diet will no doubt continue for some time. It is hard to argue, however, against the reality that most people eating the standard Western diet would benefit considerably by moving in a more plant-based direction.

If you've been eating the way most Westerners eat, the advantages of shifting toward more plant foods and fewer animal foods and a more natural diet are many and significant. You will lose weight, improve your cholesterol and other serum lipid profiles, and lower your risk for many chronic diseases including cancer, heart disease, and diabetes. You will consume less fat, less saturated fat, less animal protein, and more fruits and vegetables, all of which are important steps in the right direction. You will consume less cholesterol and be exposed to fewer environmental toxins, which is again all to the good.

As long as you don't consume too many processed and overly refined foods such as sugar, white flour, and hydrogenated fats, you'll get more than ample amounts of protein. You'll have the inner peace that comes from knowing that your diet is more cruelty-free. And you will very likely be healthier, age more gracefully, and live longer.

———

In the modern Western world, people tend to fear that no matter what choices they make, the aging process leads inescapably to deterioration, disease, and suffering. Few of us anticipate that with the passing years we will deepen not only in wisdom, but also in our capacity for joy.

I was born in 1947, which makes me a charter member of the baby boom generation. I listened to the song "My Generation" that was wildly popular in the 1960s, in which the British pop group The Who repeatedly sang "I hope I die before I get old." Ours was a generation that looked at older people with doubt and suspicion. Our motto was "Never trust anyone over thirty."

Some of us never made it through that stage. Keith Moon, drummer for The Who, died of a drug overdose in 1978. He was only thirty-one. The Who's lead singer, Roger Daltrey, claimed in 1965 that he would kill himself before reaching thirty because he didn't want to get old. In 2004, though, he was still performing the song, saying now that the song is really about an attitude, not a physical age.

What I have learned from the elders of Abkhasia, Vilcabamba, Hunza, and Okinawa is that The Who, back in the sixties, were unconsciously reinforcing a damaging cultural stereotype. I've learned that one can be old and beautiful, old and still passionately alive, old and still bursting with wonder and blooming with joy. I've come to see that old age can be a time of growth and renewal, wisdom and well-being. I've come to understand that the lives of older adults can be as full of promise and potential as those of younger people, and that different generations can relate to one another with dignity and respect.

There is a continuity to human life. Today's older persons are yesterday's children, and today's children are tomorrow's elders. The health you will experience and the opportunities you will have in your later years depend to a substantial degree on how you choose to live between now and then. The good news is that you do not have to choose between paths that all lead to sickness and pain. You can take steps that lead in a far more promising and hopeful direction.

Eating wisely is one such step, and a most important one. But what if there was more you could do to bring about a longer, healthier, and more fulfilling life? What if there was another secret you could discover, leading toward an elderhood of strength and health, beauty and joy? And what if this was something that would give your body cause to thank you every day for the rest of your life?

This "secret" has long been second nature to the Abkhasians, the Vilcabambans, the Hunzans, and the Okinawan elders. We'll take a look at it in Part Three.

# STEPS YOU CAN TAKE

Taking steps toward a better diet can make an extraordinary difference, even if you've eaten poorly for years. One reason is that although you may think of your body as a permanent structure, most of your body's tissues are actually in a constant state of renewal. The cells lining your stomach, for example, are replaced every five days, while your red blood cells last about four months. The cells in an adult human liver are replaced every three to five hundred days. Even your bones are far from permanent; the entire human skeleton renews itself about every ten years. Almost all the cells in your body are being continually regenerated, so what you eat today literally becomes your body tomorrow.

---

- Bring consciousness to the foods you eat. Ask whether they are natural, wholesome, and in alignment with the health of your body and your spirit.
- Don't pollute your body. Don't eat junk food. Go to your kitchen cupboard and get rid of any food products that no longer serve your potential to be radiantly fit and healthy.
- You don't have to count calories if you make every calorie count.
- Eat slowly, chew thoroughly, digest well. Eat just to the point of fullness without feeling stuffed. Remember that it takes twenty minutes for your stomach to register how full it is, so give it time.

• Whenever possible, shop at local farmers' markets or participate in community-supported agriculture, buying produce direct from the grower. Shop at local natural-foods stores, or at chains like Whole Foods, Wild Oats, and Trader Joe's. Always read labels so that you can select foods with the most nutritious ingredients.

• Save money and packaging by buying in bulk.

• Don't buy or eat anything that contains partially hydrogenated oil. Learn to recognize the smell of rancidity, and don't eat nuts, seeds, or grain products that carry the telltale odor.

• Keep away from high-fructose corn syrup. Replace regular ketchup with organic brands that are sweetened with fruit juice. Look for jams that are 100 percent fruit sweetened (no added sugar).

• Stay away from food dyes (blue 1, blue 2, citrus red 2, green 3, red 3, red 40, yellow 5, yellow 6, etc.).

• Drink soy milk rather than cow's milk. Switch from mayonnaise to a more healthful soy or canola version. Eat whole-soy products like tofu and tempeh rather than meat.

• Eat less meat or none at all. For protein, depend on soy foods, other beans, peas, whole grains, and nuts.

• If you eat any kind of meat, purchase products that you know to be truly free-range and organic, such as those with the Animal Compassion logo from Whole Foods.

• If you eat fish, be sure it's low in mercury, and wild, not farmed. To learn about the mercury levels in various kinds of fish, visit gotmercury.org.

• Whenever possible, select fresh fruits and vegetables rather than frozen or canned ones. If you are unable to get the fresh produce you want, then choose frozen (without added salt or sugar) over canned.

• Get to know the amazing variety of vegetables beyond French fries and iceberg lettuce. Enjoy eating a wide assortment of fresh vegetables, especially lots and lots of dark green leafy vegetables (kale, collards, mustard greens, spinach, chard, broccoli, etc.).

• Eat an abundance of fresh raw vegetables and fruits.

• Whenever possible, eat food that is in season and locally grown.

- Eat fewer products made with flour (bread, crackers, chips, pastries), and more whole grains, beans, sweet potatoes, and vegetables.
- If you eat chocolate or drink coffee, get fair-trade and organic whenever possible. And get darker forms of chocolate, because the higher the percentage of cocoa, the greater the health benefits.

---

- Buy and eat organic food.
- If possible, grow organic food. Plant collards or kale in the late summer (or early summer where growing seasons are short) so that you have fresh greens all winter.
- Add your voice to the call for genetically engineered food to be labeled.

---

- Pack your own lunch. If you make someone else's lunch, write a love note and put it in with the food.
- Bake with your children. Involve them in making wholesome food. Bake delicious whole-grain muffins with blueberries, bananas, or other fruits they love.
- Serve a green leafy salad to your kids while they are waiting for dinner—you'll be surprised by what they will eat when they are "starving." In your salads, use romaine and other lettuces rather than iceberg (they have more vitamins and minerals). Also include chopped-up carrots and other vegetables.
- Buy or make healthful desserts and healthful comfort foods.
- Put wholesome snacks such as seeds, nuts, and vegetables with hummus in a conspicuous and accessible part of the fridge.

---

- Eat many colors. Foods' natural colors are not just treats for the eye but also signs of important nutrients such as antioxidants.
- When you crave something crunchy, try raw vegetables or nuts instead of salty chips.
- Every few days, grind organic flaxseeds in an electric coffee grinder reserved for this purpose. Keep the ground seeds in the refrigerator

and sprinkle them daily on your meals. Try them on cereal and salads and in sandwiches and stews.
- Eat plenty of fresh vegetables every day. Make a big pot of vegetable soup, keep it in the fridge in a large container, and heat up small batches throughout the week.
- Eat whole grains, not refined grains. Eat baked potatoes with the skins, not French fries. Eat your own homemade vegetable soups, not the highly salted ones generally available in grocery stores. Look for brands that say "organic" and "low sodium."
- Between meals, drink lots of pure water. Avoid soft drinks and diet sodas. Herbal teas can be comforting as well as healthful, particularly on cold days.

---

- Use monounsaturated oils such as olive oil and canola oil as your primary cooking oils. Avoid heating oils to the smoking point. For the fat in your diet, eat walnuts, almonds, hazelnuts, sunflower seeds, avocados, and other nuts and seeds.
- Avoid saturated fat by staying away from dairy products and fatty meats.
- Minimize consumption of oils that are high in omega-6 fatty acids, including corn, safflower, sunflower, soybean, and cottonseed oils.
- Shun trans-fatty acids. Stay away from margarine, vegetable shortening, commercial pastries, deep-fried food, and most prepared snacks and convenience foods.

---

- Instead of eating out, invite friends over for dinner. And invite yourself over to a friend's house for dinner, offering to bring a delicious and wholesome meal.
- Patronize only restaurants that serve healthful food or at least can accommodate your preferences.
- Instead of soft drinks, buy your kids fruit smoothies from Jamba Juice or similar stores.
- When you are interacting with people who don't eat the same way as you do, never be ashamed of the steps you are taking toward greater health. Let your enthusiasm and love of life be contagious.

# PART

# 3

# THE BODY-MIND
# CONNECTION

# 9

## Stepping into Life

*If you can't fly, then run. If you can't run, then walk. If you can't walk, then crawl. But whatever you do, keep moving.*
                                                                —Dr. Martin Luther King, Jr.

What if there was a pill that would keep you fit and lean as you aged, while protecting your heart and bones? What if it was as good for your brain as for your body, if it made you stronger, more confident, less susceptible to depression? What if it improved your sleep, mood, and memory and reduced your risk of cancer, all while adding life to your years and years to your life?

A great number of studies have found that exercise can provide all these benefits and more, even for people who begin late in life.[1] We are learning that much of the physical decline that older people suffer stems not from age but from simple disuse. When we sit all day, year after year, our bones, muscles, and organ systems atrophy, and our self-confidence wanes. But the ability of exercise to revitalize and invigorate our lives is now a proven fact.

Certainly part of the secret to the exceptionally healthy aging found in Abkhasia, Vilcabamba, Hunza, and Okinawa is the extraordinary amount of regular exercise built into the routines of daily life. In each of these cultures, a high level of physical fitness is both required by and produced by the way in which people live and work.

No one is sedentary. Everyone, at every age, is continually engaged in physical activity. The elderly still chop wood and haul water, and even the oldest of the old still work in the orchards and gardens.

The vast amount of regular physical exercise incorporated into their daily lives is one of the reasons that elders in these cultures typically experience levels of physical fitness that are superior to those typically found in much younger people in the West. When it comes to strength, coordination, flexibility, reaction time, stamina, and other measures of fitness, ninety-year-olds in these societies very often surpass sixty-year-olds in the modern industrialized world.

## FIT FOR THE AGES

Not very long ago, many experts thought vigorous exercise might be okay for younger people, but it was dangerous for people over fifty. Such was the prevailing belief in the 1960s, when the epidemiologist and physician Ralph Paffenbarger embarked on the landmark College Alumni Health Study, investigating the exercise habits of more than fifty thousand University of Pennsylvania and Harvard College alumni. Dr. Paffenbarger and his associates tracked their subjects' health and activity levels for four decades and found that participants' death rates fell in direct proportion to the number of calories they burned each week. Almost invariably, the more active they were, the longer they lived.

The College Study, representing more than two million person-years of observation, is one of the largest data sets ever compiled on the subject of activity, health, and longevity. In 1996, Dr. Paffenbarger summarized the lessons learned from the College Study about the benefits of an active and fit way of life:

> The data clearly show that if you become and remain physically active, you will live longer. And the study has also provided heartening news. . . . It's never too late to change from a sedentary to an active lifestyle, nor to benefit from that change. Findings from the College Study show quite clearly that it's possible for even the most determined couch spud to become and remain active and vital well into old age, largely free of all those so-called diseases of

civilization that leave too many of us worn out by life in our later years. . . . If you become and remain active, you will not only live longer, you'll live better, look better, and feel better about yourself. You will have more vitality, you'll think more clearly, and you'll sleep better. You'll function better, and be more productive, creative and joyful.[2]

Dr. Paffenbarger was so convinced by the initial data that in 1967, at the age of forty-five, he took up jogging. Now in his eighties, with more than 150 marathons and ultramarathons to his credit, he still jogs regularly, and still teaches at both the Harvard School of Public Health and Stanford University Medical School.

Dr. Paffenbarger is far from the only physician whose study of the effects of exercise on aging has changed his life. Walter M. Bortz, M.D., is one of America's most respected authorities on aging. The former president of the American Geriatrics Society, he is a professor at Stanford University Medical School and cochaired the American Medical Association Task Force on Aging.

Dr. Bortz coined the term "disuse syndrome" to describe how a lack of physical activity can destroy health and lead to rapid premature aging. It is a well-known principle in physiology that any part of the body that falls into disuse will begin to atrophy. Bortz discovered that this effect is actually true for the body as a whole. When people become sedentary, they essentially invite their entire physiology to atrophy. As a result, a constellation of problems appears: the heart, arteries, and other parts of the cardiovascular system become more vulnerable; the muscles and skeleton become more fragile; obesity becomes a high risk; depression sets in; and systemic signs of premature aging develop.[3]

Currently in his mid-seventies, Dr. Bortz still regularly runs marathons, as does his wife. "For me," he says, "exercise is the sacrament of the commitment to living life fully."[4]

## A BRIGHTER TOMORROW

It is now widely recognized that there are benefits to all types of exercise. Aerobic exercise (such as jogging) is particularly good for preserving the heart, lungs, and brain. Stretching (such as yoga) enhances circulation, increases range of motion, and provides greater body awareness. And weight lifting improves bone density while increasing muscle strength, balance, and overall fitness, something that can be even more important for the elderly than for high school jocks. When Dr. Maria Fiatarone of Tufts University got chronically ill nursing-home residents to lift weights three times a week for two months, the results were dramatic. The participants' average walking speed nearly tripled, and their balance improved by half. Many no longer needed their canes. Their self-confidence soared.[5]

Other Tufts University researchers have shown that simple strength training exercises can help keep women from needing canes in the first place. Twenty volunteers, all past menopause and none taking estrogen, were randomly divided into two groups. Half continued life as usual, while the other half lifted weights twice a week. After a year, it was found that the women who had not done any strength training had (predictably) lost bone density, while the bone density of the weight lifters had actually increased. The women who had adopted the exercise regimen also lost fat, and many ended up measurably stronger than their daughters who were twenty or thirty years younger. Dorothy Barron, a participant who was sixty-four at the outset of the study, said the exercises gave her more energy and confidence than she had had since her youth.[6]

Can exercise prevent diabetes? A landmark study published in *The New England Journal of Medicine* in 2002 sought to find out.[7] It is widely known that an epidemic of diabetes is wreaking havoc on the health of the 18 million Americans who have the disease. But it's less well known that another 41 million Americans are living with prediabetes, a condition defined by elevated blood sugar levels that typically precedes the full-blown disease. The study, known as the Diabetes Prevention Program, took 3,234 people with prediabetes and divided them into three groups. One group took the diabetes drug metformin, another group took a placebo, and those in the third group were asked to eat less fat and reduce calories while following a regular program of moderate exercise.

The results were spectacular—so spectacular, in fact, that the researchers stopped the trial early in order that everyone in the study could take up the lifestyle program. Compared to that in the placebo group, the incidence of diabetes in the diet-and-exercise group was a whopping 58 percent lower. (Those taking the drug also reduced their risk of diabetes, but only by about half as much as did those making the lifestyle changes.) Those over the age of sixty in the diet-and-exercise group experienced the greatest improvement, lowering their risk of diabetes by a staggering 71 percent. Stunningly, nearly one-third of the people in the diet-and-exercise group actually reversed their prediabetes, seeing their blood glucose levels come down into the normal range.

How much exercise did it take to obtain these remarkable results? Participants in the diet-and-exercise group started with just ten minutes of brisk walking, five days a week, gradually moving up to thirty minutes a day. While even modest levels of exercise brought huge payoffs, researchers believe that if people were able to exercise for an hour a day, the results would be even better.

And exercise promotes better sleep, too. In a study published in *The Journal of the American Medical Association* in 1997, epidemiologist Abby C. King and her colleagues at the Stanford University School of Medicine found that people who exercised regularly slept almost an hour longer each night and fell asleep in half the time it took others.[8]

Given what we now know to be the great value of regular exercise, it's sad that many people in the industrialized world say they can't find time for it. One contemporary comedian quipped that if it weren't for the fact that the TV set and the refrigerator are so far apart, some of us wouldn't get any exercise at all.

Is it possible to exercise too much? Yes, there are some people who exercise so obsessively that they do not listen to their bodies' needs for rest and end up repeatedly injuring themselves. They become so addicted to exercise that it comes to take the place of almost everything else in their lives, including relationships with other people. Perhaps they get hooked on their own endorphins, opioid peptides that are produced in the body during long, continuous and strenuous exercise. (The word "endorphin" is an abbreviation of "endogenous morphine," which literally means "morphine produced in the body.")

In his book *Exercise Fix,* author Richard Benyo discusses exercise addiction at length. Benyo apparently knows what he's talking about. He was the second man to run across Death Valley (the lowest place in North America and one of the hottest places in the world), climb Mount Whitney (the tallest mountain in the United States outside of Alaska), and then run back.

Of course, the number of people who suffer with this problem is negligible compared to the number whose health is suffering greatly, and who will suffer all the more in the future, as a result of being too sedentary.

I have a friend who leads a very busy life and rarely exercises. You probably know people like her. She repeatedly tells me "I just don't have time for it." I notice, though, that she manages to make time to go to frequent appointments with doctors, and to pick up her prescriptions at the drugstore. She is not well, and I am afraid that if she keeps not finding time for exercise, she may all too soon find herself in a deepening health crisis that leaves her unable to do many of the things that she loves to do.

A kind of physical passivity can take people over in our society. The less you move, the harder it becomes to do so. But as Edward Stanley put it way back in 1873, "Those who think they have no time for bodily exercise will sooner or later have to find time for illness."

## A KARATE MASTER AT 96

Okinawa is the birthplace of karate. It is also the home of Seikichi Uehara, who at the age of ninety-six was still teaching a rare karate-like martial art (mutubu-udundi). And he wasn't only teaching; he was still extraordinarily proficient, as he demonstrated on January 1, 2000.

On the first day of the new millennium, Seikichi Uehara, only four years shy of 100, was featured in a New Year's Day boxing match that was televised throughout Japan. His opponent was Katsuo Tokashiki, a thirty-nine-year-old former World Boxing Association flyweight champion, also from Okinawa.[9] Quite a spectacle unfolded.

The bout began with the young boxer, nearly sixty years the junior of Seikichi Uehara, punching powerfully and repeatedly at the elder martial artist. But his blows never landed. The old master, displaying amazing flexibility and agility for a man his age, kept evading every punch the younger man threw at him. Deftly twisting and turning, he managed to avoid the lightning-fast blows of the powerful former world champion boxer. This continued for more than twenty minutes, during which time the older man never sought to strike a single blow. The young boxer, Tokashiki, was becoming increasingly exasperated and fatigued.

Eventually, a moment arrived when Tokashiki dropped his guard. At that instant, the Okinawan elder martial artist deftly landed one quick blow, knocking the boxer off his feet, and the match was over. It was his first and only punch of the match.

As the young boxer left the ring in a daze, he kept shaking his head in disbelief, muttering, "I can't believe it! The old man beat me! I couldn't hit him!"

Tokashiki was stunned, but not injured. It was clearly the intent of the elder martial artist to defeat but not to hurt him. The philosophy of the martial art of mutubu-udundi teaches avoiding confrontation, and calls for striking only after all other options are exhausted.

When Seikichi Uehara later spoke of the match to researchers conducting the Okinawa Centenarian Study, he laughed and said, "It was nothing. He was just too young and had not yet matured enough to defeat me."

The performance of this ninety-six-year-old man presents quite a contrast to the prevailing experience of aging in the West, where most people think it inevitable that as they age, their muscles will weaken, their reflexes slow, their eyesight deteriorate, and their physical coordination plummet. Seikichi Uehara is no doubt extraordinary even by Okinawan standards, but his example speaks vividly of the human potential for healthy aging.

## MEANWHILE, IN CANADA . . .

Though we don't see a lot of it in our sedentary and super-sized culture, it's entirely possible for people in the modern West to retain high levels of physical fitness if they eat well and stay active. If you're looking for a good example, you might consider Tom Spear of Calgary, Alberta, Canada. He provides another illustration that growing older doesn't have to mean falling apart.

Tom is one of the subjects who have been thoroughly studied (and whose ages have been unassailably confirmed) by the New England Centenarian Study. He celebrated his 103rd birthday by making ten jars of crab-apple jelly, then going dancing. He was still cooking and cleaning for himself and tending his huge vegetable garden, and was in his eighty-seventh accident-free year as a cab driver.[10] Although he misses his wife of seventy years, he still has much to live for. "I take great pleasure in accomplishing things," he says.

At the age of 103, Tom Spear plays eighteen holes of golf three times a week, and consistently shoots fifteen strokes under his age. The teaching professional at the golf club where Tom plays confirms that Tom can still hit a three-wood 180 yards. Featuring an accurate short game, he recently shot an 84 to win a fifty-five-and-over tournament in Calgary. Some of the "elders" he defeated in the competition were nearly fifty years younger than he was.[11]

## THE REAL JACK LALANNE

When it comes to exercise and health, the name "Jack LaLanne" has long been virtually synonymous with fitness. For many decades, Jack has inspired millions to live a healthful life.

But Jack LaLanne didn't start out as a model of health. When he was a teenager, he dropped out of school for a year because he was so ill. Shy and withdrawn, he avoided being with people. He had pimples and boils, was thin, weak, and sickly, and wore a back brace. "I also had blinding headaches every day," Jack recalls. "I wanted to escape my body because I could hardly stand the pain. My life appeared hopeless."[12]

Then he met the pioneer nutritionist Paul Bragg, who preached a new way of living, and to his credit, Jack listened.

Bragg asked Jack, "What do you eat for breakfast, lunch, and dinner?"

"Cakes, pies, and ice cream," Jack answered truthfully.

"Jack," Bragg replied, "you're a walking garbage can."

He pointed young Jack in a healthier direction. That night Jack got down on his knees by the side of his bed and prayed. He didn't say, "God, make me the strongest man in the world." Instead, he asked for a new beginning. "God, please give me the willpower to refrain from eating unhealthy foods when the urge comes over me. And please give me the strength to exercise even when I don't feel like it."[13]

Jack set out to see what he could accomplish with a good diet and exercise. He found a set of weights and began to use them. He ate only the most healthful of foods. He developed exercise equipment that evolved into what has become standard in many health spas today. In 1936, he opened the first modern health club, paying $45 a month for rent in downtown Oakland.

Jack LaLanne touted the value of exercise and nutrition long before it became fashionable. Many people thought he was a charlatan and a nut. When he encouraged the elderly to lift weights, doctors said this was terrible advice. They said it was a good way for the elderly to break bones. But now, of course, we know that weight-bearing exercise is precisely what is needed to build bone strength and *prevent* elderly bones from breaking. He was among the first to advocate weight training for women. Doctors said women who tried it would not be able to bear children. Now we know that regular exercise is one of the best preparations for childbirth. Over the years, he's been vindicated a thousandfold. His television programs have brought his ideas to hundreds of millions of people and helped change the way we all view health and fitness.

It has been said that without eccentrics, cranks, and heretics the world would not progress. I don't think Jack LaLanne is a crank, but he is most certainly an eccentric. On his sixtieth birthday, he swam from the notorious Alcatraz island prison to San Francisco while handcuffed, towing a thousand-pound boat. "Why did you do that?" people asked. Jack's response: "To give the prisoners hope." (The prison has since closed, and today Alcatraz Island is a U.S. National Park Service attraction.)

On his sixty-fifth birthday, Jack LaLanne towed sixty-five hundred pounds of wood pulp across a lake in Japan. On his seventieth birthday, he celebrated by towing seventy rowboats with seventy people on board for a mile and a half across Long Beach Harbor, all while handcuffed and with his feet shackled.

He said his purpose in these phenomenal performances was to demonstrate that a healthful lifestyle can work wonders.

Having pioneered health and fitness gyms in the United States, Jack is gratified that physical fitness and nutrition have become a huge growth industry worldwide, because he believes that the emphasis on exercise and a healthful, natural diet creates stronger, smarter, and better people. "With healthier citizens," he says, "we unburden society from sickness, and reduce the medical bills that are draining people's savings and causing so much grief."[14]

Having enjoyed his ninetieth birthday in 2004, Jack is living testimony to the value of regular exercise and a healthful lifestyle. He used to be a vegan (no meat, dairy, or eggs), but though he still eats no dairy products—"anything that comes from a cow, I don't eat"—he now occasionally eats egg whites and wild fish. Mostly, he eats organic raw fruits and vegetables. And he takes lots of vitamins.[15]

His vibrant message is that it's never too late to get in shape. "Those who begin to exercise regularly, and replace white flour, sugar, and devitalized foods with live, organic, natural foods, begin to feel better immediately," he says. He emphasizes that it takes both nutrition and exercise. "There are so many health nuts out there who eat nothing but natural foods but they don't exercise and they look terrible. Then there are other people who exercise like a son-of-a-gun but eat a lot of junk. . . . Exercise is king. Nutrition is queen. Put them together and you've got a kingdom!"[16]

Now in his nineties, Jack LaLanne is still a model of fitness and vitality. Full of life and spirit, Jack's one-minute "Jack LaLanne Tip of the Day" pieces are now shown on seventy television stations. As energetic and flamboyant as ever, he and his wife, Elaine, speak all over the world, inspiring people to help themselves to a better life, physically, mentally, and morally. Jack and Elaine have been married for fifty-three years.

Jack was recently asked if he thought he'd live to be 100. His answer was to the point. "I don't care how old I live! I just want to be *living* while I am living! I have friends who are in their eighties, and now they're in wheelchairs or they're getting Alzheimer's. Who wants that? I want to be able to do things. I want to look good. I don't want to be a drudge on my wife and kids. And I want to get my message out to people." He smiled. "I tell people, I can't afford to die. It would wreck my image."[17]

He was once asked about George Burns, the famous comedian who made it to 100 though he smoked cigars, drank alcohol, and was not health oriented. Jack, it turns out, knew George Burns well, and he answered, "George Burns was more athletic than you think he was. And he was a very social man. He loved people, he enjoyed life. He worked at living. Old George was a social lion, he got around and did things. That's the key right there. It starts with your brain."[18]

Jack LaLanne is a man of great accomplishments. But perhaps his greatest achievement is that this once painfully shy and sick young man has learned to love people and to love being alive.

# 10

## Born to Move

*The aging process has you firmly in its grasp if you never get the urge to throw a snowball.*

—Doug Larson

When George Burns was in his nineties, he received a letter saying: "My husband and I are senior citizens and we still care about each other. Is it okay to make love in the 90s?"

George replied: "I think it's best around 70 or 75. If it gets any hotter than that, I turn on the air conditioner."

Like Jack LaLanne, George Burns understood that the greatest misconception people have about the aging process is that it's synonymous with decline and illness.

Like a fish unaware of water, we move about in a world of invisible assumptions. We usually don't realize how pervasive are such negative beliefs about aging. We take them for granted. And we unconsciously pass them on to our children.

Witness, for example, "Secrets of Aging," which opened at the Museum of Science in Boston in 2000. Billed as the first comprehensive exhibit on the topic of aging, the exhibit drew more than a half-million visitors in its six months in Boston, then toured nationally to other museums throughout the United States. The most popular component of the exhibit attracted long lines of children. It was called "Face Aging."[1]

After waiting in line, each youngster sat down inside a booth and had his or her face photographed by an automatic camera. After another wait, the child's digitized portrait appeared on a TV monitor. Then, by tapping a simple keyboard, each youngster could rapidly call up simulations of what he or she would "look like" at various ages. By tapping quickly, the series of stills could be made to run almost like a movie. The series of "photos" went up to the age of sixty-nine.

Everything about the exhibit implied scientific truth. It was held in the Museum of Science, and it involved an impressive array of complex and nonhuman technologies: the photo taken by a robot eye with no human involvement, the computer-driven graphics, the "interactive" button that produced an aging effect forward and then reversed it if you went backward.

What did the children see? As the "years" went by, the computer added grotesque pouches, reddish skin, and blotches to their familiar features. Their faces sagged and distorted, becoming increasingly repulsive.

When the children emerged from the booth, they were shaken. One eight-year-old girl within the hearing of a *Boston Globe* reporter moaned, "I don't want to get old." When author Margaret Gullette interviewed children as they exited, she asked, "What did you learn?" The answer was always the same: "I don't want to get old."[2]

Whatever the people who designed the booth intended, the message that came across to the children was that regardless of the choices they might make in their lives, regardless of how they eat or whether they exercise, and regardless of the kind of people they become, they will inevitably become ugly as they age. The message they received was that with each passing year, their appearance would become, predictably and inescapably, more and more repulsive. The title of the exhibit spoke with finality, leaving no room for the impact of the way the children would live their lives. "This is the way all faces age," it told them.

In real life, of course, as people age, their faces change in concert with the way they live, the way they think, and the way they feel. As we age, our faces and bodies become historical repositories of our experience. I've known elders whose faces are scowls, bitter and mean, and I've known elders whose faces glow with wisdom, joy, and deep human beauty. Over the course of their lives, their faces have become the outer expressions of the attitudes toward life they have held and from which they have lived.

## ANOTHER APPROACH

In England, similar computer wizardry is now being used for a very different purpose. In dramatic contrast to the "Face Aging" booth, the point is to encourage children and families to adopt more healthful lifestyles. Overweight children and their parents are being shown what the youngsters will look like in middle age *if* they continue to eat junk food and not exercise. Child health experts are overseeing the experiment for a BBC3 reality TV show titled "Honey, We're Killing the Kids!"

Julie Buc is a mother whose family took part in the show. Her children, Jason, aged ten, and Joanna, aged eight, loved eating fried food and candy, and drank up to two liters of soda pop a day. They typically ate their food while watching TV, and they were seriously overweight.

A team of experts assembled by the TV program used high-tech computer graphics to show how the children would look as adults *if* they continued in their current ways. Julie said she was shocked by the images she saw. "All those years that we've been giving the children what they want has got to change," she said.

Motivated by what they saw, and assisted by a team of nutritionists provided by the TV program, the family adopted a much more healthful diet and began to exercise far more. Gone were the soft drinks, sweets, and fried foods; in their place salads, fruits, and vegetables were introduced. The family began eating their meals together, without watching TV.

How did the kids like the changes? Ten-year-old Jason said, "It's been really good eating at the table, and I think it's good for the family to tell each other what they've been doing during the day."

At the end of the project, the family father, Jimmy Buc, said, "The most important things to me are my wife and my children, and I want my children to be successful. I hope they will be now, because we have changed, and there's no way we will be going back."

## BIOMARKERS OF AGING

Shows like "Honey, We're Killing the Kids!" are needed, because all too often in modern society people believe there is nothing they can do to prevent themselves from deteriorating as they age. Burdened by such beliefs, they never find out who they could have been. They expect their passion to wane, their waistlines to enlarge, and their joy in life to diminish. Then they find themselves ensconced in lifestyles that end up producing the very outcomes they believed, falsely, to be inevitable.

As a result, as people in modern industrialized societies grow older they typically experience a predictable set of changes. They lose muscle mass and become weaker, their basal metabolic rate slows down, they lose aerobic capacity, their blood pressure rises, they lose some of their blood-sugar tolerance, their cholesterol levels worsen, their bone density decreases, and their ability to stabilize their internal body temperature is impaired. So common are these patterns of impairment that scientists now use them as measures of biological aging, called *biomarkers*.

But studies at the Human Nutrition Research Center on Aging at Tufts University have shown that the decline of these biomarkers is far from inevitable. In fact, much of it can be reversed.[3]

Take muscle strength, for example. Many people consider a decline in muscle strength to be an unavoidable part of aging. The average American begins to lose 6.6 pounds of muscle with each decade after young adulthood, and the rate of muscle loss accelerates as they get older, particularly after age forty-five. But a great deal of research has found that with proper exercise, muscle strength and size can be not only maintained but increased at almost every age.

In one study at the Human Nutrition Research Center on Aging, twelve men between the ages of sixty and seventy-two were put on regular supervised weight-training sessions three times a week for three months. They were asked to train at 80 percent of their "one repetition maximum," the heaviest weight they could lift at one try. At the end of the experiment, the strength of the men's quadriceps had more than doubled, and the strength of their hamstrings had tripled. By the end of the program, many of these older men could lift heavier boxes than could the twenty-five-year-olds working in the laboratory.[4]

What about the really old? Could they also benefit from such a program? In another study, gerontologists at Tufts University put residents of a chronic-care hospital, almost all of whom were over the age of ninety, on a weight-training program. Did this sudden introduction to exercise exhaust or kill these frail and fragile people? Hardly. Eight weeks later, wasted muscles had grown stronger by 300 percent, and both balance and coordination were much improved. Subjects who had needed assistance to walk could now get up by themselves and go to the bathroom in the middle of the night.[5]

These and many other studies are clearly showing that the prevailing belief that we should "take it easy" as we age needs to be reconsidered.

Two of the world's foremost experts on exercise, diet, and healthy aging are Irwin H. Rosenberg, M.D., and William Evans, Ph.D. Dr. Rosenberg was director of the Human Nutrition Research Center on Aging from 1986 to 2001 and is the former chairman of the Food and Nutrition Board of the National Academy of Sciences and the former president of the American Society of Clinical Nutrition. Dr. Evans served as the chief of the Human Physiology Laboratory at the Human Nutrition Research Center on Aging, is a fellow of the American College of Sports Medicine, is the author of more than 160 publications in scientific journals, and has been exercise advisor to many professional sports teams, including the New England Patriots and the Boston Bruins. In 1991, Drs. Rosenberg and Evans coauthored the book *Biomarkers: The Ten Determinants of Aging You Can Control.*

These two authorities believe that to a far greater extent than most people realize, muscle is responsible for the vitality of your body. A high muscle-to-fat ratio, they point out, causes your metabolic rate—the rate at which you burn calories—to increase. This means you can more easily burn body fat and alter your body composition even further in favor of beneficial muscle tissue. When your metabolic rate slows down, on the other hand, it becomes much more difficult to lose weight and far easier to pack on the fat. Building muscle automatically reverses this tendency, making it easier to stay lean.

The reason is that muscle burns more calories than fat, even at rest. A pound of muscle burns roughly 15 more calories a day than a pound of fat. If you lose ten pounds of fat and gain ten pounds of muscle, you would thereafter burn 150 more calories a day without increasing your exercise level. Over the course of a year, this would translate into a difference of twelve pounds of body weight.

In actuality, the difference is even greater, because when people have more muscle and less fat, they want to exercise more and find it easier to do.

But that's only the beginning. Studies have shown that exercise regimens that build muscles produce a cascade of positive health effects. Rebuilding and maintaining muscle strength helps you to preserve your aerobic capacity, to keep your blood pressure low, to retain a healthy blood-sugar tolerance, to maintain healthy cholesterol, to sustain the mineral density of your bones, and to stabilize your body's ability to regulate its internal temperature.

Aerobic capacity (also called "maximal oxygen intake" or "work capacity") is a fundamental measure of the health of your cardiopulmonary system—your heart, lungs, and circulatory mechanisms. Simply put, your aerobic capacity is your body's ability to process oxygen. It includes your ability to breathe amounts of air into your lungs for aeration of your blood, and your ability to transport oxygen effectively to all parts of your body through your bloodstream. Elders in Abkhasia, Vilcabamba, Hunza, and Okinawa retain most of their aerobic capacity, even into their nineties. But by age sixty-five, the average American has lost 30 to 40 percent of his or her aerobic capacity. Increasing your muscle-to-fat ratio increases your aerobic capacity—and the health of your entire cardiovascular system.

One of the worst things about inactivity is that it reduces your cells' oxidative capacity (the ability to burn oxygen). This is why many older people who have lived typical Western lifestyles experience chronic fatigue. But it doesn't have to be that way. As your blood circulates, carrying its vital oxygen load, it flows from your large arteries into tiny capillaries. Aging and inactivity slow down capillary growth, with the result that the supply of oxygenated blood reaching your muscles and other tissues declines. But as Drs. Rosenberg and Evans repeatedly point out, whether you're young or old, regular exercise will improve your body's capillary density. The result is a happy one: muscles awash with a rich supply of blood.

There's yet another biomarker for physiological aging that can be reversed by regular exercise: glucose tolerance and insulin sensitivity. For most people in modern society, the body's ability to use glucose in the bloodstream declines with age. As people develop more body fat and less muscle, their muscle tissue becomes less and less sensitive to insulin. As a consequence, it takes more and more insulin to have the desired effect. Once again, though, increasing your muscle-to-fat ratio can reverse this deterioration, improve your blood-sugar tolerance, keep your insulin sensitivity high, and greatly reduce the chances you'll ever develop diabetes.

Drs. Rosenberg and Evans consider creeping blood-sugar intolerance to be one of the most devastating of all the so-called age related changes. To avoid this problem, they say, keep your muscle-to-fat ratio high. And to do that, they say you should "eat much less dietary fat and more fibrous carbohydrates, such as raw vegetables and whole grains . . . and do strength-building exercises."[6]

This advice could not be more congruent with the lifestyles of the world's healthiest and most long lived peoples. The Abkhasians, Vilcabambans, Hunzans, and elder Okinawans all eat little dietary fat, basing their diets on high-fiber carbs such as raw vegetables and whole grains. They don't belong to gyms or lift weights, but their daily lives are at every stage and age full of strength-building exercise. As a result, they remain lean, strong, and healthy as they age. Even the elderly have strong muscles, carry no extra body fat, and have high muscle-to-fat ratios.

Most people in the modern world, however, gain fat as they age even if they aren't gaining weight. Their musculature shrinks while fat tissue accumulates. This is particularly true in sedentary people.

In the United States and similar societies today, the average twenty-five-year-old woman has 25 percent body fat. If she's sedentary, by the time she's sixty-five her body-fat level will rise to 45 percent. And a similar pattern holds for men. The average American man at age twenty-five has about 18 percent body fat. If he's sedentary, by sixty-five he will have nearly 40 percent body fat.[7]

But such unhealthy developments do not have to occur. Studies at the Human Nutrition Research Center on Aging at Tufts University and elsewhere have repeatedly shown that by following a low-fat, plant-based diet made up of whole natural foods, and by getting regular and vigorous physical exercise, it is entirely possible to keep your body-fat level low, your muscle-to-fat ratio high, and your weight at a healthy level.

A cautionary note: A certain amount of body fat is necessary for energy storage and to cushion your vital organs. You may have seen competitive bodybuilders who have used synthetic steroids in their effort to build gigantic muscles and reduce their body fat to an absolute minimum. They may look impressive, but they are seriously jeopardizing their health.[8]

Other than such extreme cases, though, it remains a fact that *for most of us in the industrialized world, increasing the strength of our muscles and decreasing the amount of body fat we carry around is one of the most meaningful steps we can take on the path to healthy aging.*

Based on an extraordinary body of careful scientific research, Drs. Rosenberg and Evans have come to the same conclusion as Jack LaLanne. Exercise and a good diet are the keys to a healthy and rewarding old age, and it's never too late to start. They write:

> You do have a second chance to right the wrongs you've committed against your body. Your body can be rejuvenated. You can regain vigor, vitality, muscular strength, and aerobic endurance you thought were gone forever. . . . This is possible whether you're middle-aged or pushing 80. The "markers" of biological aging can be more than altered: in the case of specific physiological functions, they can be reversed.[9]

## EXERCISE AND BONE DENSITY

As people age in the modern world, we tend to lose calcium from our bones, making our skeletons weaker, less dense, and more brittle. Placing stress on a bone repeatedly, however, causes it to get stronger. This is why people who play tennis have stronger bones in the arm they use to swing their racket than in their other arm. Similarly, many studies have shown that weight-bearing exercise (such as walking, running, cycling, and weight lifting), if continued over time, can effectively reduce the rate of bone loss, even in the population most at risk—postmenopausal women.

One ingenious study at the Human Nutrition Research Center on Aging examined the bone health of older women before and after a one-year exercise training program.[10] The women were divided into four groups:

- Group 1 walked at a brisk pace for 45 minutes, four days a week. They also took a calcium supplement, raising their total daily calcium intake to 1,200 milligrams.
- Group 2 walked exactly as much as Group 1, but took a placebo, so their daily calcium intake was only 600 milligrams.
- Group 3 did no added exercise, but took the same calcium supplement as Group 1.
- Group 4 did no added exercise, and took the placebo.

As it turned out, the exercise program made all the difference, while the calcium supplement had virtually no effect. The active women, even those with lower calcium intake, not only stopped losing bone, but actually increased their bone mineral content. The women who did not undertake the exercise, even those who consumed the extra calcium, experienced demineralization.

And this study was not an anomaly. Similar studies at other institutions have come to exactly the same conclusion. When Dr. Everett Smith at the University of Wisconsin performed a similar study over a three-year period, his results were essentially identical. The only difference was that because his study went on for three years rather than one, the amount of bone gained by those who exercised and the amount of bone lost by those who did not was magnified.[11]

How about for younger women? We now know that much of a female's bone mass is built between the ages of twelve and twenty-two and then slowly lost in the remaining decades of her life. Is exercise the key to bone strength in young women, too?

Yes. As part of the longitudinal Penn State Young Women's Health Study, Professor Tom Lloyd and his colleagues conducted a ten-year study of 80 females who were twelve years old when the study began.[12] When these young women reached the age of twenty-two, it was determined that although their daily calcium intake had varied nearly fourfold, there was almost no relationship between calcium consumption and bone strength. Exercise, on the other hand, was found to be of major significance. When the study was published in *The Journal of Pediatrics* in 2004, Professor Lloyd said that "although calcium is often cited as the most important factor for healthy bones, our study suggests that exercise is really the predominant lifestyle determinant of bone strength in young women."[13]

## WHAT ABOUT HUMAN GROWTH HORMONE?

In 1990, a researcher at the Medical College of Wisconsin, Daniel Rudman, M.D., published an article in *The New England Journal of Medicine* that has given birth to an entire industry touting human growth hormone (HGH) as a virtual fountain of youth.[14] Rudman's study, though very small, was impressive. He gave twelve healthy older men (aged 61 to 81) injections of HGH three times a week for six months. Compared to a control group of healthy men of similar age, the men receiving the HGH experienced a substantial increase in lean body mass, a major decrease in adipose tissue mass, and a significant increase in bone density. In short, their muscles became substantially larger, they lost major body fat, and their bones became notably stronger. Based on this study, there are now thousands of Internet sites touting the benefits of HGH and promising that their products will increase muscle mass, decrease fat, and retard aging.

Unfortunately, the vast majority of the Internet sites selling HGH products are not what they claim to be. For one thing, they aren't selling actual HGH, but rather remedies that are said to promote the release of HGH from the pituitary gland (where it is naturally made in the human body). Most of these agents are in fact entirely ineffective at causing any significant HGH release. Some contain glutamine, which has been shown to temporarily increase plasma HGH levels.[15] Supplemental glutamine may be of benefit to people undertaking prolonged vigorous exercise, undergoing surgery, or being treated for burns or infectious disease (all of which deplete the body's glutamine levels). But the short-lived spike of HGH you can get from consuming oral glutamine in no way approximates the natural episodic waves of HGH released by your pituitary gland. (The pituitary secretes HGH every ninety minutes or so, with increases during sleep.)

What about injections of actual HGH, such as were used by Rudman in his study? There is no doubt that such injections do in fact increase muscle mass and decrease body fat, but at a considerable cost. For one thing, the injections require a prescription, are seldom covered by health insurance, and cost more than a thousand dollars a month. Further, they commonly have disagreeable side effects, including joint pain and carpal tunnel syndrome. Plus, there is a real possibility of increased cancer risk. And besides, injected HGH does not come close to replicating the natural cycle of secretion, and any benefits are lost as soon as you stop taking it. All in all, I would say it is definitely not worth it.

The wonderful reality is that regular exercise, particularly resistance training and other weight-bearing forms of exercise, produces the same beneficial changes in the body as human growth hormone—increased muscle mass, decreased body fat, and stronger bones. Although there may be something superficially appealing about swallowing a pill or receiving an injection, the advantages of actual exercise are many, while the claims made for most HGH products are hyperbole at best, and in many cases instances of outright fraud and deception.

## THE STORY OF JIM FIXX

Exercise is tremendously important, but sometimes people try to accomplish with exercise alone what can be achieved only with a combination of exercise and nutrition. Those who believe that exercise can compensate for a high-fat diet, excess sugar consumption, or other dietary transgressions could learn from what happened to a remarkable man named Jim Fixx.

Fixx was the author of one of the most influential and successful books on exercise ever written, *The Complete Book of Running*.[16] His book topped the bestseller lists for nearly two years in the late 1970s and is widely credited for helping start the fitness revolution in the Western world.

Jim Fixx had not always been a runner. Up until his mid-thirties, he smoked two packs of cigarettes a day, loved his burgers and shakes, and weighed 220 pounds. But at age thirty-five, he stopped smoking and began running. Within a short time he was running eighty miles a week and racing marathons, and had lost all his excess weight. His belief in the healing powers of running was so great, though, that he did not think he had to change his diet much. In his bestselling book, Fixx repeatedly quoted Thomas Bassler, M.D., who was then claiming that any nonsmoker fit enough to run a complete marathon in under four hours would never suffer a fatal heart attack.

Fixx knew that his father had died of a heart attack at age forty-three. But he believed that exercise (and the improved circulation it generates) would protect him. He thought that as long as he ran daily and didn't smoke, he would stay healthy and avoid his father's fate.

Jim didn't just ignore expert advice that he needed to eat more healthfully. On at least one occasion, he went out of his way to criticize those who offered such advice. At the time, probably the world's foremost advocate of a low-fat diet as a means to open and heal clogged arteries was Nathan Pritikin. In his book titled *Diet for Runners,* Pritikin described a conversation he had with Jim Fixx that took place in January 1984:

Jim Fixx phoned me and criticized the chapter "Run and Die on the American Diet" in my book *The Pritikin Promise*. In that chapter, I said that many runners on the average American diet have died and will continue to drop dead during or shortly after long-distance events or training sessions. Jim thought the chapter was hysterical in tone and would frighten a lot of runners. I told him that was my intention. I hoped it would frighten them into changing their diets. I explained that I think it is better to be hysterical before someone dies than after. Too many men, I told Jim, had already died because they believed that anyone who could run a marathon in under four hours and who was a nonsmoker had absolute immunity from having a heart attack.[17]

Sadly, only six months after this conversation, a passing motorcyclist discovered a man lying dead beside a road in northern Vermont. He was clad only in shorts and running shoes. The man was Jim Fixx.

Jim Fixx, the nation's leading spokesperson on the health benefits of running, had tragically died of a massive heart attack while running alone on that country road. Only fifty-two years old, he paid a terrible price for his belief that he didn't have to pay much attention to nutrition, for thinking that exercise alone would protect him. An autopsy revealed that three of his coronary arteries were more than 70 percent blocked, and one was 99 percent obstructed.

You may have heard the Jim Fixx story before. He became the butt of late-night jokes as overweight comedians made fun of the fact that the running guru had died of a heart attack. Sedentary people often want to believe that exercise isn't that important. They comfort themselves by telling and retelling the Jim Fixx story, as if the moral was that there's no harm in being a couch potato. But to do that is to miss the point entirely.

The real moral of Jim Fixx's tragic death is that while exercise is wonderful and necessary for a healthy life, it cannot make up for poor eating habits.

## PHENOMENAL HEALING POWER

In May, 2005, a major study published in the *Journal of the American Medical Association* found that regular exercise reduces the death rate among women who have already had breast cancer. These findings were particularly striking because the benefits were found to occur regardless of whether women were diagnosed early or after their cancer had spread. The study found that breast cancer patients who walk or do other forms of exercise for three to five hours a week are about 50 percent less likely to die from the disease than sedentary women.

None of this would surprise a friend of mine, Ruth Heidrich, who has led an extraordinary life and come to know a great deal about the healing power of both running and nutrition. She's the author of *Senior Fitness: The Diet and Exercise Program for Maximum Health and Longevity*. I find her story dramatic and moving; here it is in her own words:

Breast cancer. These two words, this cold clinical diagnosis, were to shatter my life, then transform it. The words stirred a cauldron of red-hot emotions: rage, fear, hatred. I remember the day and moment of the dreaded diagnosis as starkly as if it happened yesterday.

It's 1982 and I'm forty-seven years old. I hate it when I feel sorry for myself. I'm a strong, self-reliant female—the equivalent of a lieutenant colonel in the U.S. Air Force. I've raised two dynamic, smart and successful children, largely on my own after the breakup of two tough marriages. I've put myself through college up to and including my doctorate. *"I am woman, I am strong, hear me roar!"* In the vernacular, I am one tough broad. Then why am I so frightened? Why am I crying? My value system, my identity, my whole worldview is shaking under the assault of this terrible revelation. And I'm really, really scared. How much time do I have left?

Infiltrating ductal carcinoma—a moderately fast-metastasizing cancer. The doctors had been following it for the three years since I had first reported a suspicious lump in my right breast. Now it had grown to the size of a golf ball. I know because I saw it. I had insisted on watching the surgery when they removed the large, red, ugly mass of deadly tissue. But because the cancer had spread through the whole breast, the surgeons told me that they needed to perform a modified radical mastectomy. As soon as I recovered from *that* surgery, they would then have to remove the other breast due to its high risk of being cancerous as well. Worse yet, the cancer had spread to my bones and left lung.

Devastated, feeling betrayed by the medical system and by my body, I enrolled in a breast cancer research study conducted by author and physician John McDougall, that required me to follow a vegan diet. I would have tried anything to help save my life. I talked to my then-husband. He thought I was crazy to think that diet had anything to do with breast cancer, and he believed I had fallen into the hands of a quack.

Around the time of my diagnosis, I saw a sporting event on television called the "Ironman Triathlon." I was captivated as I watched these superb young athletes race through a 2.4-mile swim, followed immediately by a 112-mile bike ride, then a full 26.2-mile marathon. *"I want to do that,"* I thought. Then I remembered: *"Hold on, Lady, you're a cancer patient and you're forty-seven years old—way too old to do such an event."* This wasn't just negative self-talk; it was the voice of reason. After all, no woman that old had yet attempted the Ironman. But the idea just wouldn't go away. With my new diet, I could swear I was feeling stronger, lighter, more energetic, faster, and healthier.

Of course, the doctors thought I was absolutely insane. *"You should be resting,"* they said. *"All that stress on your body isn't good for it. Running marathons (much less endurance swims and 100-mile bike rides) will depress your immune system."* That's when I stopped relying solely on the doctors for advice.

Back in those days, before most people had even heard of triathlons, there was little guidance on how to train for such grueling endurance races. So I just got out there and swam until I couldn't lift my arms, biked until I couldn't pedal anymore, ran until I couldn't run another step and lifted as many pounds as I could without injuring myself. To simulate actual racing conditions, I entered every race I could find. If there were two on the same day, so much the better, because that would force me to race when tired, a condition I knew I'd face doing the Ironman. I entered "The Run to the Sun," a 37-mile run up to the top of Haleakala, a 10,000-foot-high mountain on the island of Maui, Hawaii. I remember reaching the twenty-six-mile point and looking back at the ocean far, far, below, not believing that these two legs had already carried me the equivalent of a full marathon, straight uphill. Then I turned back toward the mountaintop, still more than ten miles beyond. My internal response was *I don't have it in me; I just can't do it.* My next thought was, *Listen, Lady, if you think this is rough, just wait until you get in the Ironman!* That technique served me well in the coming months. And competing in and winning first-place trophies in my age-group events added to the post-race highs.

I found myself getting stronger and developing muscles I never knew I had. I was passing my cancer checkups as well: The hot spots in my bones—once a source of despair because they indicated cancer—were disappearing, and the tumor in my lung stayed the same size.

The only real reminder of the cancer were the two postsurgical, angry red gashes, which left a chest that resembled a prepubescent male's. Because of all my training, I was having to shower and change clothes several times a day, so the reminders of the cancer were constant. I wanted so much to have a normal body again. Enter the plastic surgeons, who gave me a fabulous choice; I could now pick my new size. *You want a "C"?* they said. *We can do that.* I told them I wouldn't be greedy—Just give me what I had before, a nice, average "B." They also gave me something else I never thought possible: breasts that will never sag. I believe you have to look at the positive side of life, and now, at seventy years old, I can really appreciate this benefit.

Today, there's no sign of cancer in my body. I've continued my vegan, low-fat diet now for more than twenty years, and I have never been healthier or more fit in my life. To date, I have raced the Ironman Triathlon six times, plus over a hundred shorter triathlons, a total of sixty-seven marathons, plus hundreds of shorter races. In 1998, at the age of sixty-three, I was named one of the Ten Fittest Women in America by *Living Fit* magazine (the other nine were all under thirty-five years of age). My bone density has increased through my fifties and sixties, which is supposed to be 'impossible' since most people are told they will lose bone density as part of the 'natural' aging process. My VO2max, which is the measure of my body's ability to process oxygen, is one of the highest ever recorded at the Tripler Army General Hospital in Honolulu, Hawaii, where I live. My blood pressure runs 90/60, which means that my arteries are very elastic and essentially wide open. My cholesterol is under 150; I have 15 percent body fat, and my hemoglobin—the test for iron in the blood—is at the top of the charts.

I do not share this information about my physical condition to boast (although I admit I'm proud of it), but to show what can be accomplished through dedication and discipline.

Perhaps I'm an anomaly by most medical standards. And maybe a vegan diet and endurance exercise won't be a magical answer for everyone, but I stand as an example of a lifestyle change that might be worth exploring.

When will this awesome journey end? Will I have to slow down gradually, let go, cut back to walking laps around a retirement community? I really can't say. But I know this: I had cancer and it had spread; I might have folded my cards back then, but I chose life, and I'm going to live as long as I can and run the good race. Maybe only a few will take the path I've chosen, but if sharing my story helps a few more to step forward and in their own way race for life, it will have been all the more worthwhile."[18]

## CHOOSING LIFE

It's hard not to be impressed by the marvelous health and longevity of people like martial arts expert Seikichi Uehara, golfer Tom Spear, fitness guru Jack LaLanne, and triathlete Ruth Heidrich. Their lives, like the lives of the elder Okinawans and all the rest of the world's exceptionally healthy elders, dramatically demonstrate two things that modern society needs desperately to remember: *Exercise is not something to avoid. And aging is not a disease.*

Unfortunately, many people in modern societies today succumb to the belief that aging means becoming the helpless victim of a slow, torturous, and inevitable deterioration. They live in fear, believing that with each passing year they will only feel worse and suffer more. They do not exercise. They eat unhealthful foods. They shut down emotionally. Eventually, their fear becomes self-fulfilling, and they create the very tragedy they believed would occur.

You probably know many people like that. But you don't have to be one of them. You can know the joy that arises when you commit to your own greatest health and healing.

The key is to do the best you can with what you've got. Maybe it starts with taking a walk every day, or jogging a half-mile, or taking a yoga class or a dance class. Maybe it starts with playing soccer or tennis, or learning how to lift weights correctly.

What's important is that you challenge whatever would keep you from entering your life with passion and vitality. What matters is that you never let anything keep you from walking the path of your highest good. What's pivotal is that you know the power of taking a stand for what gives you life.

11

## Keeping Your Marbles

*Death is not the greatest loss in life. The greatest loss is what dies inside us while we live.*

—Norman Cousins

A healthy and vibrant body will serve you well as you age. But there is, of course, more to living well than physical health. Few things are more important than the healthy functioning of your mind. Remaining alert and clear-thinking is of great consequence throughout your life, and particularly as you move into your wisdom years.

Sadly, half of the people over age eighty-five in the United States suffer from dementia. Indeed, mental deterioration is so common among the elderly in the industrialized world today that many of us assume it is normal and inevitable as people age. In the cultures that exemplify healthy aging, in contrast, dementia is quite rare even among the oldest of the old. The authors of the Okinawa Centenarian Study report that Okinawan elders of both genders "have remarkable mental clarity even over the age of one hundred."[1]

On the one hand, an ever-increasing number of older people in modern Western societies are suffering from Alzheimer's disease and other forms of dementia, deteriorating inexorably to the point that they no longer remember who they are or recognize loved ones. On the other hand, the elders in Okinawa, Abkhasia, Vilcabamba, and Hunza are happily going about their lives in their nineties and beyond, fully present both mentally and emotionally, playing a needed and important role in their families and societies.

The difference could hardly be more poignant.

## ALZHEIMER'S DISEASE

Alzheimer's disease, the most common form of dementia, is a degenerative disorder that progressively robs its victims of memory and judgment, eventually leaving them unable to carry out even the most basic functions on their own. Named after Alois Alzheimer, the German physician who first identified the disease in 1901, the disease initially wipes out short-term memory, then layer by layer destroys connections to the past. It generally takes eight to ten years to destroy its victims' brains. At current rates, fifteen million elderly Americans will be stricken by 2050, and tens of millions of adult children will be drained by ever-mounting medical bills and endless hours of care.

The financial costs of Alzheimer's disease are staggering. The disease already costs the U.S. Medicare system three times as much as any other disease, and the costs are increasing dramatically. Medicare spending on Alzheimer's was $32 billion in 2000 and is expected to reach $50 billion by 2010, with an additional $30 billion from the U.S. Medicaid program. "If left unchecked, it is no exaggeration to say that Alzheimer's disease will destroy the health care system and bankrupt Medicare and Medicaid," says Sheldon Goldberg, president of the Alzheimer's Association.[2]

The costs of caring for people with Alzheimer's threatens to wipe out government health programs, and yet it is not the government but individuals and families who incur the vast majority of the costs. Many Americans think that Medicare covers nursing home expenses, but in fact Medicare was never intended to pay for long-term care, and generally pays only for hospital and physician expenses. And Medicaid will cover nursing home costs only after the patient's assets have been reduced to $2,000 or less. Meanwhile, nursing home costs for an Alzheimer's patient run $4,000 to $5,000 per month, and patients may need such care for many years.

## A MIND IS A TERRIBLE THING TO LOSE

The writer and artist Bobbie Wilkinson tells of an experience she had while traveling:

> I watched as she led him by the hand to the bathroom at the airport terminal. Travelers surrounded them, rushing past, and although he seemed a little bewildered, he seemed secure as long as his hand was in hers.
>
> Returning to their seats at the gate, she combed his hair and zipped his jacket. He fidgeted and asked, "Where are we going, Mommy? What time is it? When will we get to ride our plane?"
>
> I marveled at the woman's patience and love. I watched her take him by the hand when they were finally allowed to board.
>
> Upon finding my seat, I discovered that the three of us would be together. I squeezed past the two of them to my window seat, then told him how handsome he looked in his new coat. He smiled. She helped take off his jacket and buckle his seat belt. He said that he had to go to the bathroom again, and she assured him that he could last until the end of the flight. I hoped she was right.
>
> As the jet engines started, he became frightened and searched for her hand. She explained what was going on and began talking to him about their trip. He was confused about the different relatives they would be seeing, but she patiently repeated herself until he seemed to understand.
>
> He asked many more questions about the time, what day it was, how much longer until they got there—and she lovingly held his hand and gave him her full attention.
>
> We introduced ourselves and shared the usual things all mothers like to share with one another. I learned she had four children and was on her way to visit one of them.
>
> The hour passed quickly, and soon we were preparing to land. He became frightened again, and she stroked his arm, reassuringly. He said, "I love you, Mom," and she smiled and hugged him. "I love you, too, Honey."
>
> They got off the plane before I did, the mother never realizing how deeply she had touched me. I said a quiet little prayer for this

remarkable woman and for myself—that I would have enough love and strength to meet whatever challenges came my way, as this extraordinary mother clearly had.

When I last saw them, she was still holding his hand and leading her husband of 44 years to the baggage claim area.[3]

I share this painful story not to be overly dramatic, but to illustrate something with which all too many of us are unfortunately familiar. There can be love and courage in the land of dementia, as Bobbie Wilkinson witnessed, but the sad reality is that Alzheimer's exhausts the patience and endurance of even the most committed caregivers.

## WHAT CAN BE DONE?

Unfortunately, Alzheimer's disease is very difficult to treat. There are drugs (Cognex, Aricept, Exelon, Reminyl) that in some cases allow the patient to function for an extra few months. But these drugs are only palliatives that do nothing to slow the progressive neurodegeneration that ultimately leads to dementia and death. In late 2003, the U.S. Food and Drug Administration approved a new drug, memantine (Namenda), for treating patients with moderate to severe Alzheimer's. By blocking the action of the chemical glutamate, this new drug may help treat symptoms in some patients, but it does not modify the underlying pathology of the disease.

*Our inability to cure or effectively treat Alzheimer's makes prevention all the more important, and the examples of the world's most healthy and long-lived societies all the more meaningful.*

Is there anything that you can do to ensure that your mind as well as your body will remain healthy and vital? Are there practical steps you can take to help assure you of the ability to think clearly throughout the length of your days?

Absolutely.

The good news is that a tremendous amount has been learned about preventing Alzheimer's and other forms of dementia. We now know a great deal about what you can do to maintain clear thinking well past the age of 100. And we have a good understanding of what it is about the lifestyles of the world's most long-lived peoples that has consistently produced such marvelous cognitive functioning even at very advanced ages.

## THE ROLE OF EXERCISE

For one thing, the regular physical exercise that is a central part of the lifestyles of these cultures is key. You may be surprised that physical exercise could play an essential role in preventing Alzheimer's disease. But many studies have found that it can do exactly that.

For example, the value of exercise in sustaining healthy cognitive function was demonstrated in a five-year study published in *Archives of Neurology* in March 2001. The study found that people with the highest activity levels were only half as likely as inactive people to develop Alzheimer's disease and were also substantially less likely to suffer any other form of dementia or mental impairment. Even those who engaged in light or moderate exercise had significant reductions in their risks for Alzheimer's and other forms of mental decline. The study concluded that the more people exercise, the healthier their brains remain as they grow older.[4]

Three years later, in September 2004, *The Journal of the American Medical Association* published a series of studies further confirming that regular exercise helps preserve clear thinking even at advanced ages. One study found that women aged seventy and older who had higher levels of physical activity scored better on cognitive performance tests and showed less cognitive decline than women who were less active. Even walking only two hours a week at an easy pace made a marked difference, though the most benefits were found in women who walked six hours a week.[5] Another study found that older men who walked two miles a day had only half the rate of dementia found among men who walked less than a quarter-mile a day.[6]

What are the mechanisms behind these benefits? In the last decade, neuroscientists have been discovering that exercise produces a multitude of positive changes in the brain. They are finding that physical activity enhances memory, improves learning, and boosts attention, as well as increasing abilities like multi-tasking and decision-making. A large number of studies have found that exercise makes the brain more adaptive, efficient, and capable of reorganizing neural pathways based on new experiences.[7]

Exercise, of course, increases the flow of oxygen to the brain. This in turn produces a larger number of capillaries in the brain, and possibly the production of new brain cells. It also boosts brain neurotransmitters (including dopamine, serotonin, and norepinephrine) that play crucial roles in cognition.

## PREVENTING ALZHEIMER'S BY EATING WELL

As well as exercise, there is diet. The Abkhasians, Vilcabambans, Hunzans, and elder Okinawans all eat whole-foods, plant-based diets high in antioxidants. This is now known to be one of the key reasons they have such extraordinarily low rates of Alzheimer's and other forms of dementia.

Antioxidants are substances that keep you young and healthy by increasing immune function, decreasing the risk of infection and cancer, and, most important, by protecting against free-radical damage. Free radicals are cellular desperadoes that play a pivotal role in the aging process, and their damage takes a toll on virtually every organ and system in the aging human body. This in turn sets the stage for all sorts of degenerative diseases, including Alzheimer's and other forms of dementia. Antioxidants neutralize free radicals and keep them in check.

Antioxidants are found in fresh vegetables, whole grains, fresh fruits, and legumes such as soy. Carotenoids, the substances that give fruits and vegetables their deep, rich colors, are antioxidants. Vitamin C and E are also antioxidants, as are the minerals magnesium and zinc. *If your diet is high in antioxidants, your risk of many age-associated diseases—including cancer, heart disease, macular degeneration, and cataracts—decreases.*

When it comes to preventing Alzheimer's disease and other forms of senility and cognitive decline, antioxidants are extraordinarily important. It is free-radical damage that underlies the development of cognitive dysfunction, dementia, and most of the other ravages of unhealthy aging as well. And antioxidants are your body's best defense against free-radical damage. Many scientists now believe that the reason people who eat plant-based diets have far less dementia is because plant foods contain far more antioxidants. Animal-based foods, on the other hand, typically tend to activate free-radical production and cell damage.

A large number of studies published in the world's most prestigious medical journals have demonstrated the benefit of diets high in antioxidants in preventing Alzheimer's and other forms of dementia and cognitive decline. What about supplements containing antioxidants? At present, the evidence is not as substantiated, but it is certainly encouraging. In January 2004, for example, a distinguished group of medical researchers from four U.S. universities published a study in the *Archives of Neurology*, finding that people taking both vitamin C and E supplements had a 78 percent lower rate of Alzheimer's.[8] Personally, I take supplementary antioxidants daily.[9]

## HEALTHY MIND, HEALTHY YOU

Throughout history, people have seen the elderly develop certain diseases and mistakenly believed those diseases were inevitable outcomes of aging. As recently as one hundred years ago, tuberculosis was the leading cause of death in the United States, and was thought to be a natural consequence of aging. Now we know, however, that tuberculosis is an infectious disease caused by a bacteria called *Mycobacterium tuberculosis,* and is spread through the air from one person to another.

Later, arteriosclerosis was considered a hallmark of aging. But then we learned that this condition is almost entirely avoidable with a healthy diet. Fifty years ago, most people believed that heart disease was simply part of nature's script for human beings. But now we know many of the lifestyle factors that produce this illness. Even more recently, the decline in kidney function that had been attributed to the natural aging process has been found instead to be due to pathology.

Alzheimer's is so common today in the industrialized world that many have come to view it as an inevitable adjunct of aging. Most people in nursing homes are there because of Alzheimer's. But as widespread as it is, Alzheimer's is a disease. It is not normal aging. It is not a natural condition. And it is not inevitable.

If you want to lower your risk for Alzheimer's markedly, here's the central thing you need to know: *Study after study is finding that a whole-foods plant-based diet built on fresh vegetables, whole grains, and legumes—such as the diet eaten by the Abkhasians, Hunzans, Vilcabambans, and elder Okinawans—is good for brain function and dramatically lowers the incidence of Alzheimer's and other forms of dementia.*

Such diets also keep people from being overweight, keep cholesterol levels and blood pressure low, and reduce arteriosclerosis—all factors that are extremely important to retaining healthy mental functioning. In 2004, Dr. Miia Kivipelto of the Karolinska Institute in Sweden told an international conference on Alzheimer's disease in Philadelphia of his 21-year study. The study found that people who were obese in middle age were twice as likely to develop dementia when they got old as those who were of normal weight. For those who also had high cholesterol and high blood pressure in middle age, the risk of dementia was six times higher.[10]

Many other studies also speak about the relationship between diet and the most serious forms of dementia, such as Alzheimer's. They are saying that if you want to get Alzheimer's disease, eat a diet high in meat, fat, saturated fat, cholesterol, sugar, and white flour. If you don't, avoid such foods, and instead eat a diet high in fresh vegetables, whole grains, fresh fruit, and legumes, and be sure to get enough DHA and other omega-3 fats. In essence, if you want to prevent Alzheimer's disease, eat as the Abkhasians, Vilcabambans, Hunzans, and elder Okinawans do.

## THIS IS YOUR BRAIN ON MEAT

Another key to staying mentally clear as you grow older is keeping your homocysteine levels low. Homocysteine is a toxic amino acid, a breakdown product of protein metabolism, that has been strongly linked to Alzheimer's and also to heart attacks, strokes, depression, and a type of blindness. Even small elevations in homocysteine can significantly increase the risk for these conditions. Notably, the elder

Okinawans have among the lowest homocysteine levels in the world.[11]

Everyone has homocysteine in their blood, just as everyone has cholesterol. It's a matter of how much. Problems occur when levels get too high. Blood levels of homocysteine are typically higher in people whose diets are high in meat and low in leafy vegetables, whole grains, legumes, and fruits—foods that provide folic acid and other B vitamins that help the body get rid of homocysteine.

How important is it to maintain low homocysteine levels if you want to prevent Alzheimer's disease? On October 18, 1998, David Smith, M.D., and his colleagues from Oxford University presented their findings to the American Medical Association's annual Science Reporters' Conference. Their study, published in *Archives of Neurology* the following month, found that the risk of getting Alzheimer's disease was a monumental 4.5 times greater when blood homocysteine levels were in the highest one-third.[12]

Folic acid and vitamin $B_{12}$ are key factors in preventing Alzheimer's, because blood levels of homocysteine can be reduced by increasing your intake of folic acid (also called folate) and vitamin $B_{12}$. One study found that the incidence of Alzheimer's was a staggering 3.3 times greater among people whose blood folic acid levels were in the lowest one-third range, and 4.3 times greater for those with the lowest levels of $B_{12}$.[13]

In 2001, the journal *Neurology* published the results of a three-year Swedish study of 370 healthy elderly adults. The study found that those with even slightly low levels of vitamin $B_{12}$ and folic acid had twice the risk of developing Alzheimer's disease compared to those with normal levels.[14]

What is the best was to achieve the ideal scenario of a high blood folic acid level and a low blood homocysteine level? A whole-foods, plant-based diet with plenty of green leafy vegetables and ample vitamin $B_{12}$. (For people who eat this way and yet still have high homocysteine, daily supplementation with 800 mcg folic acid, 500 mcg vitamin $B_{12}$, and 50 mg vitamin $B_6$ can be helpful. The methylcobalimin form of $B_{12}$ is far more effective than the cyanocobalimin form.)

It is particularly important for vegetarians and vegans to understand that adequate levels of vitamin $B_{12}$ are necessary for folic acid to effectively carry out its functions. Vegans who do not eats foods fortified with $B_{12}$ or take $B_{12}$ supplements to ensure they get adequate vitamin $B_{12}$ are at significant risk for elevated homocysteine levels.[15]

But this is no reason to eat meat. In fact, it is meat-eaters who are most commonly at risk for high homocysteine levels, because animal foods (and meat in particular) tend to contribute to the production of homocysteine. *One study found that subjects who ate meat as their main source of protein were nearly three times as likely to develop dementia as their vegetarian counterparts.* A survey of the medical literature on diet and Alzheimer's noted how frequently a meat-centered diet raises homocysteine levels. The report was aptly titled "Losing Your Mind for the Sake of a Burger."[16]

## EAT WELL, THINK CLEARLY

In the West today, we often take for granted that aging will bring restricted short-term memory and diminished mental faculties. A visit to most nursing homes demonstrates how commonly and how markedly people in our society experience cognitive decline as they age. As one comedian described it, "First you forget names, then you forget faces, then you forget to pull your zipper up, then you forget to pull your zipper down."

But there is good science to show that many of us can experience clear thinking well into our later years. The examples of the world's healthiest and longest lived cultures and the findings of medical science are in agreement. They are both saying that there are definite steps you can take to greatly reduce your risk of Alzheimer's and many other diseases. If you want to create an elderhood of health and clear thinking:

1. Eat a healthful plant-based diet with lots of fresh vegetables, whole grains, legumes, fruits, seeds, and nuts. This is a diet that provides plenty of antioxidants and fiber and produces clean arteries enabling a rich blood supply to the brain.
2. Avoid foods that are high in fat, saturated fat, and cholesterol.

3. Keep your homocysteine levels low by making sure you consume plenty of vitamin $B_{12}$, folic acid, and vitamin $B_6$, and by keeping your meat intake to a minimum.
4. Make sure you consume plenty of DHA, the long-chain omega-3 fatty acid.
5. Get lots of regular physical exercise.

The exciting news is that if you follow the example of the longest lived and healthiest people in the world, you nurture the possibility of a very different kind of future than is the norm in the industrialized world. You can take decisive steps towards a long, vibrant life, rich in physical strength and mental clarity. Even if you have eaten poorly and not exercised for most of your life, shifting now in a healthy direction greatly improves your prospects for the remainder of your life.

## GOOD SCIENCE ON HOW TO PREVENT ALZHEIMER'S

■ Multiple studies published in *Archives of Neurology*, the *American Journal of Epidemiology*, and other medical journals have found that people who eat diets high in fat, saturated fat, and cholesterol have at least double the risk of developing Alzheimer's disease.[17]

■ In 2006, a study published in *Annals of Internal Medicine* found that older adults who exercise three or more times a week have a 30 to 40 percent lower risk of developing dementia than their more sedentary counterparts.[18]

■ Studies published in the *Journal of Alzheimer's Disease* and *The Journal of the American Medical Association* compared Alzheimer's rates to dietary variables in eleven different countries and found the highest rates of the disease among people with a high fat intake and low intake of whole grains.[19]

■ A study of three thousand Chicago residents aged sixty-five and older published in the *Journal of Neurology, Neurosurgery, and Psychiatry* in 2004 found that those with the lowest intake of dietary niacin (vitamin $B_3$) were 70 percent more likely to develop Alzheimer's than those with a higher intake, and their rate of cognitive decline was twice as fast. (Good dietary sources of niacin include whole grain wheat products and green leafy vegetables).[20]

■ A large study published in *Archives of Neurology* in 2003 found that older people can reduce their risk of developing Alzheimer's disease by eating fish, consuming fish oil, or taking DHA supplements. Participants in the study who consumed fish once a week had a 60 percent lower risk of developing the disease than did those who rarely or never ate fish. Participants whose daily intake of DHA was above 100 mg/day had an incidence of Alzheimer's which was 70 percent lower than those with an intake of 30 mg/day or less.[21]

# 12

## Confident and Clear-Thinking

*No matter what our age or condition, there are still untapped possibilities within us, and new beauty waiting to be born.*

—Dale E. Turner

Anna Morgan died in 1997, at the age of 102, as one of the most thoroughly studied elders in the history of medical science. When she was 101, her cognitive abilities were studied intensively by scientists conducting the New England Centenarian Study.[1] The researchers asked Anna if she would be willing to donate her brain to science so that they could study it.

"But I'm still using it," she answered with a smile.

Anna Morgan spent her entire adult life helping people all over the world. In the 1920s, she distributed condoms to local farmwives (an illegal activity at the time). During the Great Depression of the 1930s, she collected food for families of the unemployed. In 1952, she was called before the Ohio State Committee on Un-American Activities, who charged her with contempt when she refused to answer their questions.

"They were right," Anna said, looking back at the age of 101. "I had a very healthy contempt for the Committee."

In 1959, the U.S. Supreme Court overturned her conviction, citing the First Amendment. It was a case with profound implications for civil rights.

During her nineties, she wrote more than twelve hundred pages of memoirs, and worked on the successful effort to have a postage stamp issued to honor the black singer, actor, and human rights activist Paul Robeson. On her one hundredth birthday, she testified before Congress. At the age of 101, Anna Morgan was still busy, volunteering for groups such as Mobilization for Survival.

But what most interested scientists was her performance on highly sophisticated brain-function tests. When researchers tested her ability at the age of 101 to sustain attention, they found she was easily able to repeat seven-digit strings of numbers, and to connect long number sequences. When they gave her five-digit strings of numbers and asked her to repeat them backward, she had no difficulty doing so. She could also, when asked to do so, spell words backward.

You may have noticed that short-term memory loss is common among the elderly in the modern world, as is a corresponding diminished ability to recall information that has been recently learned. Scientists have a way of testing for this. They give their subjects six simple words and ask them to repeat the words three times. Then they sit in silence for a minute, after which they again ask the subjects to repeat the words. Anna Morgan had no difficulty doing this.

Researchers next ask their subjects to count backward from twenty, and to recite the alphabet rapidly. And then, to see to what extent distraction has diminished their subjects' recall, and to see if they have a rapid rate of forgetting, researchers ask the subjects to repeat the list of six words once more. Anna Morgan did all this perfectly.

They tested her visual-spatial capacity (how the brain makes sense of what it sees) and found that she was able to draw even complicated figures very well. They tested her abstract reasoning and conceptualization skills, and got answers they would have expected from a mentally intact person forty years younger. Again and again, with each test performed, Anna Morgan refuted the theory that old people, simply by being old, will have significantly reduced cognitive abilities.

But the most impressive part of Anna Morgan's cognitive performance was still to come. The researchers write:

> In order to evaluate subjects' recall and new learning abilities, we tell them a rather whimsical story . . . and ask subjects to repeat it. Anna Morgan's retelling of the story was very complete, as a videotape we made of the session shows. . . .
>
> To this day, our fellow neuropsychologists gasp when they see this tape of Ms. Morgan repeating the details of a story she had heard only minutes before, with practically no hesitation and few errors. Even after having told the story hundreds of times, we ourselves have difficulty in recalling all its details. But Anna Morgan had mastered most of them after hearing it only once. It impressed us that, even at 100 years old, someone could perform better on some of the most demanding cognitive tests than the people administering them did! . . . Anna Morgan had no signs of dementia, and in our estimation was as engaged in and enthusiastic about life as a high school sophomore.[2]

Anna Morgan's life was filled with contribution, purpose, and meaning, which we now know to be another key factor in avoiding Alzheimer's. Many studies have found that people who remain connected to others and continue to be mentally stimulated as they age are less likely to fall prey to dementia.

The admonition "use it or lose it" is as true for mental faculties as we age as it is for muscle strength. An idle brain will deteriorate just as surely as an unused leg. A key to cognitive health is having goals and things to look forward to, and knowing that you are doing the work you were put on this earth to do.

The elders most likely to experience dementia are those who spend their days watching television or wandering aimlessly around the mall. On the other hand, those who are contributing to the lives of others, who are engaged in some way in making the world a better or more beautiful place, not only more fully retain their cognitive faculties as they grow older, but often find themselves expanding into new levels of awareness and understanding.

## THE AMAZING GRANNY D

Consider, for example, the extraordinary American elder Doris Haddock, known far and wide as "Granny D." Born in January 1910, Granny D helped stop the planned use of hydrogen bombs in Alaska in 1960. But what brought her to widespread attention was her walk across the United States at the age of ninety, to demonstrate her concern for campaign finance reform. She walked for fourteen months, making speeches, meeting people, and being interviewed. After walking 3,200 miles, she arrived in Washington, D.C., where forty members of the U.S. Congress walked the final miles with her.

Along the way, seventeen U.S. cities declared official "Granny D Days," and another thirteen U.S. cities presented her with keys to their cities. On her ninetieth birthday, she received the prestigious Dr. Martin Luther King, Jr., Award from the Martin Luther King Coalition.

In 2004, having just completed a more than twenty-two-thousand-mile voter registration effort, ninety-four-year-old Granny D became the Democratic candidate for the U.S. Senate from New Hampshire. She ran on the same message she had long worked for: her belief that U.S. leaders have been corrupted by special-interest money and no longer represent the interests of the people. During her candidacy, she was asked whether she was too old for the office. She replied, "It is never too late, and you are never too old. I am 94, and I am healthy. I have pledged to one term, which will end when I am 101."

True to her convictions, she ran her campaign for the U.S. Senate without a dime of special-interest money from political action committees. Drivers in New Hampshire saw a series of rhyming highway signs, such as

*Her campaign cash*
*Is Fatcat free*
*She'll represent*
*Just you and me*
*Granny D for U.S. Senate*

In her mid-nineties, Granny D was not only still active and involved, she was having an extraordinary impact on American politics. She was more than lucid. She was eloquent, clear, and energetic in her efforts to restore integrity to the American political system. The fact that she did not win did not diminish the importance of her efforts, which continued to be celebrated by prominent leaders from both major U.S. political parties.

> *Doris Haddock is a true patriot, and our nation has been blessed by her remarkable life.*
>
> —former U.S. president Jimmy Carter

> *I believe she represents all that is good in America. She has taken up this struggle to clean up American politics. . . . Granny D, you exceed any small, modest contributions those of us who have labored in the vineyards of reform have made to this earth. We are grateful to you.*
>
> —Senator John McCain

## A NEW IMAGE OF AGING

At a time when nearly half of all Americans over eighty-five suffer from Alzheimer's disease, I find it heartening to think of people like Granny D and Anna Morgan. They are extraordinary women, obviously, and I don't mean to imply that you or I or anyone else should hold ourselves to such high standards or expect ourselves to be capable of such heroic achievements. But I am inspired by their joyful and healthy elderhood because it represents an entirely different image of aging than we normally hold in Western culture.

Are they genetically blessed? Probably. But these women have also made choices. Rather than bemoaning what they can no longer do, they have chosen to be filled with energy for what they *can* do. They aren't the type to seek protection from life within gated communities or behind locked doors and security systems. In their active, socially engaged lives, they remind me of many of the elders in Okinawa, as well as those in Abkhasia, Vilcabamba, and Hunza, who have remained committed, alert, and healthy into their nineties and beyond.

Scientific studies have found that attitude and social engagement are profoundly important to health. In 1984, the MacArthur Foundation Research Network on Successful Aging began one of the largest and most interesting aging studies ever undertaken. Recognizing with dismay that the field of gerontology had become preoccupied with studies of disability and disease, the Research Network began studying healthy elderly people.

A central goal of the MacArthur study was to determine what factors enable some people to retain their mental faculties as they age. The researchers found that one of the most statistically significant predictors of maintaining cognitive functioning with age is the sense of "self-efficacy." Elders who have a "can do" attitude and who remain engaged in activities as the years go along are far more likely to retain intact mental abilities.[3]

I have a friend, Kimberly Carter, who has one of the most positive attitudes about life, and about aging, of anyone I know. In her fifties, she lives every day with a great sense of gratitude and celebration, and looks forward to another fifty years of enjoying her health and her opportunities to contribute to the joy of others. She runs several miles each day, and expects to continue running every day until she reaches her mid-eighties, at which point she expects she'll switch to hiking. I asked her what might account for her optimistic attitude about aging, and she answered by speaking of the profound influence of her grandmother Amelia, who inspired in her a positive zeal for old age.

Amelia lived to be 103, and was engaged and alert to her last breath. She took a trip to Yugoslavia for her ninetieth birthday, returning home in time to remodel her kitchen and buy a new car, which she then enjoyed for another thirteen years.

Amelia walked a mile each day on her round trip to the post office. One day when she was 100 she was standing on a corner waiting to cross the street when she heard a young man whisper to his companion, "Do you think I should offer to help the old lady across the street?" Amelia looked around to see who he might be talking about! When she finally died, it was from a heart attack that occurred while she was laughing.

Amelia was born in 1882 and became one of the first women to get a Ph.D. in biology. She taught science at Bryn Mawr, and was actively engaged in just about everything: women's voting rights, public policy, alternative education, natural health care, economics, and international affairs. My friend Kimberly believes that along with her grandmother's immense common sense about healthful eating and exercise, the lifeblood of her longevity was her level of engagement. Not a day goes by that Kimberly doesn't give thanks for the gift of having known and been loved by her grandmother.

## FREE AT LAST

Those of us who have known elders whose lives have been healthy and bright with promise and hope are fortunate indeed, for we have seen the special gifts that can come with age. I have been blessed to know many men and women who, when they reach the age of fifty or sixty, begin to free themselves from cultural constraints and to express themselves in ways they had not dared to do before. They become less defined by what others think of them and more by what they think of themselves. Increasingly freed from the burden of having always to fulfill other people's expectations, their lives start to reflect a new kind of willingness to be exactly who they are. They break free from histories of physical stress, neglect, and abuse. They become more alive.

Instead of thinking of it as a tragedy when their bodies begin to creak and slow down, they accept the limitations that arise and see the transitions they are going through as opportunities to ground themselves in a deeper sense of self and a greater wisdom. Their love for others and for the world becomes more accepting. They increasingly let go of minutiae and the nonessentials of life. Their perspective shifts, details soften, and the larger panorama comes into focus. They are able to enjoy life more than they did when they were young because they have a deeper understanding of it.

Maybe you, too, have known someone like this. These are people who do not conform to a youth-obsessed culture's expectations of what their latter years will be like. Instead, their lives come to enact an entirely different vision of aging. No longer so driven by the desires that shaped the first part of their lives, their lives become more about meaning than about ambition, more about intimacy than about achieving. They experience the second half of their life as a time of deepening creativity and ripening of the soul.

In her 2005 book, *Plan B,* author Anne Lamott gives beautiful voice to this revelation of what aging can be:

I was at a wedding the other day with a lot of women in their twenties and thirties. Many wore sexy dresses, their youthful skin aglow. And even though I was twenty to thirty years older than they, a little worse for wear, a little tired, and overwhelmed by the loud music, I was smiling. . . .

Age has given me what I was looking for my entire life—it has given me *me.* It has provided time and experience and failures and triumphs and time-tested friends who have helped me step into the shape that was waiting for me. I fit into me now. I have an organic life, finally, not necessarily the one people imagined for me, or tried to get me to have. I have the life I longed for. I have become the woman I hardly dared imagine I could be. . . .

I still have terrible moments when I despair about my body— time and gravity have not made various parts of it higher and firmer. But those are just moments now—I used to have *years* when I believed I was more beautiful if I jiggled less, if all parts of my body stopped moving when I did. But I know two things now that I didn't at thirty: That when we get to heaven, we will discover that the appearance of our butts and skin was 127th on the list of what mattered on this earth. And that I am not going to live forever. Knowing these things has set me free.

I am thrilled—ish—for every gray hair and sore muscle, because of all the friends who didn't make it, who died too young of AIDS and breast cancer. . . . I have survived so much loss, as all of us have by our forties—my parents, dear friends, my pets. Rubble is the ground on which our deepest friendships are built. If you haven't already, you will lose someone you can't live without, and your heart will be badly broken, and you never completely get over the loss of a deeply beloved person. But this is also good news. The person lives forever, in your broken heart that doesn't seal back up. And you come through, and you learn to dance with a banged-up heart. . . .

Look, my feet hurt some mornings, and my body is less forgiving when I exercise more than I am used to. But I love my life more, and me more. I'm so much juicier. And as that old saying goes, it's not that I think less of myself, but that I think of myself less . . . And that feels like heaven to me.[4]

## BEING JUICIER

One of the things I love about the people I've known who have exemplified the healthiest kind of aging, be it in Okinawa, Abkhasia, or America, is that they have, like Anne Lamott, found strength and joy in their self-acceptance. I don't mean by this that they are complacent or smug. I mean that they know and respect who they are, and they have found a way of engaging with the world that brings them joy.

Some of us find our passion in activism, like Anna Morgan and Granny D. Maybe you, too, will in your own way find yourself being some kind of activist, taking a stand and speaking out on behalf of some cause or purpose. But many people find their passion and aliveness draws them down a different, less conspicuous path. Maybe you will find in your later years that you are an artist, or a teacher, or a volunteer, or a gardener, or a grandparent who becomes deeply involved with your grandchild or grandchildren. Maybe you will step into your wisdom years to discover that you have been deepened by all you have experienced. Maybe you will find new richness and growth in your self-appreciation and inner life. Maybe you will find that healthy aging can be about far more than the preservation of your youthful faculties, that it can be about the blossoming of your finest and wisest self.

I don't think it's terribly important what form your engagement with life takes, but I do think it matters that you keep finding ways to share your wisdom and to experience your courage, to live with vigor, zest, and zeal, whatever your age. For then I believe you will continue to find, in every season of your life, sources of hope and reasons for thanksgiving.

# STEPS YOU CAN TAKE

Even taking one step is significant. Each step you take makes it easier to take the next. And even small changes in your lifestyle habits continued over the course of months, years, and decades can make a profound difference.

---

- Play in the snow. Run in the rain. Dance in the moonlight. Walk barefoot in the grass. Learn to skate, or take up ballroom dancing or tennis. Try physical activities that you've always wanted to do but never have done.
- Make an exercise date with a friend. Go jogging or hiking, or work out at the gym together.
- Instead of taking a pill for stress, take a hike in the mountains. Or do yoga. Or ride a bicycle outdoors, or a stationary bike indoors near an open window.
- If possible, jog or hike on trails rather than pavement.
- To enhance sleep, exercise regularly, in bright outdoor light if possible. Experiment with exercising at different times of the day in order to find what works best for you. Try to get at least thirty minutes a day of moderate exercise. For optimal results, exercise for an hour or longer each day.
- Create an exercise program that you enjoy and that fits well into your life. Regardless of the weather, your mood, job pressures, or

anything else, get some exercise every day. Set attainable goals, follow through, and enjoy the results.

· Keep a food, mood, and exercise diary.

· Work up a sweat at least once a day.

· When you exercise regularly, give thanks for the increasing energy, confidence, and well-being you experience.

———

· Ask yourself what makes you come alive, what you love to do. Find ways to express your passion in the way you live your life.

· Draw a picture, or make a collage of photos cut from magazines, that represents how you experience your body, including all the stresses, pains, and wounds. Then draw a picture or make a collage that represents how you would like to experience your body. Make it totally glorious. Then draw a picture or make a collage that represents you taking the steps that lead from the first to the second. Put the three in a place where you will see them daily, perhaps on a bedroom or bathroom wall, where they will remind you of your intention and provide support for your journey to joy and fulfillment.

· Hold a picture in your mind of your body as healthy and whole. Write a contract with your body in which you list the specific steps you will take to improve your health. Decide how much time you want to spend directly nurturing your body through exercise. Bear in mind that the time you spend will make a world of difference in every aspect of your life. Know that it is your birthright to feel exuberantly and totally alive.

· To get in deeper touch with your body, explore some of the body-centered therapies, such as Rolfing, Hellerwork, Aston-Patterning, Alexander, Feldenkrais, Trager, Hakomi, the Rosen Method, Dreambodywork, Pilates, T'ai Chi, yoga, and others.

· Never walk away from looking at yourself in the mirror until you feel truly appreciative of your beauty. Stay there for as long as it takes. The point is not to admire some perfect curve or external image, but to appreciate yourself just the way you are.

———

- Spend time with the young. Read to children, cuddle with them, play with them. Be nourished by their wonder.
- Spend time with the old. Befriend and learn from elders. Invite older persons to tell you stories from their lives. Find older mentors who will lead you toward wisdom.
- Speak with your family or friends about the people and events that have given you a sense of the meaning and significance in your life.
- Invite a friend to gaze at the stars with you. Or watch a sunset, or a sunrise.
- Invite friends and loved ones to join you in celebrating your major life milestones. Share stories from your journey.
- Celebrate your birthday every year by doing something you've never done before.

———

- Give time or money (or both) to a cause you believe in. Support organizations and people working for a better world. Stand for the highest possibilities of humanity.
- Once in a while, go on a media fast. For a period of time, unplug the TV, turn off the radio, don't read the newspaper or magazines, and turn off your computer.
- Listen less to the voices of the media and more to the still, small voice deep within your own heart.
- In a world beset by violence, remember the importance of your peace. In a land plagued by hurry, take time to savor each moment. In a culture becoming ever more dehumanized, let people know you love them.

# PART

# 4

# WHY YOUR
# LOVE MATTERS

## 13

# What's Love Got to Do with It?

*The heart that loves is always young.*
—Greek proverb

There is an aspect of our lives that healthy traditional cultures have always understood to be of paramount importance to human happiness, well-being, and longevity: Nothing is more important, they believe, than the quality of their human relationships. As individuals and as communities they are sustained through all kinds of hardships by the boundless commitment they have to support one another, and their complete readiness to provide mutual aid at any time.

If you happen to leave your wallet on the sidewalk in Okinawa, you can fully expect to come back the next day and find it still there. If it's gone, it's probably only because some anonymous stranger who picked it up will soon return it to you, completely intact.

Similarly, in Abkhasia, people are valued over anything else. Wealth is counted not by the amount of money a person has, but by the number and quality of relationships he or she maintains. In Abkhasia, people are not said to be successful as a result of having a large bank account, much land, or many possessions. Instead, people are considered successful if they have a large and vibrant network of loyal and devoted people in their home, extended family, and community.

In Vilcabamba and Hunza, too, the sense of connectedness people have with one another and the way they relate to each other are held to be of primary significance. Generosity and sharing are the highest values. Nothing is more important than how people treat each other. After the American doctor Y. F. Schnellow returned from Hunza, he reflected on the remarkable health he had witnessed:

> One of the most noteworthy aspects of my experience in Hunza was the palpable sense of love and connection I felt among the people. They looked after each other, they rejoiced together, there was an atmosphere of friendliness everywhere. I could not help but think that it is this great affection and reciprocity they have for one another that underlies and makes possible their unparalleled health.[1]

## LOVE AND HEALTHCARE

Thirty years ago, anyone who said there were profound medical consequences to human relationships would have had their sanity questioned by modern science. And anyone blaming loneliness for physical illness would have been laughed at. But in the last few decades there has been an explosion of scientific understanding about the deep connections between interpersonal relationships and health.

As you may know, there is in Western medicine a great deal of concern about risk factors like high blood pressure, high cholesterol, smoking, and obesity—and deservedly so, for they are very often linked to serious disease. But an ever-increasing body of medical research is coming to the surprising conclusion that the quality of your relationships with other people is every bit as important to your health as these indicators—if not more so. Chronic loneliness now ranks as one of the most lethal risk factors determining who will die prematurely in modern industrialized nations.

Though the science has been accumulating for the last thirty years, many physicians have been slow to accept the idea that something as intangible as interpersonal relationships could have so much medical significance. They tend to view love as a frill or a luxury, as something that distracts from a rational approach to patient care. Western medicine still often trains physicians and other health professionals to keep emotionally distant from their patients. It's a great loss that even if health professionals are deeply caring people, they receive little approval for their kindness, their gentleness, and their empathy. Rachel Naomi Remen, M.D., describes how this affected her:

> The second day of my internship in pediatrics I went with my senior resident to tell some young parents that the automobile accident from which they had escaped without a scratch had killed their only child. Very new to this doctor thing, when they cried, I had cried with them. After it was over, the senior resident took me aside and told me that I had behaved very unprofessionally. "These people were counting on our strength," he said. I had let them down. I took his criticism very much to heart. By the time I myself was senior resident, I hadn't cried in years.
>
> During that year, a two-year-old baby, left unattended for only a moment, drowned in a bathtub. We fought to bring him back but after an hour we had to concede defeat. Taking the intern with me, I went to tell these parents that we had not been able to save their child. Overwhelmed, they began to sob. After a time, the father looked at me standing there, strong and silent in my white coat, the shaken intern by my side. "I'm sorry, Doctor," he said. "I'll get a hold of myself in a minute." I remember this man, his face wet with a father's tears, and I think of his apology with shame. Convinced by then that my grief was a useless, self-indulgent waste of time, I had made myself into the sort of person to whom one could apologize for being in pain.[2]

## EVIDENCE THAT STUNS EVEN THE SKEPTICS

It is a sad statement about modern medicine that so many physicians consider it to be their professional obligation to remain emotionally distant from their patients, when in fact the healing power of love and relationships has been documented in an ever-increasing number of well-designed scientific studies involving hundreds of thousands of people throughout the world. In his 1998 book, *Love and Survival,* Dean Ornish, M.D., describes reviewing the scientific literature and being amazed by what a powerful difference love and relationships make on the incidence of disease and premature death from virtually all causes. "I am not aware of any other factor," Ornish concluded "—not diet, not smoking, not exercise, not stress, not genetics, not drugs, not surgery—that has a greater impact on our quality of life, incidence of illness, and premature death from all causes."[3]

Dr. Ornish is not the only esteemed medical icon to be convinced of the healing power of our relationships with one another. In May 1989, a Stanford Medical School professor of psychiatry and behavioral sciences, David Spiegel, M.D., told the annual meeting of the American Psychiatric Association of an unexpected finding.[4] He and his colleagues had been studying eighty-six women with metastatic breast cancer. The women had been randomly placed into two groups. Both groups received the same medical treatment, but one group also attended weekly support group meetings. To the amazement of the researchers, the ten-year study found that the women who participated in the support group had twice the survival time of the women in the control group. They lived an average of 37 months after entering the program, compared to an average of 19 months for the other women.[5]

"I must say I was quite stunned," said Spiegel. He told the *Los Angeles Times* that he "undertook the study expecting to refute the often overstated notions about the power of mind over disease," which he said he had found "clinically as well as theoretically irritating."[6] His intention was to disprove the idea that psychosocial interventions could have medical value for women with breast cancer, partly because he was tired of being confused with Dr. Bernie Siegel, who had written several bestsellers affirming that patients' attitude and degree of social support could play a dramatic role in their medical outcomes.

The women in the support group not only lived twice as long, they also experienced fewer mood swings and less pain and fear than their counterparts. These gains came from meeting for an hour and a half a week, during which the women were encouraged to express whatever they were feeling, including (though not limited to) their fears, anger, anxiety, and depression.

The women who participated the most actively in the meetings experienced the greatest lengthening in survival time. Although all of the women in the study had been considered "terminal," three were still alive when Spiegel made his presentation twelve years after the study began. Tellingly, these women were among those who had been most involved in the sessions.

Spiegel was not the only medical professional who was astonished at the results. Dr. Troy Thompson, a professor of psychiatry at Jefferson Medical College in Philadelphia, remarked, "This is a marvelous study, a surprising study to me as well. I would have bet the mortgage of my home that it would not have come out this way."[7]

If a chemotherapy drug existed that had the ability to increase survival as greatly as participation in the emotional support group did, it would be adopted as the standard of care and administered to virtually all women with metastatic breast cancer. Pharmaceutical companies would be making billions of dollars off the drug. Patients would be paying many tens of thousands of dollars each, and would be willing to endure toxicity and reduction in quality of life from the chemotherapy in order to obtain the added years. The support group, on the other hand, cost almost nothing, and added substantially to the women's quality of life.

Could Spiegel's study have been an aberration? A few years later, Dr. F. I. Fawzy and his colleagues at the University of California at Los Angeles Medical School conducted a study similar to Spiegel's, this one dealing with the survival rates from malignant melanoma in two groups of patients. As in Spiegel's study, the patients in both groups received the same medical treatments, and were equivalent at the beginning of the study in how far their cancer had progressed. The only difference was that one group also met regularly for mutual support. Five years later, the researchers were stunned to find that individuals in the group that did not participate in the support group were three times more likely to have died than those who had the opportunity to talk to others about their experiences.[8]

I do not know of any study that has found a higher incidence of disease or mortality for people with strong social support than for those without. But many important studies tell us that people with more love in their lives and more social support have *lower* incidence and *lower* mortality from cancer and many other diseases.

I believe these studies are providing us with a glimpse into one of the deep secrets of health and longevity.

## HOW IMPORTANT LOVE CAN BE

"We cannot live for ourselves alone," wrote Herman Melville. "A thousand fibers connect us with our fellow man." Perhaps this explains why we are often moved by people caring deeply for one another. A story illustrating the point, perhaps apocryphal, is told by a friend of mine, the noted author Dan Millman:

> Many years ago, when I worked as a volunteer at Stanford Hospital, I got to know a little girl named Liza who was suffering from a rare and serious disease. Her only chance of recovery appeared to be a blood transfusion from her five-year-old brother, who had miraculously survived the same disease and had developed the antibodies needed to combat the illness. The doctor explained the situation to her little brother, and asked the boy if he would be willing to give his blood to his sister. I saw him hesitate for only a moment, before taking a deep breath and saying, "Yes, I'll do it if it will save Liza."
>
> As the transfusion progressed, he lay in a bed next to his sister and smiled, as we all did, seeing the color returning to her cheeks. Then his face grew pale and his smile faded. He looked up at the doctor and asked with a trembling voice, "Will I start to die right away?"
>
> Being young, the boy had misunderstood the doctor. He thought he was going to have to give her *all* his blood.[9]

We find it inspiring to think of a child being so selfless and generous that he would give his life for his sister. The fact that such a simple story can move our hearts is evidence that we are all capable of acting from our higher selves more often than we do, that we are all capable of more cooperation than we often think.

There are also medical implications to whether we think of others or only of ourselves, as Larry Scherwitz found out when he conducted a most unusual study. Now the director of research at California Pacific Medical Center's Institute for Health and Healing in San Francisco, Dr. Scherwitz taped the conversations of nearly six hundred men. About a third of these men were suffering from heart disease; the rest were healthy. Listening to the tapes, he counted how often each man used the words *I, me,* and *mine.* Comparing his results with the frequency of heart disease, he found that the men who used the first-person pronouns the most often had the highest risk of heart trouble. What's more, by following his subjects for several years thereafter, he found that the more a man habitually talked about himself, the greater the chance he would actually have a heart attack.[10]

Apparently, counting the times a person said "I" was an ingenious way to quantify self-absorption. It seems that the less you open your heart to others, the more your heart suffers. Dr. Scherwitz counsels: "Listen with regard when others talk. Give your time and energy to others; let others have their way; do things for reasons other than furthering your own needs."

This is sound medical advice, and it speaks also to our spiritual and emotional needs. Many religions have taught that being trapped in the illusion of separateness is the source of much of our suffering.

Modern Western society, of course, has become highly competitive. You see it perhaps most conspicuously in sports. "Winning is not the most important thing," said the famous football coach Vince Lombardi. "It's everything." Said another coach, "Show me a good loser and I'll show you a loser." I'm sure these coaches were trying to urge their players on to greater effort, but when we become hypercompetitive, we may lose touch with honor, decency, and sportsmanship. And we almost certainly lose touch with each other.

Special Olympians train long and hard for their events and are every bit as committed to winning as are athletes in other athletic competitions. The Special Olympics is not a casual social outing. These are highly organized sporting events taken very seriously by all involved. But people at the Special Olympics Washington office have verified that the following incident took place at a 1976 track and field event in Spokane, Washington:

Nine contestants, all physically or mentally disabled, assembled at the starting line for the hundred-yard dash. At the gun they all started out running as fast as they could. All, that is, except one boy who stumbled on the asphalt, tumbled over a couple of times, and began to cry. Hearing the boy cry, several of the others slowed down and paused. Then they turned around and went back. One girl with Down's syndrome bent down and kissed him, and said, "This will make it better." Then they all linked arms and walked together to the finish line. Everyone in the stadium stood, and the cheering went on for ten minutes.

Why do we find a story like this so moving? Could it be that beneath the many ways we have of being separate, we are nevertheless somehow deeply part of each other? Can children sometimes remind us of an essential part of our humanity that we so easily forget in modern society?

In societies like Okinawa, Vilcabamba, Hunza, and Abkhasia, there are many forms of healthy competition, but no one is ever shamed because of being less able. Who wins is important for the moment, but then immediately forgotten. The quality of how people treat one another is remembered long after.

## THE HEALING POWER OF RELATIONSHIPS

Most of us are conditioned to view as scientifically valid only that which can be measured in a laboratory. Something as fuzzy and ephemeral as human relationships can seem "touchy-feely," hardly the stuff of sound science. But sophisticated research has confirmed that we are social creatures to our core, and our sense of being in touch with others and feeling connected to them has enormous implications for our health and longevity.

When researchers from Case Western Reserve University in Cleveland studied almost ten thousand married men with no prior history of angina (chest pain indicating heart disease), they found that those men who had high levels of risk factors—including elevated cholesterol, high blood pressure, diabetes, and electrocardiogram abnormalities—were more than twenty times as likely to develop angina during the next five years. They were amazed to discover, though, that those men who answered "yes" to the simple question "Does your wife show you her love?" *had substantially less angina even when they had high levels of these risk factors.*[11]

In a related study, researchers followed 8,500 married men with no history of ulcers. These men were given a questionnaire to fill out, and then tracked for five years. Those men who reported a low level of love and support from their wives at the beginning of the study were found to have more than twice as many ulcers in the ensuing five years as the other men. And those who said "My wife does not love me" were almost three times as likely to develop ulcers. In this study, having the feeling that their wives didn't show them love and support was more strongly associated with ulcers than smoking, age, high blood pressure, or job stress.[12]

The medical value of intimacy, of having a loving relationship with a spouse or a very dear friend, became overwhelmingly apparent to researchers who published a study in the *British Medical Journal* in 1993.[13] For seven years, they followed 752 men. At the outset of the study, these men had been given a medical exam during which they were asked about their emotional stress. The study found that those men who had reported being under serious emotional stress at the time of their initial exam—who were experiencing financial troubles, feeling insecure at work, defending a legal action, or going through a divorce—had more than triple the risk of dying during the seven years following the initial exam. Being under these kinds of stresses at the beginning of the study turned out to be a stronger predictor of dying within the ensuing seven years than medical indicators such as high blood pressure, high concentrations of blood triglycerides (linked to coronary artery disease), or high serum cholesterol levels.

Okay, you might say, serious stress breaks people down and can even kill them. That's no surprise, but what does it have to do with love? What made this study astounding was that for those men who said at the outset of the study that they had a dependable web of intimacy—a spouse or close friends—*there turned out to be no correlation whatsoever between high stress levels and death rate.*

Loving relationships, medical science is clearly telling us, have an extraordinary ability to defuse the negative medical effects of stress. And we have some understanding of the mechanism by which this happens.

Certain hormones (cortisol and the catecholamines epinephrine and norepinephrine, which are also called adrenaline and noradrenaline) are produced in your body when you are under stress. When these chemicals are secreted and surge through your body, your immune cells are less able to perform their functions, leaving you more susceptible to disease. In this way, stress suppresses immune resistance. There may be an evolutionary wisdom operating in this suppression, in that energy is conserved, enabling your body to put a priority on handling the immediate emergency. In extreme instances this could make the difference between life and death. But if stress continues over time, your health inevitably suffers. Social support seems to neutralize the effect of stress by lowering the production of these stress hormones.

Modern research is now repeatedly finding that your relationships with others are medically potent. *Your connections with the significant people in your life—if they are positive and loving—can prevent stress-induced illness, greatly contribute to your health and healing, and add many years to your life.* This corroborates what we've seen in Okinawa, Abkhasia, Vilcabamba, and Hunza. An abundance of positive, meaningful relationships is one of the secrets of the world's healthiest and most long-lived peoples.

One of the most remarkable people I've had the good fortune to know is Eleanor Wasson. The recipient of the Lifetime Achievement Award given by Physicians for Social Responsibility for her outstanding work for world peace, Eleanor, now nearly 100 years old, is still alert, vital, strong, healthy, and actively working for a better world. I've known Eleanor for many years, and I've found her always to be an uplifting and inspiring influence on others, even under the most challenging circumstances. I talked to her shortly after the publication of her autobiography, titled *28,000 Martinis and Counting: A*

*Century of Living, Learning, and Loving.* I asked what she would consider the secret to a long and healthy life. "Having loving parents," she said. "I always felt loved as a child. I had such wonderfully loving parents that I never knew, until years later, that not everyone had that gift in their lives. And maintaining friendships. Deep and lasting friendships are precious beyond words."

## THE POWER OF LOVE

In modern society, we can get so busy that we don't take time to feel our gratitude and receive the blessings of our relationships. Too often, we fill our lives with so much activity that we don't have room left for the people who matter to us. We can make possessions more important than people.

This is a mistake that people living the traditional way of life in Abkhasia, Vilcabamba, Hunza, and Okinawa rarely make. They are not woken by alarm clocks. Instead, they often wake to the sound of others singing. Instead of going shopping, they go to visit one another. They have need of few belongings, for they belong to each other.

Sometimes we are loved more deeply than we realize, but it can take a crisis to break us out of our patterns so that we can receive the love that others have for us. Author Elizabeth Songster describes the dramatic events that helped her to comprehend the depth of her husband's love:

> It was right before Christmas. My husband, Dan, and a buddy of his, Mike, had gone [each in his own car] to a canyon near our home in Southern California to see if the vegetation, scorched by fires a few months earlier, was growing back. Dan and Mike were both members of the California Native Plant Society. They were real "plant hounds," always exploring the nearby canyons and hills to see what kind of plants they could find and photograph.
>
> That day, after Mike left [to drive home from the area where the two men were exploring], Dan decided to do a little "solo research" by hiking into Laguna Canyon, a more remote section of the area that was not often explored. He had walked into the

canyon a few miles, gotten some pictures and was starting to make his way back to his truck, when he stepped on a water-soaked patch of ground that gave way. He fell thirty-five feet down the rough slope, hitting a number of trees, before he landed on a ledge. He could tell right away that something was terribly wrong with his left leg. It lay across his other leg at an "impossible angle."

Stunned by the fall, it took Dan a little while to realize that he was too crippled to walk. Then Dan knew he was in serious trouble. Night would fall soon and not a soul knew where he was. He had to get to the main trail or he might die out there before anyone could find him. He braced the broken leg against the other leg and, resting his weight on his hands, began inching his way down the canyon.

Making slow and painful progress, Dan stopped often to rest and call for help. The only response was the eerie sound of his own voice echoing off the walls of the canyon. As the sun set, the temperature began to drop. It was cold in the hills at night and Dan knew that if he stopped for too long, he would probably lose consciousness. It was increasingly hard, but Dan forced himself after each pause to keep hauling his sore body forward on his aching hands. He continued this awful journey for another twelve hours.

Finally, his strength and determination gave out. He was utterly exhausted and couldn't move another inch. Although it seemed futile, he summoned up a last burst of strength and shouted for help.

He was astounded when he heard a voice return his call. A real voice, not another mocking and empty echo. It was Dan's stepson—my son, Jeb. He and I were out with the police and the paramedics who were searching for Dan.

Earlier, when Dan didn't come home, I had gotten worried and called Mike. At first, Mike tried to find Dan himself, driving from canyon to canyon looking for Dan's truck. Finally, he called the police and reported Dan missing.

I'd kept calm and strong until the moment Jeb said he'd heard Dan's voice. Then I dissolved into tears, finally feeling the fear and dread I'd been pushing aside for hours. It took two hours for the rescue team to bring Dan down the ravine. Then the paramedics trundled him away on a stretcher and when I got to see him at the hospital, my tears started anew. The thought of how close I came to losing this wonderful man undid me. It was only when I felt Dan's arms around me that I finally stopped sobbing.

As I sat next to his hospital bed, my eyes fastened to the face I had been so afraid I would never see again, Dan told me his story. Immediately after his slide down the canyon, when he realized the seriousness of his predicament, Dan said that he thought of me and how much he would miss me if he didn't make it back. As he lay at the bottom of the rough cliff, he groped around until he found a suitable rock. Using the rock, which was sharply pointed, he managed to carve a message to me in a large rock near where he lay. If the worst should happen, he hoped I would eventually see the rock and know that I had been with him always, held close in his heart.

I started weeping all over again. I knew how deeply I loved my husband, but I was unprepared for this, the depth of his love for me.

For somewhere deep in the wooded hills of Laguna Canyon, there is a large rock with a heart carved on its side. And in this heart are carved the words, "Elizabeth, I love you."[14]

# 14

## The Strength of the Heart

*I have met on the street a very poor man who was in love. His hat was old, his coat was out at the elbows, the water passed through his shoes, and the stars through his soul.*

—Victor Hugo

Love's mystery and wonder, of course, are not reserved only for those who are married. But there is a special way that love can touch two people in an intimate relationship who commit themselves wholeheartedly to the journey together.

Such relationships take us through whatever we need to learn to become more conscious, loving people. They open our hearts, break our hearts, and heal our hearts—sometimes all at the same time. They give us opportunities to develop courage, patience, and resilience. They teach us to be compassionate and forgiving. They give us the strength to fulfill the purposes for which we are alive.

And now modern science is recognizing that loving and intimate relationships also keep us healthy.

It is a striking fact that mortality rates for all causes of death in the United States are consistently higher for divorced, single, and widowed individuals of both sexes and all ages.[1] Such statistics explain why life insurance companies recognize people's marital status as one of the best indicators of how long they are likely to live.

## PREMATURE ANNUAL DEATH RATES PER 100,000 MEN

|           | Nonsmokers | Smokers |
|-----------|------------|---------|
| Married   | 796        | 1,560   |
| Single    | 1,074      | 2,567   |
| Widowed   | 1,396      | 2,570   |
| Divorced  | 1,420      | 2,675   |

The Hammond Report was the study that followed the smoking habits of nearly half a million Americans and led ultimately to the warning printed on every cigarette package that smoking is hazardous to your health. If you look at the table above, extracted from the Hammond Report,[2] you'll see something that may astonish you.

As you can see, the premature death rate for smokers in each category is roughly double that for nonsmokers. What I find most remarkable, though, is that the premature death rate for nonsmokers who are divorced is almost equal to that for married smokers. For men, apparently, the breakup of a marriage can be nearly as lethal as a lifelong habit of smoking.

## THE EVIDENCE CONTINUES TO MOUNT

One of the first, and still one of the most remarkable, of the many studies exploring the influence of love and social connectedness on human health was conducted by epidemiologist Dr. Lisa Berkman beginning in 1965. Now the chair of the Department of Health and Social Behavior at the Harvard School of Public Health, Dr. Berkman led an intensive study of seven thousand men and women living in Alameda County, California. She found that people who were disconnected from others were roughly three times more likely to die during the nine-year study than people with strong social ties. The kinds of social ties didn't appear to matter. What mattered was being involved in some social network, whether it was family, friends, church, volunteer groups, or marriage.

This dramatic difference in health outcome and survival rates was found to occur regardless of people's age, gender, health practices, or physical health status. But what most astounded researchers about this study was that *those with close social ties and unhealthful life-styles (such as smoking, obesity, and lack of exercise) actually lived longer than those with poor social ties but more healthful living habits.* Needless to say, people with both healthful lifestyles and close social ties lived the longest of all.[3]

Is this study some kind of aberration? No, it is not. Many other studies have come to similar conclusions. When seventeen thousand people in Sweden, for example, were examined and followed, it was found that those who were the most lonely and isolated at the beginning of the study had nearly four times the risk of dying prematurely in the ensuing six years.[4]

For another example, an analysis of the medical risks of social isolation published in the journal *Science* in 1988 concluded that lack of emotional support was a greater risk factor for disease and death than smoking.[5]

These studies and many others like them are warning us that the medical consequences of loneliness are real and can even be fatal. At the same time, they are providing us with compelling evidence of the scientific basis for the healing powers of friendship, love, and positive relationships.

Studies have even shown that having a companion animal can make a huge difference. It's no secret that children often love pets, but recent research has taken it a step further, proving that children raised with pets are less likely to become asthmatic, more likely to be kind to other children, and more likely to have healthy self-esteem once they reach their teens. Researchers are also finding that having pets positively influences children's physical and emotional development and even their scholastic achievement.[6]

One of the most celebrated "pet studies" was undertaken by Erika Friedmann and her co-workers at the University of Pennsylvania. They found an unmistakable association between pet ownership and extended survival in patients hospitalized with coronary heart disease. Those patients who had pets at home were far more likely to survive, even after accounting for differences in the extent of heart damage and other medical problems.[7]

The medical value of pets became unexpectedly apparent to researchers who were conducting the Cardiac Arrhythmia Suppression Trial. They were studying the effects of two pharmaceutical drugs (encainide and flecainide) on men who had had heart attacks and were now experiencing irregular heartbeats. Paradoxically, the drugs were found to cause an increase in cardiac deaths. At the same time, however, it was found that those patients who had dogs were only one-sixth as likely to die during the study as those who did not have dogs.[8]

Can you imagine what would have happened if the drugs rather than the dogs had been shown to cause a sixfold decrease in deaths? The drugs would be prescribed for every heart attack patient in the country with an irregular heartbeat, and drug companies would be spending hundreds of millions of dollars telling physicians and the public how great the drugs were. But because the loyalty and loving friendship of a dog cannot be bottled and sold, there has been no such publicity campaign, and most people to this day do not realize how much healing can be found in loving relationships—including ones with companion animals.

In another study called the Beta-Blocker Heart Attack Trial, researchers followed more than 2,300 men who had survived a heart attack, to see whether there would be an increase in survival for those taking a beta-blocker drug. There was, but the researchers ended up discovering something far more significant. Stunningly, those patients who had strong connections with other people were found to have only one-quarter the risk of death—even when controlling for other factors such as smoking, diet, alcohol, exercise, and weight. In fact, the decrease in death risk due to social connectedness was found to be far stronger than that for the beta-blocker drug being tested.[9]

Partly as a result of this study, physicians today widely prescribe beta-blocker drugs for people who have survived a heart attack. Ironically, doctors typically issue these prescriptions during appointments with patients that last all of fifteen minutes, during which they never mention the far greater proven importance of friendship and social support.

## HOW MUCH WE MATTER TO EACH OTHER

Rachel Naomi Remen, M.D., tells of the difference in health outcomes human relationships can make:

> Many years ago when I was a teaching pediatrician at a major medical school, I followed six young teenagers with juvenile diabetes. Most of them had diabetes since they were toddlers and had responsibly followed strict diets and given themselves injections of insulin since kindergarten. But as they became caught up in the turmoil of adolescence, desperate to be like their peer group, this disease had become a terrible burden, a mark of difference. Youngsters who had been in diabetic control since infancy now rebelled against the authority of their disease as if it were a third parent. They forgot to take their shots, ate whatever the gang ate, and were brought to the emergency room in coma or in shock, over and over again. It was frightening and frustrating, dangerous for the youngsters and draining for their parents and the entire pediatric staff.
>
> As the associate director of the clinics, this problem was brought to my door and I decided to try something simple. I formed two discussion groups, each consisting of three youngsters and the parents of the other three. Each group met to talk once a week.
>
> These groups turned out to be very powerful. Kids who could not talk to their own parents became articulate in expressing their needs and perspectives to the parents of other children. Parents who could not listen to their own children hung on every word of other people's children. And other people's children could hear them when they could not hear their own parents. People, feeling themselves understood for the first time, felt safe enough to cry and found that others cared and could comfort them. People of all ages offered each other insights and support, and behaviors began to change. Parents and their own children began to talk and listen

to each other in new ways. We were making great progress in the quality of all the family relationships, and the number of emergency room visits was actually diminishing.[10]

These children and parents were finding that they had something important to offer each other. They were discovering that our care and compassion for others often make more difference than we realize.

## TOXIC RELATIONSHIPS

Relationships are powerful, and can be enormously important to health and longevity. But as so often is true in life, there is also a shadow side to this power. While good intimate relationships are deeply supportive of health, it's also true that bad ones can cause considerable damage. Sometimes people's hearts ache with loneliness even in the company of their spouse.

In an article published in *The Journal of the American Medical Association* in 2000, a research team headed by Kristina Orth Gomer, M.D., Ph.D., found that marital discord dramatically increases the risk of cardiac death in women.[11] The study found that women with heart disease tripled their risk of recurrent heart trouble if they were involved in a stressful relationship. Realizing that many issues could cloud their results, the researchers specifically factored out age, sedentary lifestyle, estrogen status, smoking, lipid levels, education, and a host of other variables that could have altered the outcome of the study.

What is it about unhappy relationships that so undermines the health of women? Another study, presented in 2005 at the American Heart Association's Second International Conference on Women, Heart Disease, and Stroke in Orlando, Florida, provided further insight.[12] This ten-year study followed 3,600 men and women aged 18 to 77, all of whom were married or living "in a marital situation." The researchers collected data on marital discord and tracked the health of the participants to see who developed heart disease or died of any cause during the study.

The greatest health risk was seen in women who kept quiet when conflicts arose with their spouses. Though they might have thought they were keeping the peace by remaining silent in such situations, they paid dearly for it. Women who did not express themselves in marital conflicts had four times the risk of dying during the study compared to women who spoke their minds.

Men, on the other hand, suffered in their hearts when they saw their working wives burdened by job stress. Men who said that their wives came home upset fom work were nearly three times more likely to develop heart disease than men whose wives didn't work or were happy in their work.

Relationships that help you to feel acknowledged, safe, and loved are a great boon to your health. But it is also true that relationships that make you feel frightened, hurt, or despised can be poisonous.

Andrew Weil, M.D., bestselling author and director of the Program in Integrative Medicine at the University of Arizona in Tucson, relates a particularly dramatic case of healing that took place for "a bank president with chronic hypertension, whose blood pressure normalized one day after his wife filed for divorce. It dropped to 120/80 and stayed there."[13] Somehow I suspect that this man's relationship with his wife had not been a source of love, joy, and healing in his life.

In another case, author Brendan O'Regan writes of a medical journal article describing the astonishing case of a woman with metastasized cancer of the cervix who was considered close to death. Her condition changed dramatically when, in the words of the case report, "her much-hated husband suddenly died, whereupon she completely recovered."

## THE IMPORTANCE OF PARENTING

Among the most important relationships of our lives, of course, are those with our parents. One of the foremost pioneers in understanding the influence of relationships on health is James J. Lynch, Ph.D. In his 2000 book, *A Cry Unheard: New Insights into the Medical Consequences of Loneliness,* Dr. Lynch draws particular attention to the formative role of parent-child relationships.[14] It is widely recognized that the way parents treat their children can have a huge impact on whether they become confident, joyful, and responsible people, or grow up insecure, frightened, and dysfunctional. Lynch's work, however, goes further and shows that how parents treat their children has enormous medical implications.

It's thankfully becoming ever more widely recognized that physical abuse of children is harmful and indefensible. But verbal abuse can also cause great damage. Negative words can hit as hard as a fist, and can leave deep and lasting scars. It is abusive to destroy a child's sense of self-worth with such debilitating phrases as "You're hopeless," "You're good for nothing," "You can never do anything right," "You'll never amount to anything," or "I can't wait until you grow up and get out of this house."

According to Dr. Lynch, parents who use language to hurt, control, and manipulate their children rather than to reach out and be present with them cause the youngsters to feel depressed and lonely. The kids then carry these feelings with them into their interactions with others in their lives. They tend to be socially isolated, and, Lynch shows, to end up with illnesses that reduce both the quality and the length of their lives. Lynch presents a wealth of data to support his conclusion that exposure to this kind of parenting proves "toxic" precisely because it leads to premature death. Loneliness in childhood, he says, has "a significant impact on the incidence of serious disease and premature death decades later in adulthood."

When I first learned of Dr. Lynch's theories, I was skeptical. I didn't doubt that a bleak childhood environment could predict *mental* illness in adult life. But could the way our parents treated us when we were children have that much impact on our later *physical* health? But then I learned of a truly remarkable long-term study conducted at Harvard University.[15] It began in the early 1950s, when researchers randomly chose 125 undergraduate students and asked them to rank their relationships with their parents on a four-point scale as to the degree of their emotional closeness. The scale was as follows:

(1)  Very close
(2)  Warm and friendly
(3)  Tolerant
(4)  Strained and cold

Thirty-five years later, the researchers examined the medical histories of these volunteers and found that an astounding 91 percent of those who had rated their relationship with their mothers as either "tolerant" or "strained and cold" had, by the time they reached their late fifties, suffered serious medical crises. They actually had more than twice the risk of having serious diagnosed disease by that time compared to those who, thirty-five years before, had said they had either a "very close" or a "warm and friendly" relationship with their mothers. Similarly, 82 percent of participants who had rated their relationship with their fathers as either "tolerant" or "strained and cold" had developed serious diseases by midlife.

Even more amazing was that 100 percent of those who had reported that their relationships with both their parents were "strained and cold" had experienced serious medical problems by their late fifties.

There is another aspect to this study that I find fascinating. The students were asked "What kind of person is your mother?" and "What kind of person is your father?" The researchers simply counted the number of positive and negative words the students wrote down in describing their parents. A simple score reflecting the total number of positive words was found to be profoundly predictive of these students' health thirty-five years later.

The correlation between these descriptions of parental relationships and future health was independent of family history of illness, smoking, emotional stress, subsequent death or divorce of parents, and the students' marital history. And it was immensely powerful. Fully 95 percent of students who had used few positive words to describe their parents developed serious diseases in midlife, whereas only 29 percent of those who had used many positive words developed comparable diseases. I find this fascinating, because this indicates that *having had a difficult relationship with one's parents is a greater risk factor for major adult disease than smoking, obesity, and high blood pressure combined.*

I could not agree more with the surgeon and author Bernie S. Siegel, M.D., who asserts, "The greatest disease of mankind is a lack of love for children."

Could the Harvard study have been an isolated instance? Not likely, because many other studies have confirmed these findings. In a similar study, for example, researchers at Johns Hopkins Medical School asked more than thirteen hundred healthy medical students in the 1940s to fill out a questionnaire called the "Closeness to Parents Scale" to assess the quality of the students' relationships with their parents. Fifty years later, it was found that those students who had described a lack of closeness with their parents were far more likely to have developed cancer. The predictive value of parental relationships that were not close did not diminish over time, and was not explained by any other known risk factor, such as smoking, drinking, or radiation exposure. In fact, the strongest predictor of which men would get cancer decades later turned out not to be smoking or obesity, but rather the lack of a close relationship with their fathers fifty years before.[16]

## MY FATHER, MY SON

How we raise our children is so important. We've all got our wounds, of course, but if we can face them and heal them, then we have a chance not to pass them on to our children. If we are going to build a healthy and loving world, few tasks are more crucial.

When my wife, Deo, was pregnant with our son, Ocean, I was overjoyed. But I was also concerned, because I wasn't sure what kind of father I would be.

As a boy, I had been taught that to show any kind of vulnerability or suffering was a weakness. Like many males in the modern world, I had learned to equate being strong with being stoic, and to believe that to ask for help or to cry was unmanly. I had been taught that life was a battle and you had to be armored to succeed. I didn't understand why I felt so lonely. I didn't understand my feelings much at all.

My father was a very self-assured and successful man who worked long hours and provided well for his family, yet I did not grow up feeling emotionally close to him or feeling that my love made much difference to him. When he was feeling playful he would sometimes punch me in the stomach, encouraging me to tighten my abdominal muscles to brace for the blows, and then compliment me on how tightly my stomach muscles were clenched.

On the verge of becoming a father, I was coming to realize that my childhood had left me with an unwillingness to experience and show my feelings. This emotional disconnection kept others from knowing me or being close to me, and also kept me from really knowing or being close to anyone else. I was beginning to see that what I had been taught was a strength was actually a form of fear—a fear of being open, real, and connected to others.

I wanted my son to have a different kind of childhood experience from the one I had known. I wanted to be not only physically present with him, but also emotionally present. I wanted to have a relationship with him in which he could show me who he was and not have to pretend he was anything he was not, and, most important, in which he could have the experience of knowing his worthiness, knowing how important he was to me, knowing that his love mattered infinitely to me. I wanted our feelings to be a source of contact and honesty between us. But for that to happen, I had to learn how to let down my walls.

When Ocean was about eighteen months old, his mother went away for a week, and I was left solely responsible for the little guy. We got along fabulously, but slowly the effort of taking care of his every need began to wear on me. I felt sad that it wasn't easier for me, and that I was beginning to feel overwhelmed. One evening the sadness swelled inside me to the point that it filled me with grief. My own childhood wounds were clearly being reactivated. I lay down on the bed and began to cry for all the children, myself included, who have ever been raised by parents unable to affirm their value and worthiness.

Ocean was, at that moment, sitting in his high chair eating his dinner. Seeing me crying so bitterly, he began asking to be removed from his high chair. At the time, he knew how to say only a few words, but one of them was "down." As I was crying on the bed, he looked at me with great earnestness, and began saying "Down! Down!"

"I've been looking after your every need twenty-four hours a day," I wailed. "Can't you just let me cry?"

"Down! Down!" he insisted.

"Okay," I thought, "you win." I sighed, went over to the high chair, gently picked him up, and put him down on the carpet. I kissed him, then went back to the bed, lay down, and began again to cry.

My eyes were closed when I felt a gentle pressure on my chest. Startled, I opened my eyes to see Ocean's loving gaze looking down upon me. He had made his way over to the bed, climbed up on it, crawled over beside me, and placed his hand on my heart, looking into my eyes with tender concern. He had so persistently wanted down from his high chair not because he was a ball of selfish instincts and desires, but because he wanted to be close to me in my grief. He spoke, ever so gently, with deep concern pouring through his eyes:

"Johnny hurt."

This was the first time he had ever put two words together. It was the first sentence he ever spoke.

I felt relief at that moment, because I realized that I had taken a step in the journey of breaking the cycle. There would be many more steps to take, but I was beginning to discover that I could be emotionally available to my son, and that even with all my flaws and wounds, I still had much love and nurturance to give to him.

As more than thirty years have gone by since then, I've time and again been struck by Ocean's kindness and compassion. His seemingly infinite love has continued to guide and inspire me. Being his father has been an unending source of joy and the greatest privilege of my life.

## STRONG AT THE BROKEN PLACES

If you were lonely, neglected, or abused as a child, it can be an immensely difficult journey to seek love and healing within yourself. But it is possible to overcome such a hurtful legacy and reclaim your life. A key is to learn to treat yourself differently now than you were treated then, and to surround yourself with people who see and affirm your worthiness, and in whose presence you can be your whole and loving self. You don't have to continue the legacy of hopelessness that you received, and you don't have to pass it on to your own children. Instead, you can express your uniqueness and discover the healing powers of your own way of loving.

Ernest Hemingway wrote, "The world breaks everyone and afterward many are strong at the broken places." A heart that has been broken is still alive. One of the most healing things you can ever do is to find strength in your wounds and emerge with deeper wisdom, creativity, compassion, and connection to yourself and to others.

If you are able to use your pain for self-transformation rather than self-pity, if you are able to use your loss and grief to awaken new life and compassion within you, then it ceases to matter so much how cold or dysfunctional your parents might have been. If you can be the kind of parent to yourself and to the children in your life that you have always wanted, then you will learn everything you need to know about the healing power of unconditional love.

# 15

## How Then Shall We Live?

*The great tragedy of life is not that men perish, but that they cease to love.*

—W. Somerset Maugham

James W. Prescott is the founder of the Developmental Biology Program of the U.S. National Institutes of Health and Human Development. When he conducted a survey of forty-nine traditional cultures, he found that some took pleasure in killing, torturing, or mutilating their enemies, while others did not. What, he wondered, could account for the difference? The answer, he found, was "physical affection—touching, holding, and carrying." Those societies that inflicted physical punishment on their children produced brutal adults. To put it technically, a low score on the Infant Physical Affection scale correlated with a high rate of adult physical violence.[1]

And Dr. Prescott discovered something else, too. He found that those societies that lavished physical affection on their children produced happy and healthy adults. In such societies, people were more trusting of one another, and their lives were characterized by more pleasure and less violence.

One of the hallmarks of the societies that exemplify healthy aging is that children are loved, held, and cared for constantly. They are rarely if ever scolded or shamed, and the idea of striking a child is completely foreign. Those in modern society who favor corporal punishment of children believe it is necessary to teach them right from wrong. But in these societies where no child is ever hit, children are remarkably well behaved and discipline is almost never a problem. Having been treated with respect, children naturally respect their elders.

Cultures like Abkhasia, Vilcabamba, Hunza, and traditional Okinawa have no need for orphanages. This is not because parents never die. Rather it is because when they do, the children are quickly taken in by other families and by the whole community, who do all they can to be sure that the little ones not only have their basic needs met, but also feel continuously cherished, loved, and upheld.

It seems to be a defining characteristic of societies where healthy aging is the norm that people are rarely if ever abandoned or rejected. When people are in need, be they old or young, they are always taken in and cared for. People who are disabled or who have special needs are never ridiculed, shamed, or isolated, but are helped to participate as they can in everything that goes on. *One of the great secrets of these healthy cultures is that no one is ever made to feel flawed, imperfect, or unworthy of love.*

In modern society, of course, it is not always that way. Abbie Blair tells a story that speaks, I think, to the timeless human longing for a way of life in which no one need fear rejection, in which all are welcomed and all are loved:

I remember the first time I saw Freddie. He was standing in his playpen at the adoption agency where I work. He gave me a toothy grin. What a beautiful baby, I thought.

His boarding mother (the woman at the orphanage responsible for his care) gathered him into her arms. "Will you be able to find a family for Freddie?"

Then I saw it. Freddie was born without arms.

"He's so smart. He's only ten months old, and already he walks and is beginning to talk." She kissed him. "You won't forget him, Mrs. Blair? You will try?"

"I won't forget."

I went upstairs and got out my latest copy of the Hard-to-

Place list. I wrote, "Freddie is a ten-month-old white Protestant boy of English and French background. He has brown eyes, dark-brown hair and fair skin. Freddie was born without arms, but is otherwise in good health. His boarding mother feels he is of superior mentality, and he is already walking and starting to say a few words. Freddie is a warm, affectionate child who has been surrendered by his natural mother and is ready for adoption."

Yes, he's ready all right, I thought. But is there anyone ready for him?

It was 10 o'clock on a lovely late summer morning, and the agency was full of couples—couples interviews, couples meeting babies, families being born. These couples nearly always have the same dream: They want a child as much like themselves as possible, as young as possible, and most important, a child with no problems. "If he develops a problem after we get him," they say, "that is a risk we'll take just like any other parents. But to pick a baby who has a problem, that's too much."

And who can blame them?

I wasn't alone in looking for parents for Freddie. Any of the caseworkers meeting a new couple started with a hope: maybe they were for Freddie. But summer slipped into fall, and Freddie was with us for his first birthday.

And then I found them.

It started out as it always does—a new case, a new Home Study, two people who wanted a child. They were Frances and Edwin Pearson. She was 41. He was 45. She was a housewife. He was a truck driver.

I went to see them. They lived in a tiny white frame house, in a big yard full of sun and old trees. They greeted me together at the door, eager and scared to death.

Mrs. Pearson produced steaming coffee and over-warm cookies. They sat before me on the sofa, close together, holding hands. After a moment, Mrs. Pearson began. "Today is our wedding anniversary. Eighteen years."

"Good years." Mr. Pearson looked at his wife. "Except—"

"Yes," she said. "Except. Always the 'except.'" She looked around the room. "It's too neat," she said. "You know?"

I thought of my own living room with my three children.
Teenagers now. "Yes," I said, "I know."

"Perhaps we're too old?"

I smiled. "You don't think so," I said. "We don't either."

"You always think it will be this month, and then next
month," Mrs. Pearson said. "Examinations. Tests. All kinds of
things. Over and over. But nothing ever happened. You just go on
hoping and hoping, and time keeps slipping by."

"We've tried to adopt before this," Mr. Pearson said. "One
agency told us our apartment was too small, so we got this house.
Then another agency said I didn't make enough money. We had
decided that was it, but this friend told us about you, and we decided to make one last try."

"I'm glad," I said.

Mrs. Pearson glanced at her husband proudly. "Can we
choose at all?" she asked. "A boy for my husband?"

"We'll try for a boy," I said. "What kind of a boy?"

Mrs. Pearson laughed. "How many kinds are there? Just a
boy. My husband is very athletic. He played football in high
school, basketball, too, and track. He would be good for a boy."

Mr. Pearson looked at me. "I know you can't tell exactly," he
said, "but can you give us any idea how soon? We've waited so
long."

I hesitated. There is always this question.

"Next summer, maybe," said Mrs. Pearson. "We could take
him to the beach?"

"That long?" Mr. Pearson said. "Don't you have anyone at
all? There must be a boy somewhere." After a pause, he went on.
"Of course, we can't give him as much as other people. We
haven't a lot of money saved up."

"We've got a lot of love," his wife said. "We've saved up a lot
of that."

"Well," I said cautiously, "there is a little boy. He is thirteen
months old."

"Oh," Mrs. Pearson said, "just a beautiful age."

"I have a picture of him," I said, reaching for my purse. I

handed them Freddie's picture. "He is a wonderful boy," I said. "But he was born without arms."

They studied the picture in silence. He looked at her. "What do you think, Fran?"

"Kickball," said Mrs. Pearson. "You could teach him kick-ball."

"Athletics are not so important," Mr. Pearson said. "He can learn to use his head. Arms he can do without. A head, never. He can go to college. We'll save for it."

"A boy is a boy," Mrs. Pearson insisted. "He needs to play. You can teach him."

"I'll teach him. Arms aren't everything. Maybe we can get him some."

They had forgotten me. But maybe Mr. Pearson was right, I thought. Maybe sometime Freddie could be fitted with artificial arms. He did have nubs where arms should be.

"Then you might like to see him?"

They looked up. "When could we have him?"

"You think you might want him?"

Mrs. Pearson looked at me. "Might?" she said. "Might?"

"We want him," her husband said.

Mrs. Pearson went back to the picture and spoke to it. "You've been waiting for us, haven't you?"

"His name is Freddie," I said, "but you could change it."

"No," said Mrs. Pearson. "Frederick Pearson—it's good to-gether."

There were formalities, of course, and by the time we set the day it was nearly Christmas. I met the Pearsons in the waiting room. "Your son's here already," I told them. "Let's go upstairs and I'll bring him to you."

"I've got butterflies," Mrs. Pearson announced. "Suppose he doesn't like us?"

I put my hand on her arm. "I'll get him."

When I went to get little Freddie, he looked at me intently. "Going home," he said cheerfully. I carried him upstairs to the lit-tle room where the Pearsons were waiting. When I got there, I put him on his feet and opened the door. Freddie stood uncertainly, rocking a little, gazing intently at the two people before him. They drank him in with total acceptance.

Mr. Pearson knelt down. "Freddie, come here. Come to Daddy."

Freddie looked at me for a moment. Then, turning, he walked slowly toward them. "Going home," he said, and they reached out their arms and gathered him in.[2]

## LOVE AND LONELINESS

Stories like the adoption of little Freddie are so profoundly touching because they beckon to some of the deepest callings of the human spirit. They evoke the yearning for a world in which all are cared for, in which no one feels alone, unloved, or unwanted. They remind us that love is the most powerful, magical force in the universe, and remind us of our ability to love unconditionally.

Unfortunately, many in the industrialized world are without caring support in their times of need. Twenty-five percent of American households today consist of one person living alone; half of American marriages end in divorce (affecting tens of millions of children); more than a third of all U.S. births are to unmarried women, many of whom are not in committed relationships.[3] Even within many families and marriages that are intact, there is profound disconnection and loneliness.

There sadly seems to be something about the direction of modern Western civilization itself that undermines a sense of community and makes it harder to sustain positive relationships. A few years ago, when the Unitel Corporation moved a hundred telemarketing jobs out of Frostburg, Maryland, the company's vice president, Ken Carmichael, explained that the move was made because the area's residents weren't pushy enough on the phone. The problem, he said, was "the culture and the climate in western Maryland, one of helping your neighbor and being empathetic and those sorts of things."[4]

The trend toward isolation is taking place all over the industrialized world. Nearly half of all British adults are now unmarried.[5] In Germany, the divorce rate has doubled in the past fifteen years. In

Iceland, the out-of-wedlock birthrate is now 65 percent.[6] I'm sure that to some extent these statistics represent a shakeup of traditional lifestyles, and that many couples who are not married are living together in committed relationships. At the same time, these numbers also suggest the degree of isolation that is seeping into modern life and taking a terrible toll.

In almost every culture in the world, eating dinner together has been a place for families to strengthen bonds. The French in particular have long cherished mealtime as a family ritual, so much so that children have traditionally not been allowed to open the refrigerator between meals. But the days of sitting for hours around the table savoring small portions of several courses and relishing each other's company seem to have passed. Instead, it has become commonplace for the French to eat in front of their television sets, while talking on the telephone, and even alone. As McDonald's has become more popular in France than anywhere else in Europe, the average French meal, which twenty-five years ago lasted 88 minutes, has been reduced to only 38 minutes today.[7]

The French have long been known for their propensity to talk with one another, but according to the French National Bureau of Statistics, the time spent in conversations in France has declined more than 20 percent in just the past ten years. Thousands of French cafés are closing every year. Meanwhile, the number of prescriptions for mood-elevating drugs is now higher in France than anywhere else in the world.[8]

There are clearly forces at work in the modern world that separate us from one another and lead to a sense of alienation. As I've come to appreciate how crucial our relationships with each other are to our health and well-being, I've grown in compassion for the emptiness that besets so many lives. And I've better understood why even people who take excellent care of their diet and exercise can still at times fall prey to illness. The isolation and loneliness of our times are not merely emotional realities. They take a profound toll on every cell in our bodies.

How many of us numb ourselves with cigarettes, tranquilizers, drugs, alcohol, or unhealthful diets in an effort to escape how isolated we feel? How many of us become chronic workaholics or become preoccupied by other unhealthy obsessions in an attempt to avoid the inner barrenness caused by the breakdown of relationships, family, and community?

When a psychologist recorded how many times couples in cafés casually touched each other in an hour, the results were revealing. In some traditional cultures, couples touched each other as many as 180 times per hour. In the United States, on the other hand, couples touched each other only twice per hour. In London, it was zero.[9]

Of course, the issue of touching and personal space is experienced quite differently in different cultures, and this study may not be a reliable indicator of personal connection. But as human beings, we thrive when we get enough positive physical contact, and we wither when we don't. Touch is one of the most basic forms of communication between people.

On October 17, 1995, twin girls were born at Massachusetts Memorial Hospital in Worcester. They were extremely premature, and weighed only two pounds. They were placed in their respective incubators in the newborn intensive care unit. After a week, one was doing well, but the other was struggling with a host of problems including breathing difficulties, troubling blood oxygen levels, and heart rate aberrations. At least one nurse did not expect her to live. But then another hospital nurse, Gayle Kasparian, did something that was against the hospital rules. She placed the babies together in one incubator. Almost immediately, the healthier of the two baby girls wrapped an arm around her sister. When she did, it was as though a miracle had happened. The smaller baby's blood oxygen saturation levels, which had been frighteningly low, began to rise. As her breathing improved, her frantic movements subsided, her heart rate stabilized, and her temperature returned to normal. In the days and weeks that followed, she continued to improve and thrive. The doctors later said the turning point was clearly when the twins were placed together.[10]

In the years since, the cobedding of premature twins has thankfully become standard practice in more and more hospitals.

Another technique that has been found to be extremely helpful with premature infants is called "kangaroo care." The practice involves prolonged skin-to-skin contact between parent and infant, and has repeatedly been shown to have critical benefits for the little ones, producing better digestion, a steadier heart rate, improved breathing, greater contentment, and deeper sleep.

Of course, it's common sense to recognize that babies need to be held and touched. But it's not just babies. I don't think we ever outgrow the need for affectionate and respectful human contact. One of the most insightful and effective therapists I've had the pleasure to know, Virginia Satir, used to say that regardless of your age, "four hugs a day are necessary for survival, eight are good for maintenance, and twelve for growth."

Among the exceptionally healthy and long-lived peoples of the world, touching, hugging, and other forms of respectful and affectionate contact are common daily experiences throughout all phases of their lives.

Of course, these peoples still experience psychological and social struggles. They have their share of hardships, and sometimes more than their share. But they do not undergo the kind of debilitating loneliness and social turmoil that are unfortunately becoming increasingly prevalent today in the West. When they suffer, they can count on the support and friendship of others who know them deeply and are concerned for them. They have friends, neighbors, and relatives who will smile at them when they are sad, reach out to them when they feel most alone, and care for them as they age.

## ELDERS ALONE

The more I've come to understand how important caring relationships are to healthy aging, the more my heart goes out to those elders who do not have a web of connectedness with others to draw on for support. Though it is not impossible, I see how difficult it can be in modern Western culture to begin creating meaningful relationships late in life. It can be a painful and lonely experience to be old and alone, with no one who knew you before.

In New Jersey recently, an 84-year-old man died alone in his apartment. His rent, cable TV, phone, gas, and electric bill payments continued to be automatically deducted from his bank account. This went on for more than two years without anyone's realizing he had died, until a neighbor had a visit from a blind woman with a Seeing Eye dog and the dog's behavior alerted them that something was amiss next door, leading to the discovery of the man's body.

While this is an extreme instance, it is regrettably not a cultural anomaly. Today, a painfully high percentage of American elders live alone, spending their hours and days watching TV by themselves. Many residents of nursing homes go years without seeing a child. Their only human contact may be other old people and their caregivers. They may feel that they mean nothing to anyone, that no one loves them and that their love doesn't matter to anyone. Meanwhile a small but sadly growing number of American children have never met their grandparents. There is something very wrong with this picture.

And it's not just the United States. Italy has long been renowned as a family-centered society. But in 2005, Italian physicians said that thousands of Italian grandparents had spent a lonely Christmas in hospitals because their families did not want them at home. Roberto Messina, head of a Rome-based charity for elderly people, spoke of the pain experienced by elders who know they are unwanted. "The saddest thing is when an old person remains alone during visiting hours," he said. "They pull the covers up, close their eyes and pretend to be asleep, but in reality they are crying and clenching their teeth."

The loneliness of elders in the modern world today is sometimes so profound that they literally die of broken hearts. In the world's most long-lived and healthy societies, on the other hand, elders are never shut away from the unfolding of life. Instead, they are part of extended families and continually have opportunities for mutually nourishing contact with younger generations. In Okinawa, sibling rivalries can become most heated over who will get to take care of their aging parents.

An elder Abkhasian woman who was famous for knowing many curses was asked what was the most terrifying curse that can be placed on a human being. Her answer, the worst curse she could imagine, was this: "Let there be no old folks in your house to give you wise counsel, and no young people to heed their advice."[11]

## GENERATIONS TOGETHER

Although I did not know my own grandparents very well, I consider myself extremely fortunate now to live in a harmonious three-generation household. Not everyone in the contemporary world has this opportunity, of course, and I feel grateful to have so much compatibility and alignment among the members of my current family. I live with my wife, Deo (we've been married forty years), our 33-year-old son, Ocean, his wife of thirteen years, Michele, and their twin five-year-old sons, River and Bodhi. We all feel greatly enriched by the arrangement. Deo and I do not think of Michele as our daughter-in-law, but as our daughter-in-love. We couldn't love her more if she were our biological daughter.

I'm sure that raising twins is a handful and a half in the first place, but River and Bodhi were born two and a half months premature and have had many special needs. You've probably heard the expression that it takes a village to raise a child. In this kind of situation, I sometimes think we need two villages.

But with four "parents" in the house, and many friends who also help out, we seek to provide the little guys with as much undivided attention and unconditional love as we can. Deo and I both love playing with the twins, and Deo, in particular, puts in a terrific number of hours, for which Michele and Ocean are tremendously grateful. They both work from a home office, and are co-presidents of an extraordinary nonprofit organization (www.yesworld.org).

One day, Michele was reflecting on how thankful she felt to Deo and me, and how glad she is that we are here. Thinking about the huge number of hours that Deo devotes to the twins, Michele told her, "I can't believe how much money you're saving us in child care."

Deo shot me a quick smile that spoke volumes about how she didn't want Michele to feel indebted, and how greatly she always enjoys taking care of the little fellows. Then she turned to Michele and said, "That's one way to look at it. But do you have any idea how much it would cost if we had to go out and rent grandchildren?"

## CELEBRATING THE ELDERLY

Although our living arrangement—three generations under one roof—is unusual in the United States today, it is actually very common in many tribal and traditional societies. In Okinawa, Abkhasia, Vilcabamba, and Hunza, great value is placed on extended families, marriage, and children. The generations are not artificially separated, and people at every stage of life feel a part of things and have something to contribute. Grandparents, still sprightly and spirited, romp with the new generation of babies. Great-grandparents also help out with the children and enjoy the respect of younger generations. As they get even older, people are always cared for and are never left to fend for themselves.

One of the most defining features of the cultures known for the health of their elders is a profound respect for the elderly, and a commitment that all members of society—particularly those who are most vulnerable—should be as well taken care of as possible. The elder Okinawans believe that if someone fails, whether through bad luck or any other reason, there is an obligation on the part of others to help. Indeed, they have a proverb that translates as "One cannot live in this world without the support of others."

In Okinawa, the elderly are provided with excellent medical care and many other benefits at minimal cost. When I spoke to one Okinawan man in his late eighties, he told me why he thought this was a good idea: "Sure, I'm for helping the elderly. It's only right. And besides," he added with a twinkle in his eye, "I'm going to be old myself someday."

Another elderly Okinawan told me she was struck by the contrast between the way elders are treated in Okinawa and what she has learned of how they are sometimes treated in the West. "Of course we live long lives," she said. "We love life. Who wouldn't want to grow old in a place like this?"

In every culture where healthy aging is the norm, elders are revered. Not only are they fully included in the society, they are honored and celebrated. When Okinawan elders reach the age of ninety-seven, a major celebration takes place (called *kajimaya*), where people gather to honor them, rejoice in their lives, and affirm their return to having the free spirit of a child.

It has been said that the moral test of a people is how they treat those who are in the dawn of life—the children—and those who are in the twilight of life—the elderly. By this standard, the societies that have produced the greatest and most vibrant life expectancies have something profound indeed to teach us.

# STEPS YOU CAN TAKE

Each of us has our own unique ways of expressing love and building meaningful relationships. Here are some tips to help you create and sustain positive connections in your life.

---

- Be kind. You do not need to know what burdens others are carrying to know that they are heavy.
- No matter how great the faults of another person, strive to be aware also of his or her good qualities. Know that there is something worthy of commendation in almost everyone, even though it may lie dormant and as yet undiscovered.

---

- Make time for hearing your loved ones' struggles and challenges. When a friend speaks, listen with your heart rather than your judgment. You may not be able to take away another's pain, but you can hear it. Afterward, write them a card or bring them a flower to acknowledge and thank them for entrusting you with their vulnerability as well as their strength.
- If you are dealing with an illness or personal struggle that may be shared by others, join (or start) a support group where you can meet regularly to talk about your challenges, fears, hopes, and dreams among others who will understand.

- Look for opportunities to enrich the lives of others. Ask a friend if there's a way you could be a better friend to him.
- Recall someone who helped you when you needed it. Write or tell her of your appreciation. Recognize someone in your extended family or community who has provided outstanding service. Make a certificate or plaque he can put on his wall, or send her a note with flowers or food.
- For emotionally significant communications, don't use e-mail. Meet in person, talk on the phone, or write letters that you can mail or hand-deliver. People love getting letters. It can be rare to get anything special in the mail anymore.
- Learn the art of massage, so you can use your hands to touch others with healing and respect.
- Give and receive hugs daily. Lots of them.

---

- Rather than buying gifts for friends and family, give experiences. Massage their neck and shoulders. Write them poems or letters expressing your appreciation and love. Take them for a walk, clean their house, make them dinner, babysit, help them plant a spring garden, plan a picnic or other special outing to enjoy together, take them for a day exploring back country roads or an evening of theater, or find some other creative way to express your affection and caring. If you have just a minute, call and leave a message letting them know that you are thinking of them, or mention a specific quality or experience you are remembering and appreciating about them.
- Read selections from your favorite books to your family and friends. Give away copies of your favorite books. Tell others what these books have meant to you.

---

- If you want to change the way you feel about someone, change the way you treat him (or her).
- Remember that love is necessary for great relationships, but it is not sufficient. Great relationships don't just happen because you're in love. They take work, and lots of it.

- Beware of the temptation to take others, especially your spouse or intimate partner, for granted. Rather than using your relationship for convenience, use it to become a more loving person.
- Step back every now and then and take an objective look at your own behavior. If someone important to you is being defensive, ask whether you are doing anything to make them so.
- Listen before you react to anger. Look for solutions that benefit everyone.
- Nurture the friendships with which you feel at ease. Move on from those that take enormous energy and stress to maintain.
- Respect people for who they are, not for the roles they play.

―――

- Read a story to an elder who can no longer see fine print. Record your reading on tape so they can play it back and listen whenever they wish. Help an older neighbor with home tasks, such as washing windows, shoveling snow, or painting. If there is a pet in the house, offer to take the dog for a walk, clean the cat's litter box, or shop for pet food and supplies.
- Be the coach or friend or teacher who notices a child's efforts and says "Good job." Be the older friend who sees that a child is capable of more than his behavior indicates, and lifts him toward his higher potential by helping him to show good manners, kindness to others, and responsible behavior. Be the family member who is honest with a child and in so doing reminds him or her how to be truthful. Be the teacher who validates the inner life of children by asking for their ideas and opinions about topics that are important to them. Be the eccentric relative who shows a child that it is okay to be just who he or she is.
- If you don't have a young person in your life, go to your nearby day-care center and offer to read a book or help out there. Volunteer to rock babies at your local hospital. Take kids from your neighborhood on a nature hike. Walk a child to or from school.
- Express your caring for children who are not your own. Take neighboring kids to the library when you take your own child. Provide them with healthful snacks and an accepting ear, remembering how much it matters to be listened to.

- Gather with others to gain support in taking steps toward more loving relationships. Meet regularly, and decide together at each meeting on the step or steps that you will each take before the next meeting. Share both the difficulties you encounter and the successes you experience.
- Learn from people who are different from you. Greet them with true curiosity, knowing that you can stay true to yourself no matter what the differences. Do not let differences of opinion become causes of estrangement.
- Tell others what you appreciate about them. Make sure each of your friends knows that there is something special about them that you cherish. Write them cards or letters so they have something to help them remember that you value them.
- Bake extra and share. Bring good food to people who are in transition, stress, or crisis. A few times a month, double what you are making for dinner and take the extra to someone who is having an especially busy or difficult time. It doesn't have to be a complete meal—just something that lessens her load and reminds her that she is in your heart.

PART

5

THE

HUMAN

SPIRIT

# 16

## Breaking Free from the Cultural Trance

*It is no measure of health to be well adjusted to a profoundly sick
society.*

—Jiddu Krishnamurti

Today, the term "culture" is widely understood to refer to the systematic body of learned behavior which is transmitted to children from parents, schools, and communities. But not that long ago,
this concept was part of the vocabulary of only a small and technical
group of professional anthropologists. It had not yet been widely recognized that from the moment of our births, the customs into which
we are born exert an enormous influence on our experience and behavior.

This changed with the work of one of the world's most renowned
anthropologists, the bestselling author Ruth Benedict. According to
her student, friend, and colleague, Margaret Mead, Ruth Benedict's
work is the main reason that the words "in our culture" have come
to be widely used and understood. It is largely thanks to her that we
have come to understand how profoundly we are shaped by the cultures in which we live.

In his book *A Language Older Than Words,* Derrick Jensen describes how Ruth Benedict sought to understand why some cultures
are fundamentally peaceful and healthy while others are not, why

women, children, and the aged are treated well in some cultures while in others they are not, and why some cultures are cooperative while others are competitive.[1] Based on her study of more than seven hundred societies, Benedict perceived a single pattern that seemed to explain all these variations.

At one end of the continuum, she found what she called "synergistic" societies. In these cultures, behaviors that benefit the whole group are rewarded, while behaviors that harm the group as a whole are forbidden. Generosity and compassion are esteemed, while hoarding is considered shameful, and so wealth is continuously circulated through the community and not allowed to accumulate in any one person's hands. In these societies, she wrote, "if a man has meat or garden produce or horses or cattle, these give him no standing except as they pass through his hands to the tribe at large."[2] Such cultures, she said, tend to be harmonious, peaceful, healthy, and respectful of women, children, and the elderly. Individual members tend to be happy, secure, and trusting.

In these communities, children are taught to share from early in childhood. Jack Kornfield tells of a Native American ceremony in which young children are showered with food, drink, and clothing. Then members of the tribe cry out, "I'm hungry, I'm thirsty, I'm cold." From their abundance, the children are then led to distribute their bounty to others in need. Through such games, children are taught to hold the needs of the other members of their tribe to be as important as their own.

At the far opposite end of the continuum, however, Ruth Benedict found what she called "surly and nasty" cultures. In these cultures, behaviors that benefit individuals at the expense of the whole are rewarded, and those who amass wealth are esteemed. People in such societies, she found, tend to be "paranoid, mean-spirited, warlike, and abusive toward women, children and the elderly." Individual members of such societies tend to view each other as competitors or threats, to think exclusively about their own interests, and to be self-aggrandizing, insecure, suspicious, and hostile. Wealth is concentrated in the hands of the very few.

## WEALTH DISTRIBUTION AND HUMAN HEALTH

I once believed that the wealthier a society, the better would be the health of its citizens. And it's certainly true that worldwide today, those nations whose annual per capita income is below about $5,000 to $10,000 often suffer from poor sanitation and malnutrition and have the poorest health. But studies have consistently found that above that threshold, the health of nations is no longer a matter of absolute income, but is actually more a matter of the gap between the rich and the poor. Above that point, *the larger the gap between rich and poor, the less health will prevail.*[3]

Societies in which the pie gets divided in such a way that everyone gets a decent share are healthier because as well as having their basic needs met, people tend to participate in their community, trust others, and cooperate for mutual benefit. They form friendships. They care for one another. Their relationships are marked by support, trust, and sociability.

Of all nations today, Japan has the greatest life expectancy of any nation on earth (and Okinawa has for many years had the greatest life expectancy in all of Japan). How, you may wonder, does Japan manage this stellar health (which is all the more remarkable given the very high level of smoking in Japan)? A key factor may be that Japan today is economically the most equitable of all the world's affluent nations.

It hasn't always been this way. Prior to World War II, wealth distribution in Japan was harshly unequal, and life expectancy rates were hardly better than those of impoverished third-world countries. After the war, though, things began to change when General Douglas MacArthur was given the task of overseeing the nation's reconstruction. MacArthur had his faults, but he has been called "the greatest population health doctor who ever lived" by Stephen Bezruchka, M.D., who has written extensively on the medical consequences of wealth inequality.[4]

MacArthur required three fundamental things of the Japanese. First was demilitarization—Japan was forbidden to have an army. Second was democratization—his staff created the constitution that is in use in Japan to this day, providing for a representative democracy, free universal education, the right of labor unions to organize and engage in collective bargaining, the right of women to vote, and the right of everyone to a decent life. And the third was decentralization—MacArthur broke up the family dynasties that ran the huge corporations that had controlled the country. He mandated a maximum wage for business and corporate leaders. He also carried out the most successful land reform program in history. Land was purchased from landlords who had amassed huge holdings, then sold to the tenants at the same price. The tenants were given thirty-year interest-free loans to make the purchase. Essentially, he leveled the playing field. His reforms were followed by the most rapid rise in health and longevity ever documented in any major country in world history.

From a highly stratified prewar society, postwar Japan became a nation that cherished egalitarianism. When the economy ran into trouble in the early 1990s, Japanese bosses and managers took cuts in pay rather than lay off workers. As recently as 2000, the prime minister of Japan made only four times what an average worker made, and bosses made only ten times what entry-level workers made.

When Japanese prime minister Junichiro Koizumi took office in 2001, however, he initiated Reagan-like policies of spending cuts, privatization, deregulation, and tax breaks for the wealthy. As a result the gap between rich and poor, long held in check, began to grow. But still, very few Japanese wanted to see a society divided into winners and losers. The nation's major daily newspapers ran articles with titles like "Divided Japan" and "Light and Darkness," decrying policies that favored the rich at the expense of the average Japanese. Even Prime Minister Koizumi said that "Winners and losers shouldn't be trapped in those categories. If someone loses once, he should be given a second chance."

## MEANWHILE, IN THE UNITED STATES . . .

In the United States, however, things have taken a different course since World War II. At the end of the war, there were very few homeless people on U.S. streets. Even as late as 1970, homelessness in America was still rare. But since that time economic inequality in this country has grown immensely.[5] In 1998 one American (Bill Gates) achieved the dubious distinction of amassing more wealth than the combined net worth of the poorest 45 percent of U.S. households.[6] Today, many corporate executives earn more money in a couple of hours than the average factory worker makes in a year.[7] The wealthiest 1 percent of America's population owns more wealth than the bottom 90 percent combined.[8] And meanwhile, the minimum wage in the United States, adjusted for inflation, has fallen by 37 percent since 1968, and become the lowest of any industrialized nation.

This gap has had devastating health consequences. Forty-five million Americans do not have even the most basic health insurance, and many millions more are seriously underinsured. Many Americans face the risk of financial ruin and even premature death because they can't pay their medical bills. And of course, it's the poor who are hit the hardest. Today, an African American man in Harlem has a lower life expectancy than a man in Bangladesh, one of the world's most monetarily poor countries.[9]

With less than 5 percent of the world's population, the United States now accounts for nearly 50 percent of the world's spending on healthcare. Yet the United States ranks only 26th in life expectancy, and 28th in infant mortality.[10] It may be happenstance, but not a single one of the 25 countries that have longer life expectancies than the United States, nor a single one of the 27 countries that have better infant mortality rates, has as wide a wealth gap between its richest and poorest citizens.

History shows that wherever inequality of wealth distribution becomes extreme, people tend to become divided against one another, and societies tend to spend less on public health, education, and social safety nets. Large numbers of people feel chronically left out, powerless, anxious, angry, and afraid. In such societies, everyone— whether they are "haves" or "have-nots"—tends to become less trusting of their neighbors and less inclined to help others. The result is higher crime rates, increased violence, and higher rates of heart disease, depression, and many other debilitating and deadly ailments *for both rich and poor.*

Is it a coincidence that the countries ranked first and second in the world in terms of wealth equality (Japan and Sweden) are also ranked first and second in life expectancy? And is it a coincidence that the United States, which ranks last among all industrialized countries in terms of wealth equality, now ranks nearly last in life expectancy?

In the 1990s, no state in the United States generated more wealth than California. Both Silicon Valley, the epicenter of the computer industry, and Hollywood, the center stage of the world's entertainment industry, were generating new millionaires by the minute. But instead of circulating through the culture, this wealth was concentrating in the hands of an ever smaller portion of the population. The richest 1 percent of Californians now earn more per year than the bottom 60 percent combined.

Ruth Benedict found that, in cultures which value wealth accumulation more than they value wealth sharing, the wealthy tend to be less interested in the well-being of those who are less fortunate. True to her point, many of California's wealthy have tended to wall themselves off behind gated communities and barred windows and have been more inclined to spend public funds to build prisons than to improve social conditions. In an eerie mirror image, the two hottest areas in California's construction industry since 1990 have been the building of gated residential communities and the building of prisons.

Despite the valiant efforts of many concerned citizens and organizations, including the Oakland, California–based Ella Baker Center's "Books Not Bars" campaign (which advocates spending more money on lifting kids up than on locking them up), the state now has the highest youth incarceration rate in the country. There are now five times as many African American men in California prisons as there are in California state universities.

The consequences to public health have also been tragic. California used to rank near the top of the nation in health statistics, but this is unfortunately no longer the case. The state now has one of the nation's highest percentages of families without health insurance. Children living in poor neighborhoods often have no safe place to play. High rates of violent crime and infectious disease coexist with one of the nation's lowest levels of spending on public health.

Half the adults in some California cities today suffer from hypertension.[11] Three-quarters of California's children do not meet the state's minimum standards for physical fitness.[12] California has the world's fifth largest economy, but its citizens are experiencing what can happen when accumulation for the few takes precedence over the well-being of the many.

## THE TOLL

When much of society's wealth is in the hands of a small minority, the vast majority of people are left with little recourse but to spend their precious time and energy in the continuous pursuit of financial resources. This takes a toll on the health of communities, marriages, and families that is difficult to exaggerate. Many couples have little quality time with each other, and many parents have tragically little time with their children.

I have a friend, a psychotherapist, who is a single mother. Living in California where housing costs have skyrocketed in recent years, she has to work very long hours to make ends meet. One day her eight-year-old son became so frustrated with her unavailability that he said, "If I save my allowance and give it all to you, then will you have time to listen to me?"

Many of us in the hyper-competitive modern world have become so used to not having enough time for our relationships that it is hard for us to grasp what has been lost. In the world's healthiest and longest-lived cultures, relationships are held to be of primary importance. When someone is in need, others provide whenever possible. People do not lock their doors when they leave their homes. It is expected that a visitor who finds the house empty will come in and help themselves to a meal while waiting for the family to return.

If a theft occurs, it is a rare and unusual event. In many modern cities, in contrast, if a day goes by without a murder it is a remarkable occurrence.

There are of course many wonderful and hopeful things about the modern world, and I am by no means suggesting that the way to solve our problems is to abandon the quest for material progress. But I believe J.R.R. Tolkien had a point when he said, "If more of us valued food and cheer and song above hoarded gold, it would be a merrier world."

## GROSS DOMESTIC HAPPINESS

The gross domestic product (GDP) is now routinely used throughout the industrialized world as a fundamental measure of a nation's level of success. It is taken for granted that the higher the GDP, the better a country is doing. This use of the GDP has become so ubiquitous that people often don't realize there are alternatives. Unbeknownst to many of us, the small Himalayan kingdom of Bhutan has been taking a very different path, with remarkable results.

Roughly the size of Switzerland, Bhutan is the only independent Buddhist monarchy in the world, and the only country in the world that practices the Tantric form of Mahayana Buddhism as its official religion. In April 1987, Bhutan's young monarch, King Jigme Singye Wangchuck, was interviewed by the *Financial Times*. Asked about his nation's economic development, which was among the world's lowest, he replied, "Gross National Happiness is more important than Gross Domestic Product."[13]

Though Bhutan has its problems,[14] King Wangchuck's statement was not an idle remark. Under his leadership, Bhutan has made Gross National Happiness its official index for evaluating development. As a result, the guiding principles of all Bhutanese policies have been to ensure that prosperity is shared across society, that cultural traditions are honored, the environment is protected, and the government is kept responsive to the real needs of the people. While economists in the West have scoffed at the king's ideas, calling them naïve idealism, the results speak for themselves.

Though household incomes remain among the world's lowest, the people of Bhutan have created one of the world's most intriguing societies. The nation has more monks than soldiers, not a single traffic light or mall, and a profound commitment to education. Forty years ago, Bhutan had no public education system, now there are schools at all levels throughout the country. The literacy rate, which was less than 10 percent as recently as the early nineties, now tops 50 percent and continues to increase rapidly.

When the current king took the throne in 1972, there was not a single sanitary hospital in the country. Now, all Bhutanese subjects have access to free healthcare. People entering hospitals with nonacute problems can choose Western or traditional medicine. Government policies ensure that people have a great deal of free time with their families, including maternity leaves. The elderly are provided for both by their extended families and by pension programs provided by the government. In 2005, Bhutan became the first nation in the world to impose a national ban on the sale of tobacco and on smoking in public places.[15]

As Buddhists, the Bhutanese don't kill animals for food. (If a cow dies naturally, though, they will eat it.) Most of their meals are centered on red rice, accompanied by chili peppers and other vegetables, all home-grown, with occasional cheese from local cows. There is not a single McDonald's, Burger King, KFC, or Pizza Hut in the entire country.[16]

Perhaps the most remarkable part of Bhutan's commitment to Gross National Happiness is a stunning dedication to preserving the country's natural resources. While the forests of all its neighboring countries have been decimated in recent years, Bhutan retains the highest original forest cover of any nation on earth.[17] The hunting of animals is prohibited, as is fishing in the rivers. Livestock grazing, logging, and mining are strictly controlled and limited. Plastic bags are banned, as are two-stroke engines. There are stringent fuel-quality laws. The nation has an annual holiday to honor the king, but instead of pomp and parades, he has declared the holiday Social Forestry Day, and the people now spend the day planting trees. Consistent with the Buddhist doctrine of respect for all life, a constitution is currently being written which gives inalienable rights to wildlife and trees as well as to people.[18]

How has all this affected the health of the people? In a stunningly short time, the nation has experienced one of the most dramatic increases in life expectancy in world history. In 1984, life expectancy in Bhutan was 47 years. Only fourteen years later, in 1998, it had leaped to 66 years.[19]

## WHERE OUR REAL RICHES LIE

The Bhutanese would understand the Abkhasian proverb "When money speaks, the truth is silent." In the modern West, on the other hand, we've had popular TV shows like *Lifestyles of the Rich and Famous* that glorify conspicuous consumption. I've known people who like to drive around town pointing out the most expensive homes and cars. And I've seen how this kind of preoccupation affects the way they treat people. When they meet someone for the first time, they seek to assess the person's economic status, and their behavior toward that person changes according to their appraisal. Those judged to be upper class are treated with deference, while those viewed as lower class are regarded with indifference.

It is a poignant sign of our times that the largest-selling board game in the world today is Monopoly, in which the goal is to bankrupt your opponents and amass all wealth unto yourself. More than two hundred million Monopoly sets have been sold, and the game is currently produced in twenty-six languages.

We are complex people, we human beings. There is a little bit of Donald Trump in each of us, and that part of ourselves is often rewarded and reinforced in a society that measures success primarily in material terms. But there is also a little bit of Mother Teresa in us. Each of us—including, I'm sure, Donald Trump himself—has a place that understands the greater importance of our relationships with other people, with our own spirits, and with life itself.

I wonder what would happen if instead of glorifying those who excel at getting, we gave our applause and esteem to those who excel at giving? What if we recognized the many courageous people who work day in and day out not just to make the biggest buck, but to make the world a better place?

To my eyes, the people who are truly wealthy are not those whose bank accounts are the largest, but those who find something precious in every moment and rejoice in the opportunities they have to contribute to the lives of others.

Such people, whether they know it or not, are carrying on the traditions of the Abkhasians, the Vilcabambans, the Hunzans, the Okinawans, and many other peoples who have understood what extraordinary resources we can be for one another, and who use whatever financial wealth they have to make a difference in the lives of others. As one Okinawan woman told me, "Some people have more money than others. If you have more, it's so you can use it to help those who don't. If we can't help one another, then what's the point?"

## MY ROCKY ROAD

My father (Irv Robbins) and my uncle (Burt Baskin) founded and owned an ice cream company. Starting from nothing, they were extraordinarily successful. Baskin-Robbins (31 Flavors) became the world's largest ice cream company, with many thousands of stores worldwide, and annual sales measured in the billions of dollars. We had an ice-cream-cone-shaped swimming pool in our backyard, my pets were named after ice cream flavors, and I ate countless gallons of ice cream. When people nowadays hear that I no longer eat ice cream, they sometimes feel sorry for me. "Please don't," I tell them. "I ate enough ice cream during my childhood for twenty lifetimes." Sometimes I ate ice cream for breakfast.

It was my father's dream that I would someday join him in running the business, and from my earliest childhood he set about grooming me to follow in his footsteps. Like almost every child, I loved ice cream. But when my uncle Burt Baskin was only fifty-one years old, he died of a heart attack. A large man, he had always enjoyed the family product. I asked my dad if he thought the amount of ice cream my uncle ate might have contributed to his fatal heart attack. "No," my father said. "His ticker just got tired and stopped working."

I understand why my father would not have wanted to consider the possibility that ice cream might have been involved. By this point he had manufactured and sold more ice cream than any human being who had ever lived on this planet. He didn't want to think that ice cream was harming anyone, much less that it might have contributed to the death of his beloved brother-in-law and partner. Besides, not much was commonly known then, in the late 1960s, about the connection between ice cream and disease.

But I saw the connection, as I did when my dad developed diabetes and high blood pressure, and again years later when Ben

Cohen, co-founder of the ice cream company Ben & Jerry's, needed a quintuple bypass procedure at the age of forty-nine.

A single ice cream cone, of course, isn't going to harm anyone. But even though it tastes delicious, ice cream is very high in sugar and saturated fat. The medical data is overwhelmingly clear that the more sugar and saturated fat you eat, the more likely you are to experience heart disease and diabetes and to become obese.

My father had achieved the American dream. But I was called forth by a different longing. Having enough money so that you can meet your basic needs is necessary and important, but there are other things that also matter a great deal. I wanted to see if I could be part of making the world a healthier place. I wanted my steps to be guided by a reverence for life.

Along with many Americans in the 1960s, I was part of the civil rights movement. I marched and worked with Dr. Martin Luther King, Jr., and I loved and admired him immensely. When this apostle of peace and love was murdered, I felt as though a bullet had gone through my heart, too.

Along with Dr. King and many other Americans, I abhorred the violence and insanity of the war in Vietnam. Only a few months after Dr. King was killed, another man whom many of us viewed as a bringer of hope, Robert F. Kennedy, was also assassinated. These were very dark times, and I was filled with despair. In a world that seemed increasingly adrift in violence, cynicism, hopelessness, and fear, I wanted desperately to find a path to sanity and love. I wanted to be part of a fundamental global transformation, and although I didn't know exactly how to go about a task so huge and idealistic, I did know that, for me, making and selling ice cream was not part of it.

I did not find it easy, however, to explain my thoughts and feelings to my father, a conservative businessman who was proud of the many things his great wealth enabled him to buy, and who never to my knowledge went a day without reading *The Wall Street Journal*. He had come of age during the Great Depression of the 1930s, while I was becoming an adult in the 1960s. Our lives were shaped by very different times.

"It's a different world now than when you grew up," I told him.

"The environment is deteriorating rapidly under the impact of human activities. Every two seconds a child somewhere dies of hunger while elsewhere there are abundant resources going to waste. The gap between the rich and the poor is increasing. We live now under a nuclear shadow, and at any moment the unspeakable could happen. Can you see that inventing a thirty-second flavor would not be an adequate response for my life?"

This was very difficult for my father. Having worked hard his whole life, he had attained an extraordinary level of financial success, and he very much wanted to share his achievements with his only son. He thought I was being hopelessly idealistic, and he warned me sternly that idealists end up poor and miserable. But I did not feel drawn to the life he wanted me to follow. Whether it was hopelessly idealistic or not, I wanted to be part of the effort to bring about a more compassionate and healthy world. I felt called to take a stand for a thriving, just, and sustainable way of life for all.

Under the circumstances, I decided that the most courageous and life-affirming thing to do was to walk away from the family business and to leave behind all connection to my family's fortune. This felt like the most honest and liberating choice I could make. It was a choice for my integrity.

It was not a choice, however, that my father could then understand. Sadly, it was a source of distance in our relationship. He did not appreciate the path I was taking, and could not grasp why I would refuse the golden opportunity he was offering me.

I hated disappointing him, but I had to be true to myself. In 1969, my wife, Deo, and I moved to a remote part of a little island off the coast of British Columbia, Canada, where we built a one-room log cabin in which we lived for the next ten years. We grew most of our own food, and our gardens were totally organic. The money we needed came from the yoga and meditation classes I taught. We were financially poor, in many years spending less than a thousand dollars, but we didn't need a lot. We were profoundly in love. Our time was our own. And we were learning a lot about growing food, about healing, and about ourselves.

In 1973, four years into our time on the island, our son, Ocean, was born, at home and into my hands. As he grew up we continued to spend very little money, so that we could have time for each other and the other things that mattered to us. We understood what Thoreau meant by "I make myself rich by making my wants few." We celebrated simplicity.

As Ocean grew up I naturally had expectations for him, but more important to me than whether he lived up to them was that he be able to listen to himself well enough to know when my expectations were in alignment with his destiny and when they were not. The last thing I wanted to do was to tyrannize him with my own fears and unfulfilled wishes. What mattered was not whether he disappointed me, but that he not betray his own soul.

Eventually we moved back to California, and several of my books about healing ourselves and healing our world became bestsellers, giving us some measure of financial security. The press took to calling me things like "the rebel without a cone" and "the prophet of nonprofit."

Meanwhile, my father, on account of his diabetes and high blood pressure, was beginning to make major changes in his diet. Gradually he gave up eating ice cream or any other form of sugar, and he greatly decreased his intake of meat. As a result, his health improved dramatically. He liked reminding me that he was "not a card-carrying vegetarian," but he was beginning to have far more respect for the lifestyle choices I had made and the work I was doing.

A year or so after my grandtwins were born, my parents, now in their mid-eighties, came to visit us and stayed for a few days. They saw our three-generation household living together in ways that they were not accustomed to. They watched as we all shared in the joys and challenges of caring for the babies, and saw how we sought to respond to the little ones' special needs with patience and kindness.

The babies, who had been born extremely prematurely, had spent nearly the first two months of their lives in a hospital's neonatal intensive care unit, and they had come home from the hospital fragile and terrified of life. Babies born that early are often exceedingly touch-averse. We had been warned by doctors that they might never respond normally to human contact. Our response was to hold the little ones in continuous skin-to-skin contact with us virtually twenty-four hours a day, even allowing them to sleep on our bodies at night. My parents—who were products of a time when beliefs prevailed like "Spare the rod and you'll spoil the child" and "Don't pick up babies or you'll spoil them"—saw how we provided the babies with endless opportunities for physical connection. And they observed the results—the twins were growing into joyful, curious little guys who loved being cuddled.

I expected it to be difficult for my parents to see the very different way we were raising these little ones, and also for them to see how in our home the men as well as the women changed diapers, cleaned house, and made the meals. Perhaps because they were nearing the end of their lives, they seemed more accepting of our differences than I had experienced them before. I didn't realize, though, how deep the acceptance went.

At one point, my father took me aside. "When you left Baskin-Robbins," he reminisced, "I thought you were crazy."

"Yes," I replied. "I remember."

"Well," he said, speaking more slowly now and turning to face me, "I see that time has proved you were right to follow your own star."

Hearing him speak this way, I felt for the first time his blessing on my life. And when the time came for them to leave, my mother, too, said something I had never before heard her say. "You may not be rich in material things," she told us, "but it's obvious that you are rich in love." She took a deep breath. "And in the long run, that is actually more important."

## WHAT MATTERS

Although the possibility that love is what matters most in a human life and is the source of our greatest healing may seem out of step with the modern drive to become rich and famous, it is really quite an ancient understanding. The columnist Rochelle Pennington retells an old story:

> The wives who lived within the walls of the Weinsberg Castle in Germany were well aware of the riches it held: gold, silver, jewels, and wealth beyond belief.

Then the day came in 1141 A.D. when all their treasure was threatened. An enemy army had surrounded the castle and demanded the fortress, the fortune, and the lives of the men within. There was nothing to do but surrender.

Although the conquering commander had set a condition for the safe release of all women and children, the wives of Weinsberg refused to leave without having one of their conditions met, as well. They demanded that they be allowed to fill their arms with as many possessions as they could carry out with them. Knowing that the women couldn't possibly make a dent in the massive fortune, their request was honored.

When the castle gates opened, the army outside was brought to tears. Each woman carried out her husband.[20]

## THE OLDEST CULTURE ON EARTH

Of all the world's cultures, those that have endured the longest are those that have placed the highest value on human relationships, like the African Pygmies. The late Jean-Pierre Hallet, an internationally renowned ethnologist and the world's leading authority on the African Pygmies, described how easily and openly the Efé Pygmies of central Africa express their caring for one another, and the great amount of touching and affection he continually saw expressed among all the Pygmies.[21] Babies and small children are continuously held and carried. Older children and adults often touch one another. He was struck by how much the Pygmies cuddle, how frequently they hold hands or sit with an arm around a friend or place their head in another's lap.

A central understanding in the Pygmy world is that we are made for companionship and relationship. If food is scarce, the first to be fed are the children and the elders—those who are most vulnerable. After studying their religion in considerable depth, Hallet concluded that "the whole substance and meaning of the Pygmy religion is 'Be good to other people. Respect, protect and preserve.' "

Every anthropologist or ethnologist who has lived within Pygmy society has been deeply moved by their gentleness and family devotion. In Pygmy society, all children are cherished, and boys and girls are valued equally. There is no equivalent of the orphanage, since any orphaned child is immediately embraced and adopted by relatives or friendly neighbors.

Pygmy women traditionally enjoy complete freedom and equality. There is no crime, there are no police, and no one is ever punished. Every person is accustomed to being treated with respect and caring, with the result that people of all ages experience a remarkable degree of security and comfort within themselves. There is a striking absence of greed, aggression, or envy.

Their language has no word for "hatred" and no word for "war." But just as Eskimo languages have many words for different kinds of snow, the Pygmies have a considerable number of words that describe different kinds of affection and caring.

You can learn a lot about a people by discovering what they view as the greatest sins. With the Pygmies, the worst violation of their laws and commandments is to be cruel to children or old people.[22]

Author and physician Bernie Siegel is so impressed by the mental health of the Pygmies that he writes, "If we would love one generation of the world's children as the Pygmies love theirs, the planet would change and our problems disappear."[23]

Researchers who have studied the Pygmies speak not only of their emotional and spiritual health but also of their vigor and heightened sensory acuity. According to Hallet, "these healthy, delightfully happy and highly expressive people . . . have the keenest vision of any living humans."

The pygmies are not merely a life-affirming society. DNA and genetic studies have confirmed that they are the most ancient ancestral form of Homo sapiens. One anthropologist concluded that they are "older than the sphinx, older than the pyramids, older than the texts written on papyrus, camel bones, bronze, brick or stone."[24] He and many other scientists hold that the Pygmies merit the title of the earliest civilized people known to history.

Their connectedness to one another and their respect for the natural living world have sustained the Pygmies for an estimated fifty thousand years. This is a hundred times the length of time that has passed since Columbus. Sadly, though, in the last century the forest home of the Pygmies has been decimated by outside forces, and these kindhearted people have suffered greatly. It is a source of deep sorrow to me that they are today on the edge of extinction.

## HEALING MAKES OUR HEARTS HAPPY

The Pygmies are not the only ancient society whose way of life can tell us something profound about the qualities that have been essential for a culture to thrive for tens of thousands of years. The Bushmen—also known as the San people of southern Africa—are another of the world's very oldest societies, and may even be as ancient as the Pygmies. Most anthropologists are in agreement that the Bushmen have existed as a culture for at least forty thousand years, and maybe much longer.

In the 1980s, the widely viewed film *The Gods Must Be Crazy* exposed many in the modern Western world to the extraordinary sweetness, gentleness, and innocence of these people. The star of the film was a Bushman named N!xau, who prior to the making of the film had been only minimally exposed to the wider world. He had seen only three white people in his life, and he had never seen a settlement larger than the village huts of his San people. Knowing nothing about money, he let his first wages, $300 in cash, simply blow away in the wind. Many millions of people saw the film, and virtually all were captivated by his profound human warmth, radiant joyfulness, and inner peace.

We can learn a great deal from the Bushmen, as we can from the Pygmies, not only about their culture but also about human nature and who we are as human beings.[25] They have always lived with dignity and been committed to each other's health and happiness. They have been for many tens of thousands of years a thoroughly cooperative people and have lived together in almost complete harmony. They have lived in a desert so barren it is almost inconceivable that humans can survive there, but they have never responded to the scarcity and hardship of their environment by hoarding or violence. They have responded instead by sharing whatever they have. They live by the belief that an individual's well-being is inextricably inter-woven with that of the group to which he or she belongs.

A friend of mine, Tom Burt, has spent much time with the Bush-men. He told me, "When I was there, I would sit out every night close to their huts and listen to the joy in their conversations and laughter. It is remarkable how much happiness they experience in their every-day life. The unconditional love that they have for one another and for all life is a model for the rest of the world to follow."

Among the Bushmen, as among the Pygmies, there is almost com-plete equality between the sexes. There is also a shared sense of hor-ror at the thought of violence and cruelty, including toward animals. Children and elders are cherished, and youngsters are taught that their most important resource is the goodwill of their neighbors. Their primary method for treating sicknesses of all kinds is a healing dance that brings the community together and maintains the pro-found spirit of sharing that the people see as all-important.[26]

Healing dance may seem terribly primitive compared to modern healing methods such as gene manipulation and organ transplanta-tion, but before we totally reject such practices we would be wise to remember that these are a people who have thrived for tens of thou-sands of years, something I seriously doubt people of the distant fu-ture will say about our current form of civilization. When it comes to the healing power of loving human connections, the Bushmen, like the Pygmies, seem to know a great deal that modern medicine and modern society as a whole may need to relearn if we are to survive.

The Pygmies and the Bushmen, these oldest of all peoples, remind us that our capacities for mutuality, cooperation, and empathy are every bit as real and every bit as much a part of our humanity as our capacities for greed, competition, and exclusiveness. Raising their children with unlimited respect and treating each person as having infinite worth, they have survived longer than any other culture known to science. The Pygmies and Bushmen represent the living ori-gin of humanity, and as societies they embody the greatest fulfillment that I know of on earth of the biblical injunction to "love thy neigh-bor as thyself."

Unfortunately, the Bushmen's survival as a culture, like that of the

Pygmies, is now very much in jeopardy. It is tragic that these life-affirming peoples who have made so few demands on their environment, and who have been able to sustain themselves for upward of forty thousand years, are finding themselves unable to survive in our modern world.

I believe we have much to learn from these people, but I am certainly not advocating that we return to their level of technological primitivism or that we turn our back on all forms of progress. Our material and scientific development have given us much for which I am deeply grateful. If we are to survive the challenges and difficulties of the times ahead, however, I believe we will need to integrate into our use of technological advances something the Pygmies and the Bushmen, like the Abkhasians, Vilcabambans, Hunzans, and elder Okinawans have long understood: We are part of each other. We need each other. Without love in our hearts for each other and for this beautiful world, we shall perish.

## SURVIVAL OF THE FITTEST— OR, LOVE THY NEIGHBOR AS THYSELF

Down through history there have been great thinkers who have spoken of the fundamental unity underlying the human condition. They have known and taught that each of us is truly part of an extended family that includes all people everywhere. But today the future itself depends on more than just a few wise people understanding the concept. The quality of life for humanity in the future depends on ever-increasing numbers of people incorporating this understanding into their everyday lives. The health and survival of the human species in the days ahead depend on how deeply we grasp the reality of our interdependence.

Many of us tend to think that human nature is inherently competitive and destructive. We hear about "selfish genes," as if our very genetic makeup predetermines that we will be egotistic people and that we will fight with one another.[27] We're told that our species contains a built-in "killer instinct," and that it is normal and inevitable for us to wage wars and massacres. It is widely believed that we are descended from "killer apes" who needed to be brutal and ferociously aggressive to survive the hostile conditions of prehistoric times.[28] According to such notions, the natural world is an unrelenting battle for survival, and it is a romantic fallacy to believe that people can live in peace with one another and with their environment for any significant length of time. "War," said U.S. vice president Dick Cheney in 2004, is the "natural state of man."[29]

Cheney and others who think like him believe that the human condition is inherently and inexorably competitive, and that all of human experience is an expression of the Darwinian principle of "survival of the fittest." If they are correct, then given the existence of nuclear weapons, our species is almost certainly doomed. But in *The Descent of Man,* Charles Darwin mentioned the survival of the fittest only twice, and one of those times was to apologize for using what he had come to feel was an unfortunate and misleading phrase. By contrast, he wrote ninety-five times about love. In his later writings, Darwin repeatedly stressed that the "survival of the fittest" model of natural selection dropped away in importance at the level of human evolution and was replaced by moral sensitivity, education, and cooperation.[30]

We sometimes think of ourselves at root as just nattily attired chimpanzees, noting that chimps have quite a propensity for deceit, violence, theft, infanticide, even cannibalism. But it is equally true that among chimps, the toughest rivals will reconcile after a fight, stretching out their hands to each other, smiling, kissing, and hugging. And besides, there is another primate who is as genetically similar to us as the chimpanzee—the bonobo, an ape species native to the Congo. If, instead of studying chimps for clues to the origins of human behavior, we had been studying bonobos, we would have come to very different conclusions. Instead of the killer-ape model, we would have had the lover-ape model, for these primates show a phenomenal sensitivity to the well-being of others. Today, writes author Marc Barasch in his 2005 book, *Field Notes on the Compassionate Life,* "primatologists are finding in the bonobos evidence that it is not tooth-and-nail competition, but conciliation, cuddling, and cooperation that may be the central organizing principle of human evolution."[31] One of the world's leading experts on primate behavior, Frans de Waal, calls it "survival of the kindest."[32]

What kind of creature, then, are we? There are those who believe human beings are fundamentally selfish, and there are those who believe we are essentially kindly creatures who need only love to flourish; but I stand in neither camp, or maybe I should say I stand in both camps. It appears to me that we have nearly infinite potential in both directions. Part ego and part divinely inspired, we have both the potential to compete and the potential to cooperate. We can create societies like the ones Ruth Benedict called "surly and nasty," and we can create ones like those she called "synergistic." Depending on what we choose to affirm and cultivate within ourselves and our children, we can collectively turn this planet into a hell or a heaven. Whether we like it or not, and whether we accept it or not, our choices make an enormous difference. How we treat ourselves and each other always matters.

## THE REAL NEWS ON THIS PLANET

This is why I believe that the world's healthiest and most long-lived peoples offer us a vision of hope for our time. In Okinawa, Abkhasia, Vilcabamba, and Hunza, there is a deep sense of human connection and social integrity. People continually help one another and believe in one another. There are always ways for people to make amends for mistakes and be forgiven, so people are almost never discarded or rejected. Wealth is shared rather than hoarded. As one Abkhasian proverb puts it, "I am whole because you are whole."

Characterized by the great respect with which women, children and the elderly are treated, these are societies with very little violence or cruelty, no harsh punishment, and hardly any crime. Instead of envy and greed, people living in these cultures are imbued with an attitude of trust and confidence, not only in others, but in the natural world.

*In Hunza, I seemed to be in another world, a world of friendliness and good nature. Covetousness, envy and jealousy were nonexistent; no police force was needed to keep order; unlocked doors were not a temptation.*

—Dr. Allen Banik, author of *Hunza Land*

*I have been fortunate enough to travel many places and experience a wide variety of different cultures, but there is something truly unique about Okinawan culture, which I believe is largely responsible for their long lifespan. Okinawans are by far the kindest, calmest, most warm-hearted people that I have ever encountered.*

—David Puzey, longtime resident of Okinawa

*I went to visit [the Vilcabambans] because I had heard they were old. But I stayed with them because they were themselves, a most lovable people, from whom I wanted to learn. Each one seemed to believe that he would become all that he had given away. I never before experienced a people who had so little and gave so much.*

—Grace Halsell, author of *Los Viejos*

I know, of course, that it would be neither practical nor helpful for those of us in the modern world to try live exactly as the Abkhasians, Vilcabambans, Hunzans, or elder Okinawans have lived. We have different challenges, different opportunities, and different destinies, and nothing would be gained by living imitative lives. But at the same time, I believe that if we can learn something from their examples, we can become more healthy, more fully human, and more loving people. They show us that there are steps we can take to reaffirm our humanity and health even if we live in the midst of a society that, comparatively speaking, seems to believe in "every man for himself."

Today, the effort to create a web of caring, support, authenticity, and trust among your friends and family members, and in the larger human community, may be the most healing act you can undertake. To overcome the isolation and disconnectedness that pervade contemporary life means to build, nurture, and prioritize relationships grounded in the understanding that every human life is precious, and that each of us has unique gifts and forms of love to give.

As children, many of us did not grow up in an environment that provided the care and support we deserved. As adults, many of us still suffer from a lack of connection, affection, and support in our lives. We know now that this loneliness is not only a source of emotional suffering, but also has serious medical consequences.

There are few achievements more important than to move beyond this legacy of lovelessness. Your efforts in this direction will likely lead to healing and greater longevity for yourself and your loved ones. But the impact of your caring will not stop there. The ripples that fan out from your acts of befriending and cherishing will also give rise to wider realities. They will, I believe, affect the greater political and spiritual directions of our times. They will not just improve your life and the lives of those in your circle of care. They will also influence our collective future for the better.

We are far more connected with one another than we often recognize. Deeply interwoven, we contribute to wellness or disease by the way we talk to each other, and we contribute to fulfillment or frustration by how we treat one another. We are part of each other's hopes, part of each other's healing, part of each other's dreams.

The choices that we make today as to the way we treat each other, the way we raise our children, the kinds of families and communities we create, will determine how the future unfolds. If we treat each other one way, we can cultivate people driven by a death urge, who are despondent and mean. If we treat each other another way, if we encourage and uphold our essential goodness and capacity for loving connection, we can nurture a society of people who are healthy and whole and whose lives will bring healing, peace, and joy to those they touch.

I believe that the real news on this planet is love—why it exists, where it came from, and where it is going. I believe that ultimately it is the love in our lives that underlies and makes possible our greatest healing and longevity.

Whether we acknowledge it or not, we all have a choice to be either accomplices in the status quo or everyday revolutionaries. We have a choice whether to succumb to the cultural trance, eat fast food, and race by each other in the night, or to build lives of caring, substance, and healing. So much depends on that choice.

# 17

## Grief and Healing

*There will come a time when you believe everything is finished.*
*That will be the beginning.*

—Louis L'Amour

If one of the most important signs of an advanced civilization is the amount of unconditional love in the community, then modern Western culture may be more primitive than we normally think, while the Pygmies and the Bushmen may be leading the way. This makes it all the more a source of sorrow, then, that the Pygmies and Bushmen stand today on the edge of extinction.

And even more sadly, they are not alone. The modern world is becoming an increasingly inhospitable place for many traditional societies.

In Abkhasia, the idyllic isolation that the region long enjoyed, and that permitted the fabled health and longevity of its inhabitants to flourish, has been severely compromised in recent years, following the breakup of the former Soviet Union. Prior to 1993, Abkhasia had been part of Soviet Georgia, though with its own culture and beliefs. While many Abkhasians were living peacefully in the traditional lifestyle, others were beginning to abandon the old ways in favor of modernity and were taking an increasing interest in politics. After Georgia broke away from the Soviet Union in the early 1990s,

Abkhasian authorities decided to pursue their wish of becoming an autonomous republic, and declared the region's independence. Almost immediately, Georgia sent its military forces into Abkhasia in an attempt to reclaim the region. In 1993, this tragically became a devastating war in Abkhasia, resulting in more than a hundred thousand deaths while causing tremendous upheaval and destruction.

What the future will hold for Abkhasia is uncertain, but the war and related events of the past decade have grievously damaged the social and economic structure throughout the Caucasus. This is not the first time in human history that war and violence have decimated a life-affirming society, nor is it likely to be the last. I believe that those of us who are spared direct involvement in this kind of violence owe it to those who are harmed to do what we can to build a culture of peace, prosperity, and justice in the world, to lessen the likelihood that such tragic events will ever take place again.

Throughout the world today, the wisest and most long-lived cultures are having a difficult time surviving. In Okinawa, the way of life that has long produced such remarkable results for the elders is being abandoned by subsequent generations. Exposed to junk food as a result of the massive U.S. military presence, the younger residents of Okinawa have become eager consumers of fast-food burgers, soda pop, doughnuts, processed meat, and canned foods—with disastrous health consequences. And likewise in China, where the quest to emulate the American diet is leading to skyrocketing rates of obesity, cancer, and heart disease.

There are few cities left anywhere in the world today where you can walk down the street without being bombarded by advertisements promoting the sale of soft drinks. Coca-Cola, McDonald's, KFC, Baskin-Robbins, and similar multinational corporations are rapidly setting up shop wherever people have money to spend. Worldwide, Dunkin' Donuts now sells 6.4 million doughnuts each day (enough to circle the world twice).[1] And as McDonald's so proudly proclaims, the company has now sold more than one hundred billion burgers, roughly sixteen for every man, woman, and child on earth.

In some cities there are now "all you can eat by the minute" restaurants where instead of paying according to the food they eat, customers pay according to how many minutes they sit at the table. Not surprisingly, people eating at these restaurants rarely speak with one another. They are determined to eat as much as they can as quickly as possible.

It is part of the anguish of our times that a toxic food environment that causes weight gain, heart disease, cancer, and diabetes is rapidly going global, with the result that obesity and its attendant ailments are increasing today in every single nation in the world. These trends are reaching, I'm sorry to say, even into places as previously isolated and pristine as Hunza and Vilcabamba.

## RECENT DEVELOPMENTS IN HUNZA

The Hunza valley is still witness to some of the most magnificent mountain grandeur to be seen anywhere on earth. Until only a few decades ago, the only access into the Hunza valley was a harrowing trail that was at points nothing more than rocks hammered into the side of the mountain. Sometimes in the winter the Hunza River would freeze solid and could be crossed. But at other times, to get to Hunza, people had to crawl on their hands and knees across perilous rope bridges above the river's raging waters.

In the late 1960s, all this began to change. The government of Pakistan, wanting to be able to obtain help from China in case of a war with India, began creating a primitive road that could be traversed by specially equipped vehicles.

By 1973, when Alexander Leaf visited Hunza for *National Geographic,* the consequences of the road were already evident. He wrote,

> In the past, the clothes they wore had all been made from the cloth they wove of the wool from their own sheep, but now they are dressed in brightly colored cotton prints from Japan. Imported tea is replacing the traditional drinks of fruit juice. Small shops are appearing in the villages as natives turn to commerce rather than agriculture for their livelihood. The old people told us repeatedly that "no one has time for relaxation and festivities any more."[2]

The Hunzan leader lamented to Leaf,

> With the road, the young people go to Pakistan for military ser-
> vice or employment. They return and change the traditional ways
> of my people. The diet is changing and health is deteriorating.
> There are fewer old people now.[3]

Then, in 1979, this high mountain kingdom became far more accessible to the world with the completion of the paved Karakoram
Highway. One of the world's great engineering feats, the Karakoram
Highway was chiseled out of a thousand kilometers of almost verti-
cal mountain rock. Even with the work of tens of thousands of Chinese laborers, it took nearly twenty years to build. More than a
thousand men died as a result of avalanches and accidents during its
construction. Upon completion, it had an immediate impact upon the
timeless tranquility of Hunza.

A few years later, a leading Hunzan elder, Gulam Mohamad Beg,
described to an American reporter how the intrusion of the outside
world has changed things:

> Hunza is not the same since the Karakorum Highway invaded our
> quiet lives. Before, no one ever locked their doors. Theft was un-
> heard of. Before, the social pressure to be honest was strong. Be-
> sides, there was little money to steal. Now everyone chases after
> money so they can ruin their health by buying canned food from
> Karachi. Every year there is more crime. Only ten years ago, we
> had no jail and no police! But the saddest part is that Hunza peo-
> ple are forgetting their own culture. We used to share everything.
> We passed the winters by dancing all day for hours on end. Our
> life was communal and that was enough.[4]

The completion of the Karakoram Highway created an entirely
new social and economic reality for the Hunzans. As late as 1965,
these were a people who did not use money. They paid no taxes and
had no banks. All trade was barter. But now there are hotels, shops,
and a tourist industry made up primarily of people coming to see the
world's most incredible views and climb the mountains. A scholar at

the American Institute of Pakistan Studies, Dr. Julie Flowerday, calls the transformation that has occurred in Hunza in the last twenty years "as extraordinary as a cultural earthquake."

Since the construction of the road, whole new settlements have sprung up, and many Hunzans have migrated to the larger towns and villages in Pakistan. Young Hunzan men have enlisted in the Pakistani army, returning with a taste for tobacco and candy.

In recent years, Hunza has been formally annexed by Pakistan. Yet there are still some ways that Hunza retains its own culture. For example, many women in Pakistan are completely veiled, but women in Hunza do not wear veils, and they participate much more freely in wider community life than do women in most of Pakistan. The Hunzans still farm their marvelous terraces completely organically. But with each passing day, Hunza is becoming less itself and more like the rest of Pakistan. Despite its idyllic past, Hunza can no longer maintain its isolation from the larger Pakistani society.

The younger Hunzans are now beginning to westernize their diets and lifestyles. Canned meat products, candy bars, and white flour are increasingly common. Diseases that had been unknown are starting to appear.

The phenomenal health and longevity of the Hunzans, who have endured for thousands of years and withstood ten thousand avalanches in the Karakoram mountains, are sadly now beginning to be buried under the greater avalanche of modern Western civilization.

## VILCABAMBA TODAY

On the other side of the world lies another of the societies long renowned for health and longevity: Vilcabamba. As in Hunza, modernity started to come to Vilcabamba in the 1970s. By the 1990s, progress had arrived in the form of a paved highway, electricity, primitive telephones, television, and a wide array of highly processed and refined foods including Coca-Cola and candy bars.

Along with the highway came modern medical practices. Through Ecuador's Rural Medicine Program, eager young graduates arrived and began prescribing antibiotics and other drugs in Vilcabamba. Though this provided some benefits, within a few months of the arrival of the young physicians, several of the elders died of dysentery after antibiotics wiped out the friendly bacteria in their colons.[5]

As Vilcabamba has lost its isolation, attitudes too have begun to change. "Where elders used to be revered for their wisdom and experience," reflects one longtime Vilcabamban, "they have now come to be regarded simply as old. Their traditional role as oral transmitters of history and culture, the sources of wisdom in the times of crises, has eroded, and they are now regarded as anachronistic."[6]

Until very recently, the only way to get to Vilcabamba from Loja (the nearest town) was arduous, time-consuming, and treacherous. But now there is a two-lane highway with bus and taxi service from Loja. Only a few years ago, the center of Vilcabamba was a serene plaza with a small park and a church. The air was pristine. There were no cars, no electricity, no pavement. Now, the noise and exhaust of Jeeps and SUVs fills the plaza during the tourist season. There are internet cafés catering to gringo backpackers and wealthy Ecuadorians, and Vilcabamba even has its own tourist office.

The mineral-rich waters that course through town are still free for bathing, and the climate is still paradisiacal. But if you visit Vilcabamba today expecting to find a place populated by healthy centenarians, you are likely to be disappointed. You probably won't see village elders holding court or sitting in the plaza. Many of the remaining elders have moved far up into the hills. What you will see are members of the younger generation who eat candy bars, drink soda pop, and play video games. They are eager to migrate to the big city, though they often do not even begin to understand what will happen to them when they arrive, or the value of what is being lost.

It is sad to see wholesome cultures and ways of life that have thrived for countless centuries vanishing before our eyes. Sometimes, of course, leaving tradition behind is the only way that transformation and evolutionary development can occur. But I shudder to see Western consumerism becoming the dominant ethic in the world, and high-fat, high-sugar foods becoming the dominant diet.

These days, many people fear that the survival of the human race could be threatened by the breakdown of modern society as we know it. I'm beginning to wonder if our survival may be just as threatened by the *continuation* of modern society as we know it.

## LIVING WITH THE SADNESS

There is great violence and loss in our world today. Vast numbers of species are becoming extinct, as are the Bushmen and Pygmies, the oldest and perhaps the most unconditionally loving of all human societies. And many of the world's healthiest and most life-affirming traditional cultures are finding it difficult to survive in the face of the continuing spread of Western consumer culture.

These realities affect us all. If we are going to find healing in these times, we need to see what is happening, acknowledge our grief, and act on behalf of what we love.

Many of us in the Western world have been taught to deny our pain. But when we do that, we fight against the truth of ourselves, and this creates illness on many levels. One of the great unacknowledged sources of sickness in the modern world is the repression of our feelings and the resultant decline in our capacity for joy and vivacity.

Armoring ourselves to keep from experiencing loss depletes us and prevents healing from occurring. It's exhausting to continually hold in our emotions. When we avoid our pain, we tend to become dull and incapable of feeling. We become passive and resigned, not because we don't care, but because we don't grieve. We shut down because we have allowed our hearts to become so filled with loss that we have no room left to feel. Rest, exercise, play, the releasing of unrealistic expectations, all help us cope. But sometimes we really begin to heal only when we learn how to live with our pain, when we become deeply intimate with our suffering, when we learn how to grieve.

This is not always easy to do, but if we try to avoid the pain of facing what is happening and seek comfort at any cost, we are left incapable of the love and emotional connection with others that we need in order to be healthy and whole. If we repress our grief, we suffocate our hearts.

There are a thousand voices in modern society and in each of our minds seeking to distract us from the sadness in our lives. We learn early to treat suffering as an enemy to be defeated, to reject what is unpleasant, difficult, or disappointing. Often, we judge ourselves

harshly for our woundedness. But healing is not the absence of suffering. Healing is addressing our suffering and allowing it to catalyze
responses that bring us to greater wholeness and make us more fully
human. Healing begins with being who we are, with being honest
about the reality of ourselves and our world. Compassion requires
the courage to face suffering.

One of the secrets of the cultures in which people often live long,
healthy, and happy lives is that they have ways of expressing and
sharing their joys with other people, and perhaps even more important, their fears and their griefs. They recognize that we all have times
when we feel overwhelmed and defeated, when we feel terribly alone,
when we are tempted to hide in a corner and feel sorry for ourselves.
They know we all have dark nights of the soul, and they understand
that at such times it is necessary to have others to go to, others with
whom we can be emotionally vulnerable and honest. In this way,
even in the midst of our despair we are reminded that we are part of
a community, that there are others who care about us, and that we
are still part of the stream of life. Our grief becomes a source of connection to who we are, to our passion, commitment, courage, and
vulnerability.

This is enormously important for us to understand today, because
I don't think anyone could become aware of the immensity of what
is happening in our world and not feel pain for life and fear for our
collective future. Each of us has our own suffering, of course, our
personal losses and disappointments and frustrations. But the pain
inside us today goes beyond the personal. It affects each of our individual lives and also something greater. It is the future of life on earth
that now hangs in the balance.

This sorrow belongs to us all. It is in the nature of our times and
it is ours to embrace. In the depths of our shared pain, we can also
experience our shared caring, our mutual prayers, and the roots of
our capacity to act. The pain we feel is the breaking of the shell that
encloses our power to respond. Something precious can be born in
times like these. In our shared pain, we labor to bring it to birth.

We live now in a time that has been called "the great turning." In
such a time, I believe it is our task to sustain the gaze, to be attentive
both to what is dying and what is being born, to what is marred and

what is beautiful. We are called to be unafraid of pain and unafraid of joy, to remember that no feeling is final, and to affirm our power to make a difference.

We are witnesses in our times to wars, destruction, plagues, and pestilence on a biblical scale. But what we do with calamity is up to us. We can let it shatter our resolve and our sense of possibility. Or we can use the pain to deepen our commitment to all that is good and life-giving in ourselves and the world.

I believe it helps to remember that at this moment, as in every moment, babies are being born, children are playing, and people are singing. People are learning to read, people are learning to listen, and people are learning to understand themselves and others. As people are finding new ways to resolve conflicts, friendships are being made and strengthened. Right now, millions of people are taking responsibility for their health, and giving of themselves that their families and communities might thrive.

It is profoundly important today that we not give up on ourselves and on one another, that we retain faith in the possibilities of human nature. It is true that as a species we have produced what Ruth Benedict called "surly and nasty" cultures, where people are warlike and mean-spirited. But we are also a species that has produced the Pygmies and the Bushmen, the Abkhasians and the Vilcabambans, the Hunzans and the Okinawans, and countless other societies where people have lived with respect for each other and for the greater earth community.

These are not easy times to uphold ourselves and the greater human possibility, nor to feel confident in our collective future. It saddens me beyond telling that human beings can be so destructive. But I take strength from the reality that as a species we have also produced people like Dr. Martin Luther King, Jr., Nelson Mandela, Aung San Suu Kyi, and millions of others whose names are not as well known but whose lives have also demonstrated profound generosity, wisdom, and courage.

I am thinking, for example, of the hundreds of thousands of people who have worked day in and day out for decades so that we are now within a whisker of forever wiping out the last traces of both smallpox and polio from the face of the earth. And of the hundreds of millions of people worldwide who are endeavoring to create an environmentally sustainable, spiritually fulfilling, and socially just human presence on this planet.

The next time anyone tells you that who you are doesn't matter, or that your actions and love are insignificant, here's what they need to know: All who take a stand with their lives on behalf of what they cherish are part of something vast. The struggle for justice is as old as tyranny itself, and the longing for a world guided by love is as old as the human heart.

# 18

## Death and Awakening

*I know everybody has to die sooner or later. But I thought an exception would be made in my case.*

—William Saroyan

A few years ago, I received a letter from a woman in Southern California. She wrote that she and her husband had for many years avidly followed a path of health. Their lifestyle, she believed, had been exemplary. They had practiced yoga and meditated, and neither of them had let a single bite of anything containing refined sugar pass their lips. They exercised regularly and never took any drugs, not even so much as an aspirin. They had been very happy together, she said, and had believed that by eating healthful foods and undertaking other sound health practices they would never fall ill.

But now she felt bitter, angry, and cheated. In his fifties, her husband had developed cancer and died. What was the point, she lamented, of all their health diligence, when this could still happen? Despondent and feeling betrayed, she had given up any semblance of health discipline and was stuffing herself with hamburgers, candy, and the other unwholesome foods she had forgone for years. She no longer exercised, and had gained more than 70 pounds in the three years since her husband's death. She had developed diabetes and was overwhelmingly depressed.

Reading this woman's letter, I felt sorrow. I felt sad for her loss of her husband, and sad for how depressed, despondent, and bitter she had become. And I felt sad, too, that she and her husband had held the misguided belief that their diet and lifestyle could guarantee them everlasting health.

There is something innocent and childlike about believing that if you eat only healthful foods and exercise enough, you will never become ill. There is a part of all of us that would like to be able to follow some magic rule or obey some infallible authority and thereby be guaranteed freedom from all suffering. But life just doesn't work that way. Life is far more unpredictable, and far more mysterious.

I've known raw food aficionados who believe that all cooked food is unhealthful and who, when they become ill, blame it on the one piece of cooked food they've recently eaten. I've known zealous Atkins adherents who demonize carbs and then agonize because in a lapse of willpower they ate a baked potato. I've known people who believe that if they eat only pure food and take thousands of dollars' worth of supplements, they will live indefinitely.

A good diet and exercise regimen is important, and living healthfully can make a tremendous difference. But there are many other factors in our lives that also have great influence over our health. Someone may die of a skin cancer at age fifty that began as the result of a teenage sunburn.[1] Some cancers—particularly breast, uterine, ovarian, and prostate cancers—start in the womb, engendered in part by the food our mothers ate and the chemicals in their environments.[2]

We live in a world that is becoming increasingly toxic and polluted. There are many environmental exposures over which we have no control. Some diseases occur whose origins are complete mysteries, descending on people seemingly out of the blue no matter what their lifestyle. Others develop that are intimately linked to social factors such as poverty and dangerous working conditions. There are powerful forces in our world that are undermining relationships, forcing people to work insane hours, and poisoning our air and water.

Because the food we eat is one factor that we can often control, we sometimes attribute to it a degree of importance that is inconsistent with reality. Doing so can give us the illusion that we are completely in charge. We may feel that nothing bad can happen to us as long as we adhere with sufficient stringency to the dietary regimen in which we have invested such magical powers. The trouble is that even people with perfect diets sometimes get cancer. Horrible things can, and often do, happen to people who do not deserve them.

The woman who wrote to me had believed that her and her husband's lifestyle would guarantee them long lives without illness. When this belief was so painfully punctured, she was left bereft and unable to cope. Hers is a very sad story, and I tell it here not to embarrass her or find fault with her in any way, but in the hope that others might learn something from her experience.

I wrote back to her that I was sorry to learn of her loss and how much suffering she had experienced. I spoke to her of the pain and disillusionment I've known in my own life, when ideals and dreams I had believed in came crashing down around me, and of the life I had found on the other side of disillusionment and despair.

Later in the letter, I said I hoped that in time she would be able to see that it is possible to make healthy choices, not in the belief that by doing so she would never be ill or die, but because she knows that suffering occurs in every human life, and she wants to prevent as much illness as she can and alleviate as much suffering as she is able. It is possible to take responsibility for your health and life, I wrote, not to avoid everything painful in the human experience, but to lessen suffering and to enrich and illumine who you are with wisdom and love.

I wrote that her letter reminded me of something I once heard from a wise man: "If you go forward, you will die. If you go backward, you will die. It is better to go forward."

## GOING FORWARD

The point of going forward—of working to make your life a positive expression of your highest vision—is not to avoid all suffering and death, for that is not within the realm of human possibility. The point, rather, is to meet all of your life experiences, including the most difficult ones, with the greatest powers of love and healing within you. The gift of going forward is not that you will never physically decline or fall ill, but that you will be less likely to do so prematurely, and better able to enter wholly into your life and meet whatever the world brings you with grace and wisdom.

If you eat natural foods, jog, or meditate because you feel better when you do, because you feel closer to yourself and more alive, then even if you should die younger than you might wish, you will not regret having cared for yourself. If you experience a particular diet or lifestyle as a point of entry into greater presence and well-being, then whatever happens, you'll be grateful for your choices. If lifting weights or doing yoga or aerobic exercise provides you with more access to yourself, if it brings you balance and strength, if it helps you listen to your body, then even if serious illness occurs, you'll be glad you've done everything you could on behalf of your wellness, and thankful for the life you've lived.

A healthful diet and lifestyle almost always lead to a longer and healthier life. They provide increased vitality, improved resistance to disease, and a greater sense of wholeness and freedom. But even the finest exercise and diet plan cannot forever overcome the inevitability of aging. Eventually, even the best-cared-for bodies begin to weaken and no longer function as once they did.

In our appearance-oriented society, aging can seem like a misfortune. But in the process of aging, people often come to understandings that are crucial to the completion and fulfillment of their lives. They learn something about loss and acceptance. They may have to cope with enormous difficulties—a husband dying, a wife getting cancer, even the death of a child. They come to know how vulnerable everyone is. They understand there are no easy answers, and that life is hard at times for everyone.

We have so much to learn form the old. There was a cartoon in *The New Yorker* entitled "Yuppie Angst." A man is saying, "Oh no, I spilled cappuccino on my down jacket." Elders, who have seen their families and friends die, who have seen generations of children being born, can have a deeper understanding of tragedy. Closer to death, they are much more in touch with the cycles of life. They understand what makes a life worth living. They know there is little point in having low cholesterol and rock hard abs if you don't love your life.

## FINDING BEAUTY EVERYWHERE

There is a story about a mother who asked a little girl to offer grace at breakfast. Agreeing to do so, the little girl began, "We thank you, dear God, for this beautiful day."

"Bless you, my dear," said her mother, "for offering the prayer, but apparently you didn't look outdoors before you prayed. It's raining and it's a dismal day."

"Mother," responded the little girl. "Never judge a day by its weather."[3]

The little girl understood how important it is to bring our love to all our moods and experiences. This means finding the beauty and giving thanks for the opportunities in every phase of our lives. This is not always easy, but it is of immense significance.

We are all vulnerable and naked before the mysteries of life. Sometimes when we look deeply and honestly at our woundedness, we discover our power, our joy, and our will to live. We realize that we can accept imperfections, and that our lives don't have to be perfect to be precious.

A human life has its seasons, much as the earth has seasons, and each one has its own particular beauty and possibilities. When we ask life to remain perpetually spring, we turn the natural process of life into a process of loss rather than a process of celebration and appreciation.[4]

## THINGS BECOME BEAUTIFUL WHEN YOU LOVE THEM

There are those who, when they look in the mirror and see signs of aging—a new gray hair, a new wrinkle or blemish—rush to cover it up with some cream, ointment, or dye. There's nothing wrong with wanting to "look your best," but if you are at war with the aging process, you are going to lose. Those who try to pretend that they aren't aging will find themselves in an impossible race with death. As Morrie Schwartz said, "If you're always battling against getting older, you're always going to be unhappy, because it will happen anyway."

Some years ago, an advertising executive working for a large beauty products company had a bright idea. In its ads, the company began asking people to send in photographs along with brief letters about the most beautiful women they knew. Within a short time, the company had received more than a thousand photos and letters.

One particular letter caught the attention of the employee whose job it was to open and sort them, and eventually the letter made its way to the company president. It was filled with spelling and punctuation errors, and was written by a young boy living in a very rough neighborhood. He wrote of a beautiful woman who lived down the street. "I visit her every day," he wrote. "And she makes me feel like the most important kid in the world. We play checkers and she listens to my problems and gives me apples. She understands me. When I leave, she always yells out the door, for the whole world to hear, that she's proud of me."

The boy ended his letter by saying, "I don't know if you can tell by this picture, but she is the most beautiful woman I've ever seen. I hope I someday have a wife as pretty as her."

Curious, the company president asked to see the photograph that had accompanied the letter. His secretary handed it to him. It showed a smiling woman whose sparse gray hair was pulled back in a bun. She was well along in years, her face bore many wrinkles, and she was sitting in a wheelchair. Yet her eyes were luminous with kindness and joy.[5]

## THE FOUNTAIN OF YOUTH

What really matters isn't whether you color your hair or get Botox injections. What matters is that you greet the experiences of your life, including the signs of your aging, with love and acceptance rather than disdain. Every life stage has its unique gifts and powers. What's most important is that your inner beauty shine through your life.

It is no indictment of healthful paths that they lead, as all paths eventually do, to the moment that you pass from this world. Life choices that can help your days be full of accomplishment, peace, and satisfaction are no small achievement. A way of life that lengthens your years, helps mobilize your inner resources, adds to your feelings of well-being and comfort, and enables the power of your spirit to illumine your days is a great blessing.

In the world's healthiest cultures, old age is not seen as a curse, and death is not seen as an enemy. Rather, the entire arc of the human condition is seen as an ever-changing series of opportunities for growth, fulfillment, and love. When people die, their whole community comes together in celebration of the continually changing nature of life.

These cultures understand and accept the entire life cycle. Death is real and close, and people have continual opportunities to remember the transiency of life. Rituals honoring those who have previously passed on are woven into the daily life of the community.

In the modern West, on the other hand, we are conditioned not only to deny death but to view it as a failure. Even though most of us want to die at home, not in a hospital, and want to die naturally, not hooked up to life support, in the end very few of us get what we want.

What one 78-year-old man experienced in a Western hospital is all too common. After he witnessed the intubation and unsuccessful attempted resuscitation of a fellow patient, he begged to be left alone. "Listen, doctor," he implored his physician, "I don't want to die with tubes sticking out all over me. I don't want that my children should remember their father that way. All my life I tried to be a mensch, you understand? . . . Rich I wasn't, but I managed to put my sons through college. I wanted to be able to hold my head up, to have dignity, even though I didn't have much money and didn't speak good English. Now I'm dying. Okay. I'm not complaining, I'm old and tired and have seen enough of life, believe me. But I still want to be a man, not a vegetable that someone comes and waters every day—not like him."

Although this man was a competent adult and made his wishes clear, they were not honored. He was "coded," tagged by hospital personnel to be resuscitated at all costs. Eventually, he managed to disconnect himself from the machinery, leaving a handwritten note to his physician: "Death is not the enemy, Doctor. Inhumanity is."[6]

It's now been forty years since the birth of the hospice movement, with its emphasis on helping people die with dignity and peace, often in the comfort of their homes. But in Western medicine, the end of life remains hypermedicalized. When someone approaches death, we still typically fight it every step of the way.

## LEARNING TO HONOR DEATH

Some of us have a particularly hard time accepting death. Immediately after U.S. baseball star and national icon Ted Williams died in 2002, his spinal cord was severed and his head was separated from his body. Then both his head and body were coated in a glycerin-based solution, placed in a pool of liquid nitrogen, brought to a temperature of minus 206.5 degrees Centigrade, and stored in this cryogenically frozen state. This procedure, which cost hundreds of thousands of dollars, was done at the behest of Williams's son, who wanted to believe that his father might someday, when medical science had become far more advanced, be brought back to life.

Most of us find that our difficulties with accepting death take less dramatic forms, but for all of us, facing death can be very hard. "Even the wise fear death," said the Buddha. "Life clings to life." There may be some of us who have overcome this fear, but most of us are afraid of dying. There is no shame in this, for it is part of our nature. We all experience the desire to push death away, to pretend life will go on forever. But still, every day on earth, hundreds of thousands of people die.

This rhythm is as steady as a heartbeat, continuing unabated day and night, winter and summer, everywhere that human beings live. Stephen Levine, who has spent decades counseling the terminally ill, reminds us that some people die from starvation while others die from overeating. Some die of thirst, others by drowning. Some die while still children. Others die of old age. Some people die in confusion, suffering from a life that remains to some degree unlived, from a death they cannot accept. Others die in surrender with their minds open and their hearts at peace.[7]

We often make an artificial distinction between "the dying," by which we mean those who have some idea of the limit that has been placed on their lives, and the rest of us, who have no idea how much time we have left. Thinking this way enables us to avoid thinking about our own dying. If we think about dying people as a separate group, we can imagine that we are not dying. We can pretend that it isn't happening to us. But every day that passes brings us steadily closer to our death. It is happening to each of us, and it is happening to everyone we know and everyone we love.

There is a story in the Buddhist tradition of a woman whose only son dies. Consumed with grief, she carries the body of her dead child from house to house, asking for medicine to cure him. Some people react with pity, others shun her, but all sense that the pain of losing her son has been too much for her and has driven her insane. Eventually, the woman goes to the Buddha and cries out, "Lord, give me the medicine that will bring back my son!"

Buddha answers, "I will help you. But first please bring me a handful of mustard seeds." The mother is overjoyed, and says she will do so immediately, when the Buddha adds, "But each mustard seed must come from a home which has not known death, from a house where no one has lost a child, a husband, a parent, or a friend."

The mother again goes from house to house in the village, asking for mustard seeds. Everyone is eager to provide the seeds, but when she asks, "Did a son or daughter, a father or mother, die in your family?" they answer her, "Alas, yes," and tell her of the loved ones they have lost. She searches for days, but can find no house in which some beloved person has not died.

Finally, the woman finds herself on a roadside, feeling weary and hopeless. She watches the lights of the town as they flicker and then are extinguished at the end of the day. At last the darkness of the night reigns everywhere, and she sits contemplating the immutable fate of humanity.

When she returns to the Buddha, he says to her: "The life of mortals in this world is troubled and brief and combined with pain. For there is not any means by which those who have been born can avoid dying." Allowing her pain now to be what it is, the mother buries her son in the forest. No longer denying the truth, she vows to devote the remainder of her life to the nurturance of compassion and wisdom in the world.

## GOING HOME

When Rachel Naomi Remen, M.D., was director of the pediatric in-patient division at Mount Zion Hospital in San Francisco, she heard angry voices coming from inside her office as she arrived for work one day. Several of the staff nurses and resident doctors had gathered there and were very upset. Apparently, someone had told a five-year-old boy who was in the end stages of leukemia that he was going home that day. He had told a nurse to pack his things, pointing with excitement to his tiny suitcase in the closet. "I'm going home today," he had told her. Remen describes the scene:

> The nurse was horrified. Who could have promised this terribly sick little boy that he could go home when he had no platelets or white cells? When everyone knew he was so fragile he could bleed to death from the slightest injury? She asked the other nurses on her shift and the previous shift if they had told the child he might go home. No one had said a word to him.
>
> The outraged nurses then accused the young doctors. The doctors were incensed at the suggestion that it was one of them who had callously promised such an impossible thing. The discussion had grown more heated and was moved to the privacy of my office. "Could he go home by ambulance, just for an hour?" they asked me, unwilling to disappoint him and destroy his hopes. It seemed too dangerous. "Did anybody ask him who told him he could go home?" I said. Of course, no one had wanted to talk to him about that. . . .
>
> A few hours later the child said he was tired. He lay down, pulling his sheet over his head, and quietly slipped away. The staff took his death hard. He was a love of a little boy and they had cared for him for a long time. Yet many told me privately how relieved they were that he had died before he had discovered that someone had lied to him and he couldn't go home.[8]

Conditioned to think of death as the enemy, members of the hospital staff did not consider that the child might actually have been profoundly attuned, sensing that he was, indeed, "going home" that day.

Our society has taught us to fear death, but there are other possible ways to look at it. "Death is not extinguishing the light," wrote the Indian poet and visionary Rabindranath Tagore. "It is putting out the lamp because dawn has come."

Kahlil Gibran, a Lebanese poet and philosopher, was long known and beloved for his work by millions of Arabic-speaking people. In the last twenty years of his life, Gibran lived in the United States and began to write in English. In his book *The Prophet*, he wrote,

> *For what is it to die,*
> *but to stand naked in the wind and to melt into the sun?*
> *And what is it to cease breathing,*
> *but to free the breath from its restless tides,*
> *that it may rise and expand and seek God unencumbered?*
> *Only when you drink from the river of silence shall you indeed*
> *sing.*
> *And when you have reached the mountain top, then shall you begin*
> *to climb.*
> *And when the earth shall claim your limbs, then shall you truly*
> *dance.*[9]

## AWAKENING

Our culture's attitude, in which death is seen as a failure, either of the doctor or the patient, is at odds with that of almost every traditional culture. But it has insinuated itself deeply into all of us. Could it be the denial of death in our culture that underlies our fear of aging and our lack of respect for the elderly?

How would our lives be different if we could realize that tomorrow isn't promised to anyone? How would our lives change if we understood that time is only lent to us, that our days are but a trust handed into our temporary keeping?

If we were to grasp fully that someday we too shall die, would it help us to answer the poet Mary Oliver's question, "What is it you plan to do with your one wild and precious life?"

It has been said that there are two very important days in each human life. One is the day we are born. The other is the day we know why we were born. I have known many people who have never experienced that second day, who have never understood the purpose of their lives, and so have come to their deaths not knowing whether they have really lived. The Methodist bishop Gerald Kennedy once described the most tragic kind of funeral service a minister is called upon to conduct:

> It is not the kind that would seem obviously to be tragic. It is not the service for a youth whose life has been snuffed out before he has even reached maturity, nor is it for the infant who never gets a chance at living. Rather, it is for those who have never learned to live, who come to their final hours with no friends and have contributed nothing with the time and talents entrusted to them.[10]

Similarly, Dr. Martin Luther King, Jr., once said, "The worst of all tragedies is not to die young, but to live until I am 75 and yet not ever truly have lived." Though Dr. King was assassinated at the age of only thirty-nine, he knew one of the great secrets of the human experience: It doesn't really matter much at what age you pass from this world. The quality of a human life cannot be measured in years. What really matters is how much love, wisdom, and courage you have brought to the life you were given.

Finding the fountain of youth is not about living forever. It's about allowing your life to be guided by the beauty of your soul. It's about finding the fountain of joy and the fountain of life. It's about living so fully that you know you have really lived. It's about loving so fully that you know you have really loved.

May you find the fountain of youth, not as an exotic place somewhere hidden and remote, but within yourself, as the very way you walk through life. May your sorrow as well as your joy be a doorway into your greater heart. May you find your way through the fathomless mystery of your life to the source of all that is good and true.

When you were born, you cried and the world rejoiced. May you live so that when you die, the world will cry and you will rejoice.

# STEPS YOU CAN TAKE

- Talk about what matters to you. Even if your voice trembles, speak the truth as you see it.
- Laugh often. Cry when needed. Be humbled by the vastness of the universe.
- Celebrate transitions. Create rituals to affirm how you want to experience and enjoy each new stage of your life.
- Celebrate the summer and winter solstices and the spring and autumn equinoxes. Notice the special gifts and beauties each season brings.
- Take pleasure in small things. Defy the myth that more is always better. Rejoice in the power of humility. Remember that small is beautiful.
- Know how much is enough. Honor the yearning for a slower pace of life with more time for joyful relationships, fulfilling work, and living your dreams. Live simply so that others may simply live.
- Give away everything that is cluttering your life. Have nothing in your house that is not useful or beautiful.
- Always remember that it is the small, simple things you do every day that bring light to this world.

---

- Consider what you would want to do if you knew you had only six months to live. See how many of these things you can do in the next two years.

- Whatever your stage of life, create an affirmation or visualization that reflects your goals for yourself. Twice a day, as you wake up in the morning and as you fall asleep at night, mentally repeat your affirmation or visualization, and engage your imagination on behalf of making your goals your reality.
- Never let the fact that you cannot be what you would *like* to be prevent you from being and appreciating what you *can* be.
- Stand for your vision of what is possible, and never underestimate your power to make a difference.
- Sing, even if you think you can't.
- Never be ashamed of the privileges that have come into your life. Never be ashamed of the gifts that have been given to you. Use them for the good of us all.

---

- Get enough sleep. Remember your dreams and share them. Keep a dream journal. Over time, watch for recurring images or themes. See what you can learn from them.
- Take time to meditate, write poetry, or keep a journal.
- Share a story with family or friends, or write in your journal, about a time when you were humbled, soothed, or awed by something in the natural world.
- Give thanks for your life, for your health, and for this beautiful earth.
- Sit quietly in nature and listen. Respect all life.
- Pet cats, dogs, and other animals. And hug people—lots. You are never too old to ask for a hug, and never too old to offer one.

---

- Sit with someone who is dying. Meditate, pray, sing, or read to them.
- Become a hospice volunteer.
- Support the family or partner of someone in your community who is nearing death. Bring food, run errands, clean his/her house, massage his/her shoulders.

---

- Speak to those who are close to you about the major illnesses of your life. Honor the insights into yourself and your way of life that you have gleaned from being sick.
- If you are faced with a serious health challenge, get the best medical care you can, and make sure you take time to honor and care for your mind, heart, and spirit as well as your body. Rather than seeing the crisis as merely an obstacle to be overcome, use it as an opportunity to discover what is most important in your life. Hold what is frightened, painful, and neglected in yourself with the tenderness and compassion with which you would hold a newborn baby. Remember that you do not have to do anything or be anything in order to be happy and worthy of love.
- If you have suffered a major loss, keep a grief journal. Write down whatever you are feeling, as a daily exercise in self-exploration and expression. Write about whatever you are experiencing, including anger or despair if those feelings arise.

---

- Identify an ancestor or some historical figure in whose lineage you feel yourself to be, and do something to pay tribute to his or her spirit.
- Celebrate death days as well as birthdays. On the anniversary of a loved one's death, create a way to remember her and to honor how her spirit lives on in you. Set up an altar of remembrance, using photos, letters, and objects that carry memories.
- Write in your journal or talk to friends or family about your death. Describe your vision of how you want to die.
- Remember that at the end of your days on this earth, the question will not be how much you have, but how much you have given; not how much you have won, but how much you have loved.

---

- Celebrate your uniqueness, realizing that there is no one in this entire world with your talents, your eyes or your heart, your fingerprints or your dreams.
- Give yourself unlimited permission to be healthy, happy, and at peace.
- Remember that one who forgets the language of gratitude can never be on speaking terms with happiness.

# Acknowledgments

The older I get, the more I realize how dependent I am on the love and support of others. At one time in my life, I thought it was a weakness to be dependent on other people. But I have come to see it very differently.

A nineteenth-century rabbi, Menachem Mendel, said, "Human beings are God's language." By this I think he meant that in answer to our needs and prayers, God sends us people. Friends, lovers, family members, neighbors, even those who appear to be our opponents or enemies, each of them helps to make us who we are.

Words cannot convey my immense gratitude to the people whose steadfast love and presence made it possible for me to write this book during a very challenging period of my life. This book would not have been even remotely possible without their help.

I thank Deo Robbins, my wife of forty years, for the vastness of her caring. I thank our son, Ocean Robbins, for being there for me when I needed him, time and again. I thank our daughter-in-love, Michele Robbins, for holding the space so deeply for all to prosper and be well. These three people continually inspire me with their commitment to life and to love. I am profoundly privileged to share my life with them.

I thank Doug Abrams for his belief in me, and for his deep willingness to learn and grow and share his passion. He is my friend as well as my literary agent, and I have been extraordinarily fortunate to have his help in the creation of this book.

I thank Caroline Sutton, the book's editor at Random House. Her keen perception and deep understanding have contributed marvelously to its fruition. And I thank her and the team at Random House for the strength of their belief in me and in this book.

I thank my team of "ruthless readers," the friends and colleagues who read the manuscript at various stages and made so many fine suggestions. In particular I thank Kimberly Carter, John Borders, and John Astin, who gave deep attention to the manuscript and whose reflections have been invaluable. I also thank Bob Stahl, Michael Klaper, Tom Burt, Patti Breitman, and Jeff and Sabrina Nelson for the quality of their attention, insights, and feedback. We all need friends who will tell us not only what we want to hear, but what we *need* to hear in order to grow. This book would not be what it is without their honesty and clarity.

I thank Don Weaver for his intrepid help in sharing with me many hard-to-find and out-of-print publications.

There are many other people whose love and attention have made it possible for me to write this book and to thrive. I thank Craig Schindler, Katchie Egger, Ann Mortifee, and Jessica Simkovic, each of whose love has meant and means the world to me. And so many others. You know who you are. I am blessed to have you in my heart and life.

I thank you, dear reader, for joining me in the search for a way of life that finds health in honoring the human spirit and our interdependence with one another and the whole earth community.

In a brightly lit room, a lighted candle is a lovely decoration and symbol. In a completely dark room, a lighted candle is far more than that—it enables us to see. Similarly, in these dark times when there is so much suffering and violence in our world, each person who keeps the flame of spirit lit with the search for truth and compassion is a blessing to us all.

Thank you for all your efforts, including those that may have seemed wasted, to bring love and wisdom to your life and to our troubled world. I appreciate every step you have taken, and every step you will yet take, toward a wiser, healthier, and more just world.

May all be fed. May all be healed. May all be loved.

# Resource Guide

John Robbins invites you to visit www.healthyat100.org for tools, leading-edge information, and a comprehensive resource guide to help you live and share the message of this book. When you visit, you will find:

- Organizations, websites, links, books, and tools to help you thrive
- Reviews of books and films you might want to know about
- Information about Healthy at 100 support groups and study groups
- Ongoing updates about the issues in this book and the latest learnings of medical science
- More information about John Robbins' life, work, and insights
- The opportunity to connect with an emerging community of peers who can support you on a healing journey
- Information about events with John Robbins and how to contact him

Please visit www.healthyat100.org.

# Notes

## INTRODUCTION

1. "Writer's Plot to 'End Pain,' " Associated Press, *The Australian* Feb. 25, 2005.
2. B. R. Levy et al., "Longevity Increased by Positive Self-Perceptions of Aging," *Journal of Personality and Social Psychology* 2002, 83(2):261–70. See also M. B. Brewer, V. Dull, and L. Lui, "Perceptions of the elderly: Stereotypes as prototypes," *Journal of Personality and Social Psychology* 1981, 41:656–70; B. Levy, "Improving memory in old age by implicit self-stereotyping," *Journal of Personality and Social Psychology* 1996, 71:1092–1107; B. R. Levy, O. Ashman, and I. Dror, "To be or not to be: The effects of aging self-stereotypes on the will-to-live," *Omega: Journal of Death and Dying* 1999–2000, 40:409–20; B. Levy, J. Hausdorff, R. Hencke, and J. Wei, "Reducing cardiovascular stress with positive self-stereotypes of aging," *Journals of Gerontology* 2000, 55:205–13.
3. Ken Dychtwald, *Age Power: How the 21st Century Will Be Ruled by the New Old* (Jeremy P. Tarcher, 1999).
4. According to an analysis by Peter R. Uhlenberg, a professor at the University of North Carolina, cited in Tamar Levin, "Financially Set, Grandparents Help Keep Families Afloat, Too," *New York Times* July 14, 2005.
5. Marla Dickerson, "Old News Travels South: Experts say a wave of senior citizens is poised to hit Latin America," *Los Angeles Times* Nov. 1, 2004.
6. Ibid.

## CHAPTER ONE: ABKHASIA: ANCIENTS OF THE CAUCASUS

1. Alexander Leaf, "Every day is a gift when you are over 100," *National Geographic* 1973, 143(1):93–119. See also Leaf, "Getting Old," *Scientific American* 1973, 229:45–52, and "Long-lived Populations: Extreme Old Age," *Journal of the American Geriatrics Society* 1982, 30(8):485–87.
2. Alexander Leaf, *Youth in Old Age* (McGraw-Hill, 1975), p. 3.
3. Ibid. p. 18.

4. "161 Years Old and Growing Strong," *Life* Sept. 16, 1966, pp. 121–27.

5. Alexander Leaf, op. cit., pp. 8–9.

6. Ibid. pp. v, 8.

7. Ibid. p. 14.

8. Ibid. pp. 20–22.

9. Ibid.

10. Zhores Medvedev, "Caucasus and Altay Longevity: A Biological or Social Problem?" *The Gerontologist* Vol. 14 No. 5, Oct. 1974, and "Aging and Longevity," *The Gerontologist* Vol. 15 No. 3, June 1975. See also Medvedev, "Age Structure of Soviet Populations in the Caucasus: Facts and Myths," in *The Biology of Human Ageing,* edited by A. H. Bittles and K. J. Collins, Society for the Study of Human Biology, Symposium 25 (Cambridge University Press, 1986), pp. 181–200.

11. Shoto Gogoghian assisted Alexander Leaf in finding the oldest Abkhasians, who were scattered in villages and collective farms. For a discussion of Gogoghian's views, see Dan Georgakas, *The Methuselah Factors: Learning from the World's Longest Living People* (Academy Chicago Publishers, 1995), pp. 37–66.

12. G. N. Schinava, N. N. Sachuk, and Sh. D. Gogohiya, "On the Physical Condition of the Aged People of the Abkhasian ASSR," *Soviet Medicine 5,* 1964.

13. Nikos Baibas et al., "Residence in mountainous compared with lowland areas in relation to total and coronary mortality," *Journal of Epidemiology and Community Health* 2005, 59:274–78.

14. Sula Benet, *Abkhasians: The Long-Living People of the Caucasus* (Holt, Rinehart and Winston, 1974), p. 20.

15. Alexander Leaf, op. cit., p. 112.

16. Sula Benet, *Abkhasians.*

17. Sula Benet, *How to Live to Be 100: The Lifestyle of the People of the Caucasus* (New York: Dial Press, 1976), p. 42.

18. Ibid. p. 42.

19. Sula Benet, *Abkhasians,* p. 3.

20. Ibid. p. 9.

21. Ibid. p. 3.

22. Ibid. p. 14.

23. Ibid. p. 105.

24. Ibid. p. 9.

25. Ibid. p. 30.

26. Every year, half a million Americans have facial cosmetic surgery, and every week, makeover shows glamorize the procedures. For a more realistic view, see Jill Scharff and Jaedene Levy, *The Facelift Diaries: What It's Really Like to Have a Facelift* (Booksurge, 2004).

27. The singer/comedian Laura Ainsworth talks about this and many other examples of the pressure and the struggle to stay young in her satirical musical show *My Ship Has Sailed.*

28. Dan Georgakas, op. cit., p. 50.

29. Sula Benet, *Abkhasians,* p. 9.

30. Ibid. pp. 95–97.

31. Ibid. p. 69.

32. Ibid. pp. 34, 69.

33. Ibid. p. 71. See also Sula Benet, *How to Live,* p. 154.
34. Ibid. p. 107.
35. Ibid. p. 32.
36. Dan Georgakas, op. cit., p. 51.
37. Sula Benet, *Abkhasians,* p. 22.
38. Ibid. p. 21.
39. Ibid. p. 35.

## CHAPTER TWO: VILCABAMBA: THE VALLEY OF ETERNAL YOUTH

1. Morton Walker, *Secrets of Long Life* (Devin-Adair, 1984), cited in *Vilcabamba: The Sacred Valley of the Centenarians* (CIS Publishing, 2004), pp. 31–32.
2. Alexander Leaf, *Youth in Old Age* (McGraw-Hill, 1975), pp. 51–52.
3. Eugene H. Payne, "Islands of Immunity: Medicine's Most Amazing Mystery," *Reader's Digest* Nov. 1954.
4. "90, 100, 130 . . . who's counting?" *The Guardian* Feb. 15, 2003.
5. Michael James, *New York Times* Sept. 28, 1956.
6. Grace Halsell, *Los Viejos: Secrets of Long Life from the Sacred Valley* (Rodale Books, 1976), p. 13. See also Alexander Leaf, op. cit., p. 217.
7. David Davies, *The Centenarians of the Andes* (Anchor Press / Doubleday, 1975), and "A Shangri-La in Ecuador," *New Scientist* 1973, 57:226–38.
8. *Vilcabamba: The Sacred Valley of the Centenarians* (CIS Publishing, 2004), pp. 25–26.
9. N. Okudaira et al., "Sleep Apnea and Nocturnal Myoclonus in Elderly Persons in Vilcabamba, Ecuador," *Journals of Gerontology* 1983, 38:436–38.
10. Steve Silk, "In the Valley of the Ancient Ones in the Southern Ecuador Village of Vilcabamba, Centenarians Are Common, Thanks to a Fertile Climate, Peaceful Setting and the Mineral-Rich Agua d'Oro," *Los Angeles Times* Dec. 12, 1993, p. 13.
11. Steven N. Austad, *Why We Age: What Science Is Discovering About the Body's Journey Through Life* (John Wiley & Sons, 1997), p. 24.
12. R. Mazess and S. Forman, "Longevity and Age Exaggeration in Vilcabamba, Ecuador," *Journals of Gerontology* 1979, 34(1):94–98. See also R. Mazess and R. Mathisen, "Lack of Unusual Longevity in Vilcabamba, Ecuador," *Human Biology* 1982, 54(3):517–24, and R. Mazess, "Health and Longevity in Vilcabamba, Ecuador," *Journal of the American Medical Association* 1978, 240(10):1781 (letter).
13. Guillermo Vela Chiriboga, *The Secrets of Vilcabamba (Secretos de Vilcabamba para vivir siempre joven)* (Corporación de Estudios y Publicaciones, 1989).
14. Ibid.
15. Grace Halsell, *Los Viejos.*
16. Grace Halsell, *Soul Sister* (Crossroads International Publishing, 1999).
17. Grace Halsell, *Bessie Yellowhair* (Morrow, 1973).
18. Grace Halsell, *The Illegals* (Stein and Day, 1978).
19. Grace Halsell, *In Their Shoes* (Texas Christian University Press, 1996).
20. Grace Halsell, *Los Viejos,* pp. 16, 20.
21. Ibid. pp. 7–8.
22. Ibid. p. 154.
23. Ibid. p. 66.

24. Ibid. p. 157.
25. Ibid. p. 157.
26. Ibid. p. 144.
27. Ibid. p. 142.
28. Ibid. pp. 150–51.
29. Ibid. p. 151.
30. Ibid. p. 25.
31. Dale Turner, *Different Seasons* (High Tide Press, 1997), p. 136.
32. Grace Halsell, *Los Viejos*, p. 41.
33. Ibid. p. 45.
34. Ibid. p. 99.
35. Ibid. p. 98.
36. Barrie Robinson, *Ageism* (University of California at Berkeley School of Social Welfare, 1994).

## CHAPTER THREE: HUNZA: A PEOPLE WHO DANCE IN THEIR NINETIES

1. For a graphic portrayal of the difficulty involved in reaching Hunza, see the video *Health Secrets of the Shangri-La—Hunza,* produced by Renee Taylor.
2. Alexander Leaf, *Youth in Old Age* (McGraw-Hill, 1975), p. 35.
3. Ibid. p. 39.
4. Robert McCarrison, *Studies in Deficiency Diseases* (Henry Frowde and Hodder & Stoughton, 1921), and Robert McCarrison and H. M. Sinclair, *Nutrition and Health* (Faber and Faber, 1961). See also Robert McCarrison, "Faulty Food in Relation to Gastro-Intestinal Disorder," Sixth Mellon Lecture delivered to the Society for Biological Research, University of Pittsburgh School of Medicine, Nov. 18, 1921, and "The Relationship of Diet to the Physical Efficiency of Indian Races," *The Practitioner* Jan. 1925, pp. 90–100.
5. *American Heart Journal* Dec. 1964. See also Brian Goodwin, *How the Leopard Changed Its Spots: The Evolution of Complexity* (Princeton University Press, 1994), p. 207.
6. Jay M. Hoffman, *Hunza: Secrets of the World's Healthiest and Oldest Living People* (New Win Publishing, 1968), pp. 1–2.
7. Eric Shipton, *Mountains of Tartary* (Hodder & Stoughton, 1951).
8. J. I. Rodale, *The Healthy Hunzas* (Rodale Press, 1948), p. 123.
9. Captain C. Y. Morris, *Journal of the Royal Geographical Society* June 1928.
10. R.C.F. Schomberg, *Between the Oxus and the Indus* (Martin Hopkinson, 1935).
11. J. I. Rodale, op. cit., p. 188.
12. R.C.F. Schomberg, op. cit.
13. Allen E. Banik and Renee Taylor, *Hunza Land: The Fabulous Health and Youth Wonderland of the World* (Whitehorn Publishing, 1960), p. 146.
14. Ibid. pp. 102, 142–43, 173, inside front cover.
15. Ibid. p. 140.
16. Senator Charles Percy, "You Live to Be 100 in Hunza," *San Francisco Chronicle* (n.d.).
17. Jay M. Hoffman, op. cit., pp. 51–52.
18. J. I. Rodale, op. cit.
19. Jay M. Hoffman, op. cit., p. 35.

20. J. I. Rodale, op. cit., pp. 44, 93.

21. Ibid. p. 80.

22. Vernon Gill Carter and Tom Dale, *Topsoil and Civilization* (University of Oklahoma Press, 1975).

23. Data for Abkhasia are derived from Sula Benet, *Abkhasians: The Long-Living People of the Caucasus* (Holt, Rinehart and Winston, 1974), pp. 21–26, and other sources. Data for Vilcabamba are derived from an analysis by Dr. Guillermo Vela Chiriboga, a nutritionist from Quito, Ecuador, cited in Leaf, *Youth in Old Age*, p. 74, and from Grace Halsell, *Los Viejos: Secrets of Long Life from the Sacred Valley* (Rodale Press, 1976), p. 13, and other sources. Data for Hunza are derived from a nutritional survey of the diets of male adults in Hunza by Dr. Maqsood Ali, cited in Leaf, *Youth in Old Age*, p. 74. Leaf also provided data (p. 73) demonstrating the well-known fact that the diets of women and the elderly are much lower in calories than those of men and younger adults. Ali's survey was of adult males in Hunza of all ages. Vela Chiriboga, studying only the elderly and including women, found the average daily diet in Vilcabamba yielded 1,200 calories. In order for the table to show the caloric consumption of adult males of all ages in each culture, I have adjusted Vela Chiriboga's daily caloric consumption figures upward in accord with well-established ratios.

24. Jay M. Hoffman, op. cit., p. 54.

25. John Clark, a geologist and author of the 1957 book *Hunza: Lost Kingdom of the Himalayas,* says he lived in Hunza for thirty-five months in the late 1940s and saw rickets, scurvy, pneumonia, and malaria. He says further that eye problems such as trachoma, conjunctivitis, and blindness were common. I find it hard to credit Clark's claims, however, because I don't see how an optometrist such as Banik could possibly have missed the eye problems Clark asserts were common. Nor can I understand how Clark could claim that the Hunzan diet "has no vitamin A" when he knew the major role apricots and carrots play. Carrots and apricots are excellent sources of beta-carotene, which the human body readily converts into vitamin A. And most important, there is the testimony of Lieutenant Colonel D.L.R. Lorimer, who lived in Hunza for more than five years and who, unlike Clark, spoke the native language. His 1935 book *The Burushaski Language* is the classic description of the Hunzan language and culture of that period.

    J. I. Rodale's book *The Healthy Hunzas* begins with the words "This book must immediately express, as it reveals on many a page, the immeasurable debt of gratitude which I owe to Lieutenant Colonel D.L.R. Lorimer for having read its manuscript and for having furnished me with more than forty closely typewritten pages of comment thereon, a critical exposition that could easily have been a slender volume in itself. Inasmuch as I adopted a large majority of his technical suggestions, I can safely present *The Healthy Hunzas* with the conviction that it is an authoritative piece of work." Rodale and Lorimer speak of "the phenomenally unique good health of the Hunzas. They do not number in their midst isolated or sporadic cases of physical perfection, nor are they a select school of a few hundred laboratory specimens. They are a group of 20,000 people, none of whom dies of cancer or drops dead with heart disease. In fact, heart trouble is completely unknown in that country. Feeblemindedness and mental debilitations which are dangerously rampant in the United States are likewise alien to the vigorous Hunzas" (Rodale, *The Healthy Hunzas*, pp. 31–32).

There are still many unanswered and perhaps unanswerable questions about Hunza. The culture and its people have regrettably not been studied with the rigor necessary to form definitive conclusions, and recent developments have altered the traditional culture irretrievably. However, even the ultimate Hunza skeptic, John Clark, wrote that the people of Hunza "did not suffer from many of the diseases common to our civilization." He said there was no cancer, no mental illness, no stomach ulcers, appendicitis, or gout, and that heart disease was extremely rare. (John Clark, "Hunza in the Himalayas: Storied Shangri-La undergoes scrutiny," *Vegetarian Voice* April/June 1979.)

26. Dale Turner, *Different Seasons* (High Tide Press, 1997), p. 112.

## CHAPTER FOUR: THE CENTENARIANS OF OKINAWA

1. Bradley J. Willcox, D. Craig Willcox, and Makoto Suzuki, *The Okinawa Program: Learn the Secrets to Health and Longevity* (Three Rivers Press, 2001).
2. Ibid. p. 5.
3. B. J. Willcox, D. C. Willcox, and M. Suzuki, "Evidence-based Extreme Longevity: The Case of Okinawa, Japan," *Journal of the American Geriatrics Society* 2001, 49(4):397. See also their "Built to last? Past Medical History of Okinawan-Japanese Centenarians," *Journal of the American Geriatrics Society* 2002, 50(4):394.
4. Thomas T. Perls, "Centenarians: The older you get the healthier you have been," *Lancet* 1999, 354:652.
5. Thomas T. Perls and Margery Hutter Silver, *Living to 100: Lessons in Living to Your Maximum Potential at Any Age* (Basic Books, 1999), p. 47.
6. Bradley J. Willcox, D. Craig Willcox, and Makoto Suzuki, *The Okinawa Diet Plan* (Clarkson Potter, 2004), p. 2.
7. Bradley J. Willcox et al., *The Okinawa Program*, p. 12.
8. Ibid. p. 1.
9. N. Ogawa, "Japan's limits to growth and welfare," in T. Kuroda, ed., "Population Aging in Japan: Problems and Policy Issues in the 21st Century," International Symposium on an Aging Society: Strategies for 21st Century Japan, Jihon University, Population Research Institute, 1982, cited in Bradley J. Willcox et al., *The Okinawa Program*, p. 2.
10. Bradley J. Willcox et al., *The Okinawa Program*, p. 1.
11. Ibid. p. 9.
12. Ibid. p. 6.
13. Ibid. p. 14.
14. R. Bonita, "Cardiovascular disease in Okinawa," *Lancet* 1993, 341:1185.
15. Bradley J. Willcox et al., *The Okinawa Program*, op. cit., pp. 18, 19.
16. K. Y. Kinjo et al., "An epidemiological analysis of cardiovascular diseases in Okinawa, Japan," *Hypertension Review* 1992, 15(2):111–19. Cited in Willcox and Suzuki, *The Okinawa Program*, pp. 427–28.
17. Bradley J. Willcox et al., *The Okinawa Program*, p. 38.
18. Ibid. p. 35.
19. *Okinawa: Cold War Island*, edited by Chalmers Johnson (Japan Policy Research Institute, 1999), p. 274.
20. P. Ross et al., "A comparison of hip fracture incidence among native Japanese,

Japanese-Americans, and American Caucasians," *American Journal of Epidemiology* 1991, 133:801–9. See also Bradley J. Willcox et al., *The Okinawa Program*, p. 43.

21. M. Suzuki and N. Hirose, "Endocrine Function of Centenarians," in H. Tauchi et al., eds., *Japanese Centenarians: Medical Research for the Final Stages of Human Aging* (Aichi, Japan: Aichi Medical University, 1997) cited in Bradley J. Willcox et al., *The Okinawa Program*, pp. 436–37.

22. M. Shores et al., "Low testosterone is associated with decreased function and increased mortality risk: A preliminary study of men in a geriatric rehabilitation unit," *Journal of the American Geriatrics Society* 2004, 52(12):2077–81.

23. S. Moffat et al., "Free testosterone and risk for Alzheimer's disease in older men," *Neurology* 2004, 62(1):188–93; V. Henderson et al., "Testosterone and Alzheimer's disease: Is it men's turn now?" *Neurology* 2004, 62(1):170–71.

24. Bradley J. Willcox et al., *The Okinawa Program*, p. 43. See also p. 59.

25. Ibid. p. 43. See also p. 86.

26. Richard Weindruch and Rajinder Sohal, "Caloric Intake and Aging," *New England Journal of Medicine* 1997, 337(14):986–94.

27. Kagawa's work is cited in Roy Walford, *Beyond the 120-Year Diet: How to Double Your Vital Years* (Four Walls Eight Windows, 2000), p. 89.

28. Roy Walford, op. cit., pp. 13, 45.

29. T. E. Meyer et al., "Long-term caloric restriction ameliorates the decline in diastolic function in humans," *Journal of the American College of Cardiology* 2006, 47(2):398–402.

30. Jim Salter, "Study: Low-Calorie Diet Keeps Heart Young," Associated Press, Jan. 12, 2006.

31. Roy Walford, op. cit., p. 17.

## CHAPTER FIVE: EAT WELL, LIVE LONG

1. Bradley J. Willcox, D. Craig Willcox, and Makoto Suzuki, *The Okinawa Program: Learn the Secrets to Health and Longevity* (Three Rivers Press, 2001), pp. 43, 71.

2. Ibid. p. 69.

3. Joanne Slavin et al., "The Role of Whole Grains in Disease Prevention," *Journal of the American Dietetic Association* 2001, 101:780–85. See also D. R. Jacobs et al., "Whole-grain intake and cancer: An expanded review and meta-analysis," *Nutrition and Cancer* 1998, 30:85–96.

4. D. R. Jacobs et al., "Is whole-grain intake associated with reduced total and cause-specific death rates in older women? The Iowa Women's Health Study," *American Journal of Public Health* 1999, 89(3):322–29. See also S. Liu, "Intake of refined carbohydrates and whole grain foods in relation to risk of type 2 diabetes mellitus and coronary heart disease," *Journal of the American College of Nutrition* 2002, 21(4):298–306; D. R. Jacobs et al., "Reduced mortality among whole grain bread eaters in men and women in the Norwegian County Study," *European Journal of Clinical Nutrition* 2001, 55(2):137–43; J. L. Slavin et al., "The role of whole grains in disease prevention," *Journal of the American Dietetic Association* 2001, 101(7):780–85.

5. James E. Tillotson, director of Tufts University's Food Policy Institute, calcu-

lates that the average American drinks the equivalent of a 55–gallon drum of soda every year. Cited in Emma Ross and Joseph Verrengia, "Obesity Becoming Major Global Problem," Associated Press, May 8, 2004.

6. James E. Tillotson, "Food Brands: Friend or Foe?" *Nutrition Today* 2002, 37:78–80.

7. "Twinkies Maker Seeking Chapter 11 Protection," Associated Press, Sept. 22, 2004; "Bankrupt Bakery to Close Plants," *San Francisco Chronicle* June 10, 2005.

8. James Bates, "Marvin H. Davis 1925–2004; Billionare Oilman, Real Estate Mogul Once Owned Fox Studio," *Los Angeles Times* Sept. 26, 2004, p. A-1.

9. "Death Rate from Obesity Gains Fast on Smoking," *New York Times* March 10, 2004, p. A-16.

10. R. Sturm, "The effects of obesity, smoking and problem drinking on chronic medical problems and health care costs," *Health Affairs* 2002, 21:245–53; R. Sturm and K. Wells, "Does obesity contribute as much to morbidity as poverty or smoking?" *Public Health Reports* 2001, 115:229–95.

11. Ibid.

12. Ruth Patterson et al., "A comprehensive examination of health conditions associated with obesity in older adults," *American Journal of Preventive Medicine* 2004, 27(5):385–90.

13. Timothy B. McCall, *Examining Your Doctor: A Patient's Guide to Avoiding Harmful Medical Care* (Carol Publishing Group, 1995), p. 242.

14. Carol Lynn Mithers, "From Baby Fat to Obesity: Why Kids Even as Young as Two Are Developing Weight Problems," *Parenting* Oct. 2001.

15. Kelly D. Brownell, *Food Fight: The Inside Story of the Food Industry, America's Obesity Crisis, and What We Can Do About It* (Contemporary Books, 2004), p. 41.

16. Ibid. p. 54.

17. Ibid.

18. Peter Menzel and Faith D'Aluisio, *Hungry Planet: What the World Eats* (Ten Speed Press, 2005), p. 223.

19. Ibid.

20. "Children in Britain 'choking on their own fat,' says obesity report," London, Agence France-Presse worldwide news service, May 26, 2004. See also House of Commons Health Committee, "Obesity," Third Report of Session 2003–04, Vol. 1.

21. Janet Adamy, "Some food makers trim low-carb plans as trend slows," *Wall Street Journal* July 12, 2004, p. B-1.

22. "USA: Low-carb diets appeal to over half the population," March 19, 2004, www.just-food.com/news_detail.asp?art=57042.

23. Arne Astrup, "Atkins and other low-carb diets: hoax or an effective tool for weight loss?" *The Lancet* 2004, 364:897–99. See also G. D. Foster et al., "A randomized trial of a low-carbohydrate diet for obesity," *New England Journal of Medicine* 2003, 348(21):2082–90; L. Stern et al., "The Effects of Low-Carbohydrate versus Conventional Weight Loss Diets in Severely Obese Adults," *Annals of Internal Medicine* 2004, 140(10):778–85.

24. E. C. Westman et al., "Effect of 6–month adherence to a very low carbohydrate diet program," *American Journal of Medicine* 2002, 113:30–36.

25. M. L. Dansinger et al., "Comparison of the Atkins, Ornish, Weight-Watchers,

and Zone diets for weight loss and heart disease risk reduction: a randomized trial," *Journal of the American Medical Association* 2005, 293(1):43–53.

26. R. M. Fleming, "The effect of high-protein diets on coronary blood flow," *Angiology* 2000, 51(10):817–26.

27. *Medical Opinion* 1(1972):13, cited in Michael Greger, "The Skinny on Atkins," *Dr. Greger's Nutrition Newsletter* June 2004.

28. Cited in Michael Greger, *Carbophobia: The Scary Truth About America's Low-Carb Craze,* (Lantern Books, 2005), p. ix.

29. *Maryland State Medical Journal* 1974:70, cited in Michael Greger, "The Skinny on Atkins," *Dr. Greger's Nutrition Newsletter* June 2004.

30. *Chicago Tribune,* Oct. 18, 1999. See also www.atkinsexposed.org/atkins/25/Atkins_Nightmare_Diet.htm.

31. Robert Davis, "Weight loss doctor dies at 72 from head injuries," *USA Today* April 17, 2003.

32. Elizabeth Cohen, CNN Medical Unit, "Heart Association to warn against low-carb diets," CNN, March 20, 2001.

33. Ibid.

34. Arthur Agatston, *The South Beach Diet* (Rodale Press, 2003), pp. 115, 94–95.

35. "Low-carb king Atkins files Chapter 11: Company owes $300 million in outstanding principal and interest," CNN.com, Associated Press, August 1, 2005.

36. Daniel DeNoon, "More Carbs, More Exercise = Weight Loss: Studies Link High-Fiber Carbs, Low Weight," *WebMD Medical News* March 5, 2004. See also P. K. Newby et al., "Risk of overweight and obesity among semivegetarian, lactovegetarian, and vegan women," *American Journal of Clinical Nutrition* June 2005, 81:1267–74.

37. Bradley J. Willcox et al., *The Okinawa Program,* p. 74.

38. John W. Rowe and Robert L. Kahn, *Successful Aging* (Dell, 1998), pp. 28–30.

39. George E. Vaillant, *Aging Well: Surprising Guideposts to a Happier Life—from the Landmark Harvard Study of Adult Development* (Little, Brown, 2002), p. 203.

40. S. Mizushima et al., "The relationship of dietary factors to cardiovascular diseases among Japanese in Okinawa and Japanese immigrants, originally from Okinawa, in Brazil," *Hypertension Research* 1992, 15:45–55. See also Y. Moriguchi, "Japanese centenarians living outside Japan," in H. Tauchi et al., eds., *Japanese Centenarians: Medical Research for the Final Stages of Human Aging* (Aichi, Japan: Institute for Medical Science of Aging, 1999), pp. 85–94.

41. David Allen and Chiyomi Sumida, "Okinawans picking up dangerous dining habits," *Stars and Stripes* Nov. 17, 2002. See also Norimitsu Onishi, "On U.S. Fast Food, More Okinawans Growing Super-Sized," *New York Times* March 30, 2004, and "Love of U.S. food shortening Okinawans' lives—Life expectancy among island's young men takes a big dive," *New York Times* April 4, 2004.

42. Spam is also popular in South Korea, Hawaii, the Philippines, Guam, and Saipan—all places (like Okinawa) where the U.S. military has had a dominant presence.

## CHAPTER SIX: NUTRITION AND THE HEALTH OF HUMANITY

1. Weston A. Price, *Nutrition and Physical Degeneration* (Keats Publishing, 1939).

2. Ibid. pp. 170–71.

3. Ibid. pp. 174, 179.

4. Ibid. p. 186.

5. Ibid. p. 182.

6. Ibid. p. 48.

7. Ralph W. Moss, "Cancer: A Disease of Civilization?" *Moss Reports* July 23, 2002.

8. Ibid.

9. Ibid.

10. Vilhjalmur Steffansson, *Cancer: A Disease of Civilization?* (Hill and Wang, 1960).

11. K. Hill and A. M. Hurtado, "Hunter-Gatherers of the New World," *American Scientist* 1989, 77:437–44.

12. The Masai tribes are cattle-raising nomads whose diet is high in animal fat and cholesterol. Some people cite the low level of atherosclerosis among the Masai as evidence that eating animal fats and cholesterol does not cause coronary heart disease. However, the Masai have the benefit of a unique genetic endowment that affects their cholesterol synthesis. Roy Walford, *Beyond the 120–Year Diet: How to Double Your Vital Years* (Four Walls Eight Windows, 2000), p. 106. Furthermore, the Masai eat a large variety of wild, indigenous plants that tend to reduce cholesterol levels. Timothy Johns, a Canadian ethnobotanist who has studied the Masai diet and lifestyle, believes their high intake of wild plants helps explain why the Masai do not suffer from heart disease despite eating so much saturated fat.

13. Weston A. Price, op. cit., pp. 134, 139. Today, the Masai still place enormous value on martial prowess. Laurence Frank, who has worked in Kenya's Masai Mara National Reserve for most of the last twenty years and is a recognized authority on developments there, says that "typically, a young [Masai] male achieves manhood by killing a warrior from another tribe during a cattle raid. Failing that, he'll kill a lion. That's how he proves himself worthy of taking wives." Glen Martin, "The lion, once king of African savanna, suffers alarming decline in population," *San Francisco Chronicle* Oct. 6, 2005.

14. Weston A. Price, op. cit., p. 54.

## CHAPTER SEVEN: THE MOST COMPREHENSIVE STUDY OF NUTRITION EVER CONDUCTED

1. William S. Kovinski, "The Great Malls of China," *Los Angeles Times* June 29, 2005.

2. T. Colin Campbell, *The China Study: The Most Comprehensive Study of Nutrition Ever Conducted, and the Startling Implications for Diet, Weight Loss, and Long-Term Health* (Benbella Books, 2004).

3. J. Y. Li et al., "Atlas of cancer mortality in the People's Republic of China: An aid for cancer control and research," *International Journal of Epidemiology* 1981, 10:127–33.

4. T. Colin Campbell, op. cit., p. 71.

5. Quoted in ibid., p. 7.

6. Ibid. p. 77.

7. T. Colin Campbell and Christine Cox, *The China Project: Revealing the Relationship Between Diet and Disease* (New Century Nutrition, 1996), p. 8.

8. T. Colin Campbell, op. cit., p. 79.

9. T. Colin Campbell and Christine Cox, op. cit., p. 13.

10. T. Colin Campbell, op. cit., pp. 80–81.

11. Ibid., pp. 69–110.

12. J. M. Chan and E. L. Giovannucci, "Dairy products, calcium, and vitamin D and risk of prostate cancer," *Epidemiology Review* 2001, 23(1):87–92.

13. B. K. Jacobsen et al., "Does High Soy Milk Intake Reduce Prostate Cancer Incidence?" *Cancer Causes, Control* 1998, 9:553–57. See also Health Professionals Follow-up Study, reported in "Dairy Products Linked to Prostate Cancer," Associated Press, April 5, 2000.

14. World Cancer Research Fund and American Institute for Cancer Research, *Food, Nutrition and the Prevention of Cancer: A Global Perspective*, 1997.

15. Ibid. p. 509.

16. In 1974, total meat consumption in China was less than 1 million tons, while in the United States it was 23 million tons. In 2005, meat consumption in China had risen to 64 million tons; in the United States, it had risen to 38 million tons. "Annual Consumption and Use of Key Resources and Consumer Products in the United States and China," in Lester R. Brown, "China Replacing the United States as World's Leading Consumer," Earth Policy Institute Eco-Economy Update, Feb. 16, 2005.

17. Clay Chandler, "Inside the New China," *Fortune* Oct. 4, 2004, p. 98.

18. Elaine Kurtenbach, "Urban China Struggles with Battle of the Bulge: High fat snacks are overwhelming the nation's lean, traditional diet. As a result, the country is seeing a rise in obesity," *Los Angeles Times* July 18, 2004.

19. Ibid.

20. Ibid.

21. Marc Santora, "East Meets West, Adding Pounds and Peril," *New York Times* Jan. 12, 2006.

## CHAPTER EIGHT: THE ROAD TO HEALTH AND HEALING

1. Dean Ornish et al., "Can lifestyle changes reverse coronary heart disease? The lifestyle heart trial," *The Lancet* 1990, 336(8708):129–33.

2. Caldwell B. Esselstyn, "Updating a 12-Year Experience with Arrest and Reversal Therapy for Coronary Heart Disease," *American Journal of Cardiology* 1999, 84:339–41. See also Caldwell B. Esselstyn, "Resolving the Coronary Artery Disease Epidemic Through Plant-Based Nutrition," *Preventive Cardiology* Fall 2001, pp. 171–77, and C. B. Esselstyn et al., "A Strategy to Arrest and Reverse Coronary Artery Disease: A 5-year longitudinal study of a single physician's practice," *Journal of Family Practice* 1995, 41(6):560–68.

3. Caldwell Esselstyn, "Making the Change," www.heartattackproof.com/morethan04_change.htm.

4. Quoted in Roberto Suro, "Hearts and minds," *New York Times Magazine* Dec. 29, 1991, p. 18.

5. Dan Buettner, "The Secrets of Long Life," *National Geographic* Nov. 2005, pp. 2–26.

6. Bradley J. Willcox, D. Craig Willcox, and Makoto Suzuki, *The Okinawa Program: Learn the Secrets to Health and Longevity* (Three Rivers Press, 2001), p. 132.
7. Thompson, Lillian, "Mammalian Lignan Production from Various Foods," *Nutrition and Cancer* 1991, 16(1):43–51.
8. "Toxic warnings grow for U.S. fish," Associated Press, August 25, 2004.
9. There is now evidence that EPA and DHA are highly effective in preventing sudden cardiac death, death from heart disease, and certain arrhythmias. Investigations involving individual heart cells have shown that EPA plus DHA prolong the refractory state of the cells by interacting with fast-acting sodium channels and L-type calcium channels. The cardioprotective effect of EPA plus DHA is thus intimately associated with the degree to which these two fatty acids are incorporated into the heart tissue (myocardium). It is also widely recognized that DHA is of crucial importance in the proper development of a fetus's brain, retina, and central nervous system. See J. Fernstrom, "Can nutrient supplements modify brain function?" *American Journal of Clinical Nutrition* 2000, 71(6):1669S–73S.
10. I am indebted to Michael Greger, M.D., for this phrase.
11. Anne Platt McGinn, "Blue Revolution—The Promises and Pitfalls of Fish Farming," *World Watch* March/April 1998, pp. 9–10.
12. Juliet Eilperin, "Farmed Salmon Raise Concerns: Study cites high levels of chemical fire retardants," *Washington Post* August 11, 2004.
13. Ronald Hites et al., "Global Assessment of Organic Contaminants in Farmed Salmon," *Science* Jan. 2004 (303):9. See also Kenneth Weiss, "Farm-Raised Salmon Linked to Pollutants," *Los Angeles Times* Jan. 8, 2004.
14. Michael Janofsky, "Report: Most fish in U.S. waters tainted by mercury," *New York Times* August 4, 2004.
15. Jane Kay, "Rich folks eating fish feed on mercury too," *San Francisco Chronicle* Nov. 5, 2002.
16. Ibid.
17. Sam Roe and Michael Hawthorne, "Toxic Risk on Your Plate," *Chicago Tribune* Dec. 11, 2005.
18. Ibid.
19. R. A. Myers and B. Worm, "Rapid worldwide depletion of predatory fish communities," *Nature* 2003, (423):280–83.
20. C. Stripp et al., "Fish intake is positively associated with breast cancer incidence rise," *Journal of Nutrition* 2003, 133(11):3664–69.
21. J. T. Salonen et al., "Intake of mercury from fish, lipid peroxidation, and the risk of myocardial infarction and coronary, cardiovascular, and any death in Eastern Finnish Men," *Circulation* 1995, 91:937.
22. J. T. Salonen et al., "Fish intake and the risk of coronary disease," *New England Journal of Medicine* 1995, 333:937.
23. For recipes using flax oil and ground flax seed, I recommend *Flax: The Super Food* by Barb Bloomfield, Judy Brown, and Siegfried Gursche (The Book Publishing Company, Summertown, Tenn., 2000).
24. Thomas T. Perls and Margery Hutter Silver, *Living to 100: Lessons in Living to Your Maximum Potential at Any Age* (Basic Books, 1999), p. 97.
25. Ibid. p. 98.

## CHAPTER NINE: STEPPING INTO LIFE

1. J. E. Manson et al., "Walking compared with vigorous exercise for the prevention of cardiovascular events in women," *New England Journal of Medicine* 2002, 347(10):716–25; W. E. Kraus et al., "Effects of the amount and intensity of exercise on plasma lipoproteins," *New England Journal of Medicine* 2002, 347(19):1483–92; A. L. Dunn et al., "Comparison of lifestyle and structured interventions to increase physical activity and cardiorespiratory fitness: A randomized trial," *Journal of the American Medical Association* 1999, 281(4):327–34; S. N. Blair et al., "The fitness, obesity and health equation: Is physical activity the common denominator?" *Journal of the American Medical Association* 2004, 292(10):1232–34; T. R. Wessel et al., "Relationship of physical fitness vs. body mass index with coronary artery disease and cardiovascular events in women," *Journal of the American Medical Association* 2004, 292(10):1179–87; A. L. Dunn et al., "Physical activity dose-response effects on outcomes of depression and anxiety," *Medicine and Science in Sports and Exercise* 2001, 33(6 Supplement):S587–97.
2. Ralph S. Paffenbarger and Eric Olsen, *LifeFit: An Effective Program for Optimal Health and a Longer Life* (Human Kinetics, 1992), p. vii.
3. Walter M. Bortz, *We Live Too Short and Die Too Long: How to Achieve and Enjoy Your Natural 100–Year-Plus Life Span* (Bantam, 1991), pp. 135–36. See also Walter M. Bortz, *Dare to Be 100* (Simon & Schuster, 1996).
4. Walter M. Bortz, *We Live Too Short*, p. 200.
5. Geoffrey Cowley, "How to live to 100," *Newsweek* June 30, 1997.
6. Ibid.
7. Diabetes Prevention Program Research Group, "Reduction in the incidence of type 2 diabetes with lifestyle intervention or metformin," *New England Journal of Medicine* Feb. 7, 2002, 346(6):393–403.
8. A. C. King et al., "Moderate intensity exercise and self-rated quality of sleep in older adults: A randomized controlled trial," *Journal of the American Medical Association* 1997, 277(1):32–37.
9. Bradley J. Willcox, D. Craig Willcox, and Makoto Suzuki, *The Okinawa Program: Learn the Secrets to Health and Longevity* (Three Rivers Press, 2001), p. 180.
10. P. J. Wade, "Canadian Homeowner and Veteran Celebrates 103rd!" *Realty Times* Nov. 9, 1999.
11. Thomas T. Perls and Margery Hutter Silver, *Living to 100: Lessons in Living to Your Maximum Potential at Any Age* (Basic Books, 1999), pp. 109, 153.
12. Patricia Bragg, "A Cheerleader for Fitness," in *Chicken Soup to Inspire the Body and Soul* (Health Communications, 2003), pp. 292–94.
13. Ibid.
14. Dennis Hughes, "Interview with Jack LaLanne: Legendary Fitness Expert, Health Pioneer, Diet and Nutrition Innovator," *Share Guide* 2003.
15. Ibid.
16. Ibid.
17. Ibid.
18. Ibid.

CHAPTER TEN: BORN TO MOVE

1. Margaret Morganroth Gullette, *Aged by Culture* (University of Chicago Press, 2004), pp. 3–6. See also "Secrets of Aging Explores the Science Behind the Universal Experience of Aging," *Senior Journal,* Boston, Feb. 10, 2005; Abigail Trafford, "Aging: The View from Below," *Washington Post* Nov. 23, 2004; Margaret Morganroth Gullette, "Trapped in Decline Culture," *In These Times* Oct. 2, 2004.
2. Margaret Morganroth Gullette, *Aged by Culture,* p. 4.
3. William Evans and Irwin H. Rosenberg, *Biomarkers: The 10 Determinants of Aging You Can Control* (Simon & Schuster, 1991).
4. Ibid. p. 49–50.
5. Ibid. p. 50–51.
6. Ibid. p. 70.
7. Ibid. p. 53.
8. Arnold Schwarzenegger, who became governor of California in 2004, was a seven-time winner of bodybuilding's top prize, the Mr. Olympia contest. When he underwent heart surgery at age forty-nine, he admitted using steroids during his career, but denied they had anything to do with his heart problems. In 1989, Schwarzenegger and a partner created the Arnold Classic, an annual bodybuilding competition in Columbus, Ohio, for elite bodybuilders. Only fourteen competitors are invited each year. In 2005, two of the invited competitors, Victor Martinez and Craig Titus, had served time in jail on steroid-related offenses, and Titus was indicted for murder in 2006. The following is only a partial list of the men who have competed in the Arnold Classic and suffered serious health problems:

    Mohammed "Momo" Benaziza died in his hotel room in the Netherlands in Oct. 1992 after competing in the Holland Grand Prix contest.

    Paul Dillett, a Canadian competitor, froze on stage while hitting a double-bicep pose at the Arnold Classic in 1994. It took several men to move Dillett into a horizontal position and carry him off stage.

    Andreas Munzer, an Austrian like his idol, Schwarzenegger, died of multiple organ failure twelve days after competing in the 1996 Arnold Classic.

    Kenny "Flex" Wheeler won the Arnold show four times. He underwent a kidney transplant in 2003.

    Don Long, who competed in Schwarzenegger's show in 1997 through 1999, also underwent a kidney transplant.

    Mike Matarazzo, a three-time Arnold competitor who lives in Modesto, California, underwent a triple bypass heart operation at age thirty-nine.
9. William Evans and Irwin H. Rosenberg, op. cit., p. 15.
10. M. E. Nelson et al., "A One Year Walking Program and Increased Dietary Calcium in Postmenopausal Women: Effects on Bones," *Medicine and Science in Sports and Exercise* 1990, 22(Supplement):377.
11. E. L. Smith et al., "Physical Activity and Calcium Modalities for Bone Mineral Increase in Aged Women," *Medicine and Science in Sports and Exercise* 1981, 13:60–64.
12. Tom Lloyd et al., "Lifestyle factors and the development of bone mass and bone strength in young women," *Pediatrics* 2004, 144:786–82.

13. "Exercise More Critical Than Calcium," press release from Penn State University. See also A. J. Lanou et al., "Calcium, dairy products, and bone health in children and young adults: A reevaluation of the evidence," *Pediatrics* 2005, 115(3):736–43. This study found "Neither increased consumption of dairy products, specifically, nor total dietary calcium consumption has shown even a modest consistent benefit for child or young adult bone health."

14. Daniel Rudman et al., "Effects of Human Growth Hormone in Men over 60 Years Old," *New England Journal of Medicine* 1990, 323:1–6.

15. T. C. Welbourne, "Increased Plasma Bicarbonate and Growth Hormone After an Oral Glutamine Load," *American Journal of Clinical Nutrition* 1995, 61(5):1058–61.

16. James F. Fixx, *The Complete Book of Running* (Random House, 1977).

17. Nathan Pritikin, *Diet for Runners* (Simon & Schuster, 1985), cited in Timothy J. Smith, *Renewal: The Anti-Aging Revolution* (Rodale Press, 1998), p. 459.

18. A version of Ruth Heidrich's story appeared in Jack Canfield et al., *Chicken Soup to Inspire the Body and Soul* (Health Communications, 2003), pp. 13–17. See also Ruth E. Heidrich, *Senior Fitness: The Diet and Exercise Program for Maximum Health and Longevity* (Lantern Books, 2005).

## CHAPTER ELEVEN: KEEPING YOUR MARBLES

1. Bradley J. Willcox, D. Craig Willcox, and Makoto Suzuki, *The Okinawa Program: Learn the Secrets to Health and Longevity* (Three Rivers Press, 2001), p. 46. See also C. Ogura et al., "Prevalence of senile dementia in Okinawa, Japan," *International Journal of Epidemiology* 1995, 24:373–80.

2. John Fauber, "Huge Increase in Alzheimer's Seen: Doctors warn that growing numbers threaten nation's health care system," *Milwaukee Journal Sentinel* August 18, 2003.

3. Bobbie Wilkinson, "The Travelers," in *Chicken Soup for the Caregiver's Soul* (Health Communications, 2004), pp. 71–72.

4. Danielle Laurin et al., "Physical Activity and Risk of Cognitive Impairment and Dementia in Elderly Persons," *Archives of Neurology* 2001, 58:498–504.

5. Jennifer Weuve et al., "Physical Activity, Including Walking, and Cognitive Function in Older Women," *Journal of the American Medical Association* 2004, 292:1454–61.

6. Robert D. Abbott et al., "Walking and Dementia in Physically Capable Elderly Men," *Journal of the American Medical Association* 2004, 292:1447–53.

7. Shari Roan, "To sharpen the brain, first hone the body: Mental benefits include better memory and learning; dementia may be slowed," *Los Angeles Times* Jan. 9, 2006.

8. P. P. Zandi et al., "Reduced Risk of Alzheimer's disease in users of antioxidant vitamin supplements," *Archives of Neurology* 2004, 61:82–88.

9. The formula I take is called Renewal Antioxidants, and is manufactured by Source Naturals.

10. Miia Kivipelto, "Body Mass Index: Clustering of Vascular Risk Factors and the Risk of Dementia: A Longitudinal, Population-Based Study," presented at the 9th International Conference on Alzheimer's Disease and Related Disorders, Philadelphia, July 19, 2004.

11. G. Alfthan et al., "Homocysteine and cardiovascular disease mortality," *The Lancet* 1997, 349:397. See also B. J. Willcox et al., "Homocysteine levels in Okinawan-Japanese," *Journal of Investigative Medicine* 2000, 43(2):205A.

12. R. Clarke et al., "Folate, vitamin $B_{12}$, and serum total homocysteine levels in confirmed Alzheimer disease," *Archives of Neurology* 1998, 55:1449–55.

13. Ibid.

14. H. X. Wang et al., Vitamin $B_{12}$ and folate in relation to the development of Alzheimer's disease," *Neurology* 2001, 56(9):1188–94.

15. It was once thought that because plant-based diets are higher in folate and vitamin $B_6$, they would produce lower homocysteine levels. And indeed, one 2000 study showed that subjects who adopted a vegan diet saw their homocysteine levels drop between 13 percent and 20 percent in just one week. D. J. DeRose et al., "Vegan diet–based lifestyle program rapidly lowers homocysteine levels," *Preventive Medicine* 2000, 30:225–33. Recently, however, a number of studies have found *long-term* vegans to have dangerously elevated blood homocysteine levels. This does not seem to occur in vegans or vegetarians whose intake of vitamin $B_{12}$ is adequate. In fact, vegans and vegetarians with a sufficient intake of $B_{12}$ typically have homocysteine levels that are *lower* than those of people eating the standard Western diet.

    How much vitamin $B_{12}$ is needed? Government recommendations call for at least 1.5 mcg per day, an amount adequate to prevent classic $B_{12}$ deficiency symptoms but usually not sufficient to keep homocysteine levels low. Current research suggests that 5–10 mcg per day are needed to keep blood $B_{12}$ levels high enough to keep homocysteine in check. Since vitamin $B_{12}$ is not found in plant foods, vegetarians and vegans must often rely on supplementary forms of this vitamin. If the primary source of vitamin $B_{12}$ is a *daily* supplement, at least 10 mcg should be taken to ensure adequate absorption. If the primary source is a *weekly* supplement, at least 2,000 mcg should be taken, because at higher doses the absorption rate significantly decreases. See Stephen Walsh, "Homocysteine and Health," *The Vegan* Winter 2002.

16. Jeff Nelson, "Losing Your Mind for the Sake of a Burger" (www.vegsource .com/articles/alzheimers_homocysteine.htm). A study of subjects who ate meat as their primary protein source found that they were nearly three times as likely to develop dementia as their vegetarian counterparts. See P. Giem et al., "The incidence of dementia and intake of animal products: Preliminary findings from the Adventist Health Study," *Neuroepidemiology* 1993, 12:28–36.

17. M. C. Morris et al., "Dietary fats and the risk of incident Alzheimer's disease," *Archives of Neurology* 2003, 60(2):194–200; S. Kalmijn et al., "Polyunsaturated fatty acids, antioxidants, and cognitive function in older men," *American Journal of Epidemiology* 1997, 145(1):33–41; J. A. Luchsinger et al., "Caloric intake and the risk of Alzheimer's disease," *Archives of Neurology* 2002, 59(8):1258–63. M. J. Engelhart et al., "Diet and risk of dementia: does fat matter? The Rotterdam Study," *Neurology* 2002, 59(12):1915–21.

18. E. Larson, "Exercise Associated with Reduced Risk of Dementia in Older Adults," *Annals of Internal Medicine* 2006, 144:73–81.

19. W. B. Grant, "Dietary links to Alzheimer's disease: 1999 Update," *Journal of Alzheimer's Disease* 1999; (1):197–201, and "Incidence of dementia and Alzheimer's disease in Nigeria and the United States," *Journal of the American Medical Association* 2001, 285:2448.

20. M. C. Morris et al., "Dietary niacin and the risk of incident Alzheimer's disease and of cognitive decline," *Journal of Neurology, Neurosurgery, and Psychiatry* 2004, 75(8):1093–99.
21. M. C. Morris et al., "Consumption of fish and omega-3 fatty acids and risk of incident of Alzheimer's disease," *Archives of Neurology* 2003, 60:940–46.

## CHAPTER TWELVE: CONFIDENT AND CLEAR-THINKING

1. Thomas T. Perls and Margery Hutter Silver, *Living to 100: Lessons in Living to Your Maximum Potential at Any Age* (Basic Books, 1999), pp. 36–46.
2. Ibid. pp. 45–46.
3. John W. Rowe and Robert L. Kahn, *Successful Aging* (Dell, 1998), pp. 132–34, 138–39, 166, 244–45.
4. Anne Lamott, *Plan B: Further Thoughts on Faith* (Riverhead Books, 2005), pp. 171–76.

## CHAPTER THIRTEEN: WHAT'S LOVE GOT TO DO WITH IT?

1. Y. F. Schnellow, "Is Hunzan Health a Myth?" in G. Rinehart, ed., *Great Adventures in Medicine* (Healing Books, 1972), pp. 36–69.
2. Rachel Naomi Remen, *Kitchen Table Wisdom: Stories That Heal* (Riverhead Books, 1996), p. 53.
3. Dean Ornish, *Love and Survival: The Scientific Basis for the Healing Power of Intimacy* (Harper Collins, 1998), p. 3.
4. Michael Lerner, *Choices in Healing: Integrating the Best of Conventional and Complementary Approaches to Cancer* (MIT Press, 1994), pp. 154–58.
5. D. Spiegel et al., "Effect of psychosocial treatment on survival of patients with metastatic breast cancer," *The Lancet* 1989, ii:888–91. See also David Spiegel, *Living Beyond Limits: New Hope and Help for Facing Life-Threatening Illness* (Times Books, 1993).
6. Janny Scott, "Study Says Cancer Survival Rates Rise with Group Therapy," *Los Angeles Times* May 11, 1998.
7. Ibid.
8. F. I. Fawzy et al., "Malignant melanoma: Effects of an early structured psychiatric intervention, coping, and affective state of recurrence and survival six years later," *Archives of General Psychiatry* 1993, 50:681–89.
9. Dan Millman, *Sacred Journey of the Peaceful Warrior* (H. J. Kramer, 1991), p. 89.
10. Larry Scherwitz et al., "Type A Behavior, Self-Involvement, and Coronary Atherosclerosis," *Psychosomatic Medicine* 1983, (45):47–57.
11. J. H. Medalie and U. Goldbourt, "Angina pectoris among 10,000 men. II. Psychosocial and other risk factors as evidenced by a multivariate analysis of a five-year incidence study," *American Journal of Medicine* 1976, 60(6):910–21.
12. J. H. Medalie et al., "The importance of biopsychosocial factors in the development of duodenal ulcer in a cohort of middle-aged men," *American Journal of Medicine* 1992, 136(10):1280–87.
13. The Swedish Study: Annika Rosengren et al., "Stressful Life Events, Social Support, and Mortality in Men Born in 1933," *British Medical Journal* Oct. 19, 1993.

14. This story by Elizabeth Songster appeared in Jack Canfield et al., *Chicken Soup for the Couple's Soul* (Health Communications, 1999), pp. 187–89.

## CHAPTER FOURTEEN: THE STRENGTH OF THE HEART

1. A great number of studies have found that married people live longer and have lower mortality for almost every major cause of death than those who are single, divorced, separated, or widowed. Numerous studies have also found that married people have a lower incidence of disease, a better chance of survival after diagnosis, and a quicker recovery. The difference is particularly pronounced for men. See C. F. Ortmeyer, "Variations in mortality, morbidity, and health care by marital status," in L. L. Erhardt and J. E. Beln, eds., *Mortality and Morbidity in the United States* (Harvard University Press, 1974), pp. 159–84. In their 2000 book, *The Case for Marriage: Why Married People Are Happier, Healthier and Better Off Financially* (Doubleday), Linda Waite and Maggie Gallagher cite studies showing that unmarried men are more likely to engage in unhealthful behaviors including excessive drinking, smoking, drug abuse, poor nutritional habits, and lack of exercise. In his classic 1979 book, *Broken Heart: The Medical Consequences of Loneliness* (Basic Books), James Lynch cites studies finding that single white males are seven times more likely to develop cirrhosis of the liver and ten times more likely to get tuberculosis than married men.

2. Harold Morowitz, "Hiding in the Hammond Report," *Hospital Practice* August 1975, pp. 35–39.

3. L. F. Berkman and S. L. Syme, "Social networks, host resistance, and mortality: A nine-year follow-up study of Alameda County residents," *American Journal of Epidemiology* 1979, 109:186–204.

4. Kristina Orth-Gomer and J. V. Johnson, "Social network interaction and mortality: A six year follow-up study of a random sample of the Swedish population," *Journal of Chronic Diseases* 1987, 40(10):949–57.

5. J. S. House, K. R. Landis, and D. Umberson, "Social relationships and health," *Science* 1988, 241:540–45.

6. Larry Dossey, "The Healing Power of Pets: A Look at Animal-Assisted Therapy," *Alternative Therapies in Health and Medicine* July 1997, p. 816.

7. E. Friedmann et al., "Animal companions and one-year survival of patients discharged from a coronary care unit," *Public Health Reports* 1980, 95:307–12. See also A. H. Katcher et al., "Looking, talking and blood pressure: The physiological consequences of interaction with the living environment," in *New Perspectives on Our Lives with Companion Animals,* edited by A. Katcher and A. Beck (University of Pennsylvania Press, 1983).

8. E. Friedmann and S. A. Thomas, "Pet ownership, social support, and one-year survival after acute myocardial infarction in the Cardiac Arrhythmia Suppression Trial (CAST)," *American Journal of Cardiology* 1995, 76:1213–17.

9. W. Ruberman et al., "Psychosocial influences on mortality after myocardial infarction," *New England Journal of Medicine* 1984, 311(9):552–59.

10. Rachel Naomi Remen, *Kitchen Table Wisdom: Stories That Heal* (Riverhead Books, 1996), pp. 226–28.

11. Kristina Orth-Gomer et al., "Marital Stress Worsens Prognosis in Women with

Coronary Heart Disease," *Journal of the American Medical Association* 2000, 284:3008–14.

12. Kathleen Doheny, "Women Who Bite Their Tongues Risk Their Lives: Avoiding conflict with husbands boosts the likelihood of death, a new study finds," *HealthDay* Feb. 17, 2005.

13. Andrew Weil, *Spontaneous Healing: How to Discover and Enhance Your Body's Natural Ability to Maintain and Heal Itself* (Alfred A. Knopf, 1995), pp. 98–99.

14. James J. Lynch, *A Cry Unheard: New Insights into the Medical Consequences of Loneliness* (Bancroft Press, 2000).

15. L. G. Russek and G. E. Schwartz, "Narrative descriptions of parental love and caring predict health status in midlife: A 35-year follow-up of the Harvard Mastery of Stress study," *Alternative Therapies in Health and Medicine* 1996, 2:55–62; L. G. Russek and G. E. Schwartz, "Perceptions of parental caring predict health status in midlife: A 35-year follow-up of the Harvard Mastery of Stress study," *Psychosomatic Medicine* 1997, 59(2):144–49; Daniel H. Funkenstein, *Mastery of Stress* (Harvard University Press, 1957).

16. C. B. Thomas and K. Duszynski, "Closeness to parents and the family constellation in a prospective study of five disease states: suicide, mental illness, malignant tumor, hypertension, and coronary heart disease," *Johns Hopkins Medical Journal* 1974, 134:251.

## CHAPTER FIFTEEN: HOW THEN SHALL WE LIVE?

1. James W. Prescott, "Body Pleasure and the Origins of Violence," *Bulletin of the Atomic Scientists* Nov. 1975, pp. 10–20. See also James W. Prescott et al., "Early Somatosensory Deprivation as an Ontogenetic Process in Abnormal Development of the Brain and Behavior," in eds., I. E. Goldsmith and J. Moor-Jankowski, *Medical Primatology* (Karger, 1971), pp. 357–75, and Howard Bloom, *The Lucifer Principle: A Scientific Expedition into the Forces of History* (Atlantic Monthly Press, 1995), p. 239. Bloom points out that a classic example of this principle is Margaret Mead's contrast between the Arapesh and the Mundugamor of New Guinea. See Margaret Mead, *Male and Female: A Study of the Sexes in a Changing World* (Dell, 1968), pp. 76–77, 86–88, 117, 134–35.

2. Abbie Blair's story about Freddie's adoption is from the Dec. 1964 *Reader's Digest* and was reprinted in *Stories for the Heart,* compiled by Alice Gray (Portland: Multnomah Press, 1996 edition), pp. 188–92.

3. James J. Lynch, *A Cry Unheard: New Insights into the Medical Consequences of Loneliness* (Bancroft Press, 2000), p. 2.

4. "Townspeople too nice for company," *Hannibal Courier-Post* March 13, 1999.

5. James J. Lynch, op. cit., p. 10.

6. Ibid., p. 11.

7. Elaine Sciolino, "France Battles a Problem that Grows and Grows: Fat," *New York Times* Jan. 25, 2006.

8. James J. Lynch, op. cit., p. 10.

9. S. M. Jourard, "An exploratory study of body-accessibility," *British Journal of Social and Clinical Psychology* 1966, 84(1–4):205–17.

10. When last heard from, the twins, Kyrie and Brielle Jackson, were healthy

preschoolers. A photo of their healing embrace, taken by Chris Christo of the *Worcester Telegram and Gazette,* has become world famous. Widely circulated on the Internet, it has also been featured in *Life* magazine and *Reader's Digest.*

11. Sula Benet, *How to Live to Be 100: The Lifestyle of the People of the Caucasus* (New York: Dial Press, 1976), p. 161.

## CHAPTER SIXTEEN: BREAKING FREE FROM THE CULTURAL TRANCE

1. Derrick Jensen, *A Language Older Than Words* (Chelsea Green Publishing, 2000), pp. 211–13.

2. Ruth Benedict, "Patterns of the Good Culture," *American Anthropologist* 1970, Vol. 72.

3. Stephen Bezruchka, "Social hierarchy and the health Olympics," *Canadian Medical Association Journal* June 12, 2001. See also Ichiro Kawachi and Bruce P. Kennedy, *Health of Nations: Why Inequality Is Harmful to Your Health* (New Press, 2002), and Population Health Forum, "Advocating for action toward a healthier society."

4. Stephen Bezruchka, "Poverty is bad for the health of Americans," keynote address, Statewide Poverty Action Network Action Summit, Dec. 6, 2003, Seattle, Washington. See also Stephen Bezruchka, "Sick of It All: Economic equality— good for what ails you," *Real Change News,* Seattle, Oct. 15, 2000.

5. Many commentators have noted that the relative wealth equality in the United States in the 1960s and 1970s did not occur by accident. It was created by what has been called the "Great Compression" of incomes that took place during World War II, and then, as Paul Krugman wrote in *The New York Times,* "sustained for a generation by social norms that favored equality, strong labor unions and progressive taxation." Krugman notes, however, "Since the 1970s, all of these sustaining forces have lost their power. Since 1980, in particular, U.S. government policies have consistently favored the wealthy at the expense of working families—and under the current [George W. Bush] administration, that favoritism has become extreme and relentless. From tax cuts that favor the rich to bankruptcy 'reform' that punishes the unlucky, almost every domestic policy seems intended to accelerate our march back to the robber baron era." Paul Krugman, "Losing Our Country," *New York Times* June 10, 2005.

6. Jeff Gates, *Democracy at Risk: Rescuing Main Street from Wall Street* (Perseus Publishing, 2000), pp. 21–22.

7. In 2004, Scott Lee, Jr., Wal-Mart's chief executive, was paid $17.5 million. Every two weeks he was paid about as much as his average employee would earn in a lifetime. See Paul Krugman, "Always Low Wages, Always," *New York Times* May 13, 2005.

8. Chuck Collins et al., ed., *The Wealth Inequality Reader* (Dollars & Sense Economic Affairs Bureau, 2005), p. 6. The United States entered the new millennium with the most unequal distribution of wealth since the eve of the Great Depression. For every additional dollar earned by those in the the bottom 90 percent of the population between 1950 and 1970, those in the top 0.01 percent earned an additional $162. That gap has since skyrocketed: For every additional dollar earned by each taxpayer in the bottom 90 percent between 1990 and 2002, each taxpayer in the top bracket brought in an extra $18,000. Meanwhile, from 1980 to 2002, the share of total income earned by the top 0.1 per-

cent of earners more than doubled, while the share of the bottom 90 percent declined. David Cay Johnston, "Richest Are Leaving Even the Rich Far Behind," *New York Times* June 5, 2005. In an accompanying editorial, *The New York Times* wrote: "It is hard to imagine anyone supporting the notion of taking money from programs like Medicaid and college-tuition assistance, increasing the tax burden of the vast majority of working Americans, sending the country into crushing debt—and giving the proceeds to people who are so fantastically rich that they don't know what to do with the money they already have. Yet that is just what is happening under the Bush administration. Forget the middle class and the upper-middle class. Even the merely wealthy are being left behind in the dust by the small slice of super-rich Americans." "The Bush Economy," editorial, *New York Times* June 7, 2005. See also Bob Herbert, "The Mobility Myth," *New York Times* June 6, 2005.

9. James Marone (Brown University) and Lawrence Jacobs (Minnesota State University), cited in Robin McKie, "Lifespan Crisis Hits Supersize America," *The Guardian* Sept. 19, 2004.

10. United Nations Development Program, *Human Development Report* 2004.

11. Jesus Sanchez, "High Blood Pressure Rates Hit Peaks and Valleys in California," *Los Angeles Times* Nov. 22, 2004.

12. "Three-quarters of state's pupils fail fitness test," *Santa Cruz Sentinel* Nov. 25, 2004, p. A-1.

13. Cited in Jeff Greenwald, "Happy Land," *Yoga Journal* July/August 2004.

14. One-third the size of its neighbor Nepal, Bhutan is far less populated. While Nepal has 25 million people, Bhutan has less than a tenth that many. To protect from being inundated by Nepalese refugees, Bhutan has cultivated an obsessive nationalism. Even Nepalese refugees whose families have lived in Bhutan for generations are not considered to be Bhutanese citizens, and have far fewer rights and privileges. Indeed, many were forced to leave Bhutan in the late 1980s, after census figures showed they would eventually overtake the country. Some of these former residents of Bhutan now live in dingy camps in southern Nepal. And even for Bhutanese subjects, the traditional way of life may not long survive. Television arrived in Bhutan in 2002. Children in this devoutly Buddhist country are now watching *Baywatch* and Worldwide Wrestling and beginning to clamor for Western consumer products (Jeff Greenwald, ibid.).

15. Stephen Herrera, "Zen and the art of happiness," *Ode* Dec. 2005, p. 63.

16. Peter Menzel and Faith D'Aluisio, *Hungry Planet: What the World Eats* (Ten Speed Press, 2005), pp. 36–45.

17. According to Harry Marshall, Producer/Director of the U.S. Public Broadcasting System (PBS) film "The Living Edens: Bhutan," 1997.

18. Jeff Greenwald, op. cit.

19. Andrew C. Revkin, "A New Measure of Well-Being from a Happy Little Kingdom," *New York Times* Oct. 4, 2005.

20. Rochelle M. Pennington, "For Richer or Poorer," *Stories for the Heart*, compiled by Alice Gray (Portland: Multnomah Press, 1997 edition), p. 156.

21. Jean-Pierre Hallet, *Pygmy Kitabu: A Revealing Account of the Origin and Legends of the African Pygmies* (Random House, 1973).

22. Ibid. p. 65.

23. Bernie S. Siegel, *Peace, Love and Healing* (Harper Perennial, 1989), p. 178.

24. Jean-Pierre Hallet, op. cit., p. 70.

25. Elizabeth Marshall Thomas, *The Harmless People* (Vintage Books, 1958); Colin M. Turnbull, *The Forest People* (Simon & Schuster, 1961); Richard Katz, Megan Biesele, and Verna St. Denis, *Healing Makes Our Hearts Happy* (Inner Traditions, 1997).

26. Richard Katz et al., op. cit.

27. *The Selfish Gene* is the title of a controversial book published in 1976 by Oxford University zoologist Richard Dawkins. According to Dawkins's gene-centered view of evolution, biological organisms, including humans, are vehicles used by their genes for making more copies of those genes, regardless of the effect they might have on individuals or species. Rather than thinking about organisms using genes to reproduce themselves, Dawkins proposed we look at it the other way around. Similar to the idea that a chicken is merely an egg's way of making more eggs, his view suggests that "our" genes build and maintain us in order to make more genes. Although we tend to see ourselves as masters of our genetic endowment, according to Dawkins we are in reality merely its servants. The concept of the "selfish gene" has led many to conclude that the world revolves around savage competition, ruthless exploitation, and deceit. Yet Dawkins goes to great pains to point out that acts of apparent altruism do exist in nature. Bees commit suicide when they sting in order to protect the hive. Birds will likewise give their lives to protect the flock. The revised edition of Dawkins's book, published in 1990, contains a new chapter entitled "Nice Guys Finish First."

28. This concept was popularized by anthropologist Raymond Dart, who interpreted fossil remains in Africa as evidence that man is a killer ape. Many other anthropologists have likewise theorized that our earliest human ancestors were hunters and possessed a killer instinct. But this is far from proven. In fact, according to Robert W. Sussman, who recently served as the editor of *American Anthropologist,* "when you really examine the fossil and living nonhuman primate evidence, that is just not the case." Sussman is the author and editor of numerous books, including *Man the Hunted, The Origins and Nature of Sociality, Primate Ecology and Social Structure,* and *The Biological Basis of Human Behavior.* In February 2006, he presented his findings to the American Association for the Advancement of Science's Annual Meeting. Based on extensive study of fossil evidence dating back nearly seven million years, he said, the idea that many contemporary human traits developed out of hunting for prey and killing competitors is incorrect. Rather, the evidence indicates that many human traits, including those of cooperation and socialization, developed as a result of being a prey species and out of early humans' need to avoid predators.

  One of the most intriguing scientific statements on the subject was compiled by a collection of scientists and scholars from a number of disciplines in Seville, Spain, in 1986. Their statement, known as the Seville Statement on Violence, was adopted by UNESCO at the twenty-fifth session of the United Nations General Conference, and has been endorsed by hundreds of major scientific organizations. According to the statement, "It is scientifically incorrect to say that we have inherited a tendency to make war from our animal ancestors. . . . Warfare . . . is a product of culture. . . . War is . . . not inevitable. . . . There are cultures which have not engaged in wars for centuries. . . . It is scientifically incorrect to say that war or any other violent behavior is genetically programmed into our human nature. . . . It is scientifically incorrect to say that

in the course of human evolution there has been a selection for aggressive behavior. . . . In all well-studied species, status within the group is achieved by the
ability to cooperate and to fulfill social functions. . . . It is scientifically incorrect
to say that humans have a 'violent brain.' . . . How we act is shaped by how we
have been conditioned and socialized. There is nothing in our neurophysiology
that compels us to react violently."

29. On the other hand, R. Brian Ferguson, a professor of anthropology at Rutgers
University, contends that before about ten thousand years ago, war was virtually nonexistent. See Jack Lucentini, "Bones Reveal Some Truth in 'Noble Savage Myth,' " *Washington Post* April 15, 2002.

30. The Darwin Project (www.thedarwinproject.com), started by the psychologist
and evolutionary systems scientist David Loye, has a council of more than fifty
leading American, European, and Asian scientists and educators. The Project
points out "*In The Descent of Man,* Charles Darwin wrote only twice of 'survival of the fittest'—but 95 times about love! 92 times about moral sensitivity.
And 200 times about brain and mind. Suppression over 100 years of the real
Darwin has led to the social, political, economic, scientific, educational, moral
and spiritual mess we are in today." One of the Darwin Project's goals is to shift
teaching in schools at all levels and in the media away from fixation on the
"old" survival-of-the-fittest Darwinian model to the long-ignored full Darwinian theory, in which Darwin stressed that at the level of human evolution it was
not natural selection but cooperation (which was called mutuality and mutal
aid in his time) that was primary. See David Loye, *Darwin's Unfolding Revolution,* available at www.benjaminfranklinpress.com.

31. Marc Ian Barasch, *Field Notes on the Compassionate Life: A Search for the
Soul of Kindness* (Rodale Press, 2005), p. 35.

32. Ibid. p. 35.

## CHAPTER SEVENTEEN: GRIEF AND HEALING

1. Kelly D. Brownell, *Food Fight: The Inside Story of the Food Industry, America's
Obesity Crisis, and What We Can Do About It* (Contemporary Books, 2004),
p. 27.

2. Alexander Leaf, *Youth in Old Age* (McGraw-Hill, 1975), p. 38.

3. Ibid. pp. 33–34.

4. Quoted in Michael Winn, "Hunza: Shangri-La of Islam," *Aramco World*
Jan./Feb. 1983, Vol. 34 No 1.

5. *Vilcabamba: The Sacred Valley of the Centenarians* (CIS Publishing, 2004),
pp. 28, 30.

6. Ibid. p. 28.

## CHAPTER EIGHTEEN: DEATH AND AWAKENING

1. R. Saladi et al., "The causes of skin cancer: A comprehensive review," *Drugs
Today* 2005, 41(1):37–53.

2. Marla Cone, "Estrogen Imitator in Womb May Lead to Cancer in Men, Study
Finds," *Los Angeles Times* May 3, 2005. In 2005, the Environmental Working
Group released a report based on tests of ten samples of umbilical-cord blood
taken by the American Red Cross. They found an average of 287 contaminants

in the blood, including mercury, fire retardants, pesticides, and gasoline byproducts.

3. Dale Turner, *Different Seasons* (High Tide Press, 1997), pp. 81–82.

4. Rachel Naomi Remen makes this point beautifully in her wonderful book, *Kitchen Table Wisdom: Stories That Heal* (Riverhead Books, 1996 edition), p. 93.

5. Carla Muir, "Beauty Contest," in *Stories for the Heart,* compiled by Alice Gray (Portland: Multnomah Press, 1996), p. 104.

6. Sandra Bertman, *Facing Death* (Taylor & Francis, 1991), p. 4.

7. Stephen Levine, *Who Dies? An Investigation of Conscious Living and Conscious Dying* (Anchor Books, 1982), p. 1.

8. Rachel Naomi Remen, op. cit., pp. 93–97.

9. Kahlil Gibran, *The Prophet* (Alfred A. Knopf, 1959), p. 80.

10. Quoted in Dale Turner, op. cit., p. 153.

# Index

## ABOUT THE AUTHOR

Widely considered one of the world's leading experts on the dietary link between the environment and health, JOHN ROBBINS is the author of the million-copy bestseller *Diet for a New America*. His work has been the subject of cover stories and feature articles in the *San Francisco Chronicle,* the *Los Angeles Times, The Washington Post, The New York Times,* and *People* magazine. Robbins has been a featured and keynote speaker at hundreds of major conferences, including those sponsored by the Sierra Club and UNICEF, and is the recipient of many awards, including the Rachel Carson Award and the Albert Schweitzer Humanitarian Award. He is the founder of EarthSave International (a nonprofit organization dedicated to healthy food choices, preservation of the environment, and a more compassionate world). Robbins lives with his wife, Deo, their son, Ocean, and daughter-in-love, Michele, and their grandtwins, River and Bodhi, outside of Santa Cruz, California.

## ABOUT THE TYPE

This book was set in Sabon, a typeface designed by the well-known German typographer Jan Tschichold (1902–74). Sabon's design is based upon the original letter forms of Claude Garamond and was created specifically to be used for three sources: foundry type for hand composition, Linotype, and Monotype. Tschichold named his typeface for the famous Frankfurt typefounder Jacques Sabon, who died in 1580.